The Pulmonary Circulation: Moving from Passive to Active Control

To our colleagues and students from whom we have learned, and our patients and children who shall so benefit.

The Pulmonary Circulation: Moving from Passive to Active Control

Edited by

Michael R. Pinsky

Director and Professor of Research
Division of Anesthesiology and Critical Care
University of Pittsburgh
Pittsburgh, Pennsylvania, USA

Jean-François Dhainaut

Department of Clinical Pharmacology and
Critical Care Medicine
Cochin Port Royal University Hospital
Paris, France

Antonio Artigas

Associate Professor of
Cellular Biology and Physiology
Department Autonomus University of Barcelona
and
Director of Intensive Care Medicine
Consorci Hospitalari del Parc Tauli
Sabadell, Spain

W.B. Saunders Company Ltd
London Philadelphia Toronto Sydney Tokyo

W. B. Saunders Company Ltd 24–28 Oval Road
London NW1 7DX

The Curtis Center
Independence Square West
Philadelphia, PA 19106–3399, USA

Harcourt Brace & Company
55 Horner Avenue
Toronto, Ontario M8Z 4X6, Canada

Harcourt Brace & Company, Australia
30–52 Smidmore Street
Marrickville, NSW 2204, Australia

Harcourt Brace & Company, Japan
Ichibancho Central Building, 22–1 Ichibancho
Chiyoda-ku, Tokyo 102, Japan

This book is printed on acid free paper

A catalogue record for this book is available from the British Library

ISBN 0–7020–2201–2

Typeset by Phoenix Photosetting, Chatham, Kent
Printed in Great Britain by Hartnolls Limited, Bodmin, Cornwall

Table of Contents

Contributors vii

Preface xi

Abbreviations xiii

Introduction: The Pulmonary Circulation: Evolving Concepts of Control and Interaction 1
M. R. PINSKY

Part I The Pulmonary Endothelium: A Local and Global Endocrine Organ

1 Endogenous Nitric Oxide Production in the Respiratory System 9
C. G. FROSTELL

2 Nitric Oxide as the Principal Endothelium-Dependent Relaxing Factor 17
J. T. REEVES & S. H. ABMAN

3 Interaction Between Vasodilating Substances and Lung Function 33
P. J. SCHENARTS & D. L. TRABER

4 Mediators of Vasoconstriction: Endothelin and Other Endogenous Compounds 57
C. S. R. GANDHI & W. D. WATKINS

Part II The Pulmonary Endothelium – Smooth Muscle Interface: Hypoxia and Vasomotor Tone

5 Modulation of Pulmonary Vascular Tone in ARDS: The Role of the Endothelium 77
N. P. CURZEN & T. W. EVANS

6 Pathophysiology of the Perinatal Pulmonary Circulation 107
J.-C. MERCIER, J. P. KINSELLA, A. T. DINH-XUAN &
S. H. ABMAN

7 Role of Nitric Oxide in Hypoxic Pulmonary Vasoconstriction 125
A. T. DINH-XUAN & J.-C. MERCIER

8 Role of Nitric Oxide in Chronic Obstructive Pulmonary Disease 139
J. A. BARBERA

9 Effect of Inhaled Nitric Oxide on Right Ventricular Function 147
R. ROSSAINT, U. KAISERS & I. SCHULZE-NEICK

10 Cardiopulmonary Response to Home Oxygen Therapy: Nasal Prongs Versus Oxygen-Saving Devices 157
C. DOMINGO & E. DOMINGO

11 Pulmonary Blood Flow in Lung Transplant Recipients 171
K. H. LEE, M. R. PINSKY & A. BOUJOUKOS

Part III Pulmonary Blood Flow

12 Acute Respiratory Failure: Pressure–Flow Relations and Nitric Oxide 175
R. NAEIJE

13 Effect of Combined Inhaled Nitric Oxide and Pulmonary Vasoconstriction Enhancement 189
S. BELOUCIF & D. M. PAYEN

14 Factors Predicting the Response to Inhaled Nitric Oxide in Acute Respiratory Failure 203
J. J. ROUBY

15 Pulmonary Vascular Tone in Ventilated Patients with Chronic Obstructive Pulmonary Disease 229
F. BAIGORRI, A. DE MONTE, D. JOSEPH, L. BLANCH &
A. ARTIGAS

Part IV The Alveolar Interface: Doorway to the Circulation

16 Consequences of Leukocyte Migration in the Lungs: A Reappraisal 241
T. R. MARTIN

17 Pulmonary Edema and Alveolar Overdistension 253
D. DREYFUSS & G. SAUMON

18 Role of Arachidonic Acid Metabolites in Vascular and Airway Tone During States of Systemic Inflammation 261
G. R. BERNARD

19 Pulmonary Edema Reabsorption: New Therapeutic Strategies 271
L. OPPENHEIMER, A. SMIT & A. PALOMAR

Index 283

Contributors

Steven H. Abman MD
Division of Pulmonary
Children's Hospital
University of Colorado Health Sciences Center
Denver, Colorado
USA

Francisco Baigorri MD PhD
Intensive Care Department
Consorci Hospitalari del Parc Tauli
Sabadell
Spain

Joan Albert Barberà
Servei de Pneumologia i Al.lèrgia Respiratoria, Hospital Clinic
Universitat de Barcelona
Barcelona
Spain

Sadek Beloucif MD
Department of Anaesthesiology & Intensive Care
Lariboisière University Hospital
Paris
France

Gordon R. Bernard MD
Professor of Medicine
Pulmonary and Critical Care Medicine Department
Vanderbilt University
Medical Center North
Nashville, Tennessee
USA

Lluis Blanch MD PhD
Intensive Care Department
Consorci Hospitalari del Parc Tauli
Sabadell
Spain

A. Boujoukos
Department of Anesthesiology and Critical Care Medicine
University of Pittsburgh
Pittsburgh, Pennsylvania
USA

Nicholas P. Curzen BM, MRCP
Unit of Critical Care
National Heart & Lung Institute & Royal Brompton Hospital
London
UK

Amato De Monte MD
Intensive Care Department
Consorci Hospitalari del Parc Tauli
Sabadell
Spain

A. T. Dinh Xuan MD, PhD
Laboratoire de Physiologie, Explorations Fontionelles
Hôpital Cochin
Paris
France

Christian Domingo MD, FCCP
Servei de S. Pneumologia
Consorci Hospitalari Parc del Tauli
Sabadell
Spain

Enric Domingo MD, FCCP
Servei de Cardiologia Ciutat Sanitària Vall d'Hebrón
Autonomus University
Barcelona
Spain

Didier Dreyfuss
Service de Réanimation Médicale
Hôpital Louis Mourier
Colombes and INSERM U82
Faculté Xavier Bichat
Paris
France

Timothy W. Evans BSc, MD FRCP PhD
National Heart & Lung Institute & Royal Brompton Hospital
London
UK

Claes G. Frostell MD, PhD
Department of Anaesthesia and Intensive Care
Karolinska Institute at Danderyd Hospital
Danderyd
Sweden

Shekhar Chandrashekhar R. Ghandi PhD
Department of Anesthesiology
University of Pittsburgh Medical Center
Pittsburgh, Pennsylvania
USA

Domenec Joseph MD
Intensive Care Department
Consorci Hospitalari del Parc Tauli
Sabadell
Spain

U. Kaisers
Klinik für Anaesthesiologie und Operative Intensivmedizin
Virchow-Klinikum
Medizinische Fakultät der Humboldt Universität
Berlin
Germany

John P. Kinsella MD
Division of Neonatology
Children's Hospital
Denver
USA

Kang H. Lee MA MBBChir MRCP
Department of Medicine
National University Hospital
Singapore
Republic of Singapore

Thomas R. Martin MD
Department of Veterans Affairs
Pulmonary/Critical Care Medicine
Seattle VA Medical Center
Seattle, Washington
USA

Jean-Christophe Mercier MD
Service de Réanimation Pédiatrique
Hôpital Robert-Debré
Paris
France

Robert Naeije MD, PhD
Department of Intensive Care
Erasme University Hospital
Brussels
Belgium

L. Oppenheimer MD, PhD
Department of Surgery
University of Manitoba
Winnipeg, Manitoba
Canada

A. Palomar MD
Department of Surgery
University of Manitoba
Winnipeg, Manitoba
Canada

Didier M. Payen MD, PhD
Department of Anaesthesiology & Intensive Care
Lariboisière University Hospital
Paris
France

John T. Reeves MD
Developmental Lung Biology Laboratory, B-131
Department of Pediatrics
University of Colorado
Health Sciences Center
Denver, Colorado
USA

R. Rossaint
Klinik für Anaesthesiologie und Operative Intensivmedizin
Virchow-Klinikum
Medizinische Fakultät der Humboldt Universität
Berlin
Germany

J. J. Rouby
Surgical Critical Care Unit
Department of Anesthesiology
La Pité-Salpétrière Hospital
University of Paris VI
Paris
France

Georges Saumon
Service de Réanimation Médicale
Hôpital Louis Mourier
Colombes and INSERM U82
Faculté Xavier Bichat
Paris
France

Paul J. Schenarts MD
Investigational Intensive Care Unit
Department of Anaesthesiology and Surgery
The University of Texas Medical Branch
Galveston, Texas
USA

I. Schulze-Neick
Kinderkardiologie
Deutsches Herzentrum Berlin
Berlin
Germany

A. Smit MD
Department of Surgery
University of Manitoba
Winnipeg, Manitoba
Canada

Daniel L. Traber PhD
Investigational Intensive Care Unit
Department of Anaesthesiology
The University of Texas Medical Branch
Shriners Burns Institute
Galveston, Texas
USA

W. David Watkins MD, PhD
Department of Anesthesiology
Montefiore University Hospital
University of Pittsburgh Medical Center
Pittsburgh, Pennsylvania
USA

Preface

Much has been learned about the pulmonary circulation over the past 15 years. So much so that physicians who graduated prior to that time would not be able to describe the mechanisms involved in determining vasomotor tone, ventilation–perfusion matching, pulmonary edema formation and resolution, and pulmonary hypertension if they had not been able to keep up with the literature. Regrettably for the physician struggling to maintain a broad knowledge base in medicine, all fields of medicine have witnessed similar growth. Thus the need for ongoing publications focusing on specific topics, which have as their strengths their up-to-date information, related subject matter among chapters and common themes and goals. This book is such a volume.

Our understanding of the interaction among the various vascular beds of the body continues to evolve. Perhaps no specific circulation has more far reaching associations than the pulmonary circulation because all the blood flow of the body must pass across its surface each circulation. Furthermore, changes in pulmonary blood flow, unlike that of other organs, must balance fluid surface forces allowing alveolar stability while maintaining maximal surface area for blood and air to meet for gas exchange. Gone are the days when we thought that the pulmonary circulation was a passive circuit, dilating and distending as perfusion pressure rose so as to keep pulmonary vascular pressure constant, with only alveolar pressure to limit this blood flow. Furthermore, the pulmonary circulation has the largest single vascular endothelium which works overtime as a metabolic organ, altering vasoactive substance function and determining to a large extent the tone of the entire periphery. As novel new insights surface in our continuing investigation of this 'lessor' circulation, important changes in our understanding of the pathophysiology of disease and its treatment arise.

This volume and the symposium it represents focused on these important issues and a diverse group of experts was assembled with the express purpose of solidifying these insights into common presentation. The span of the topics within is, by the nature of science today, broad, and thus not easily summarized by a single thought, process or application. The chapters of this volume are divided into four sections. The initial section addresses the important role that the vascular endothelium plays as an endocrine organ. The vascular endothelium is central in the metabolic control of both vasodilating and vasoconstricting substances. As in the rest of the body, nitric oxide plays an important role, but here it helps to define resting vasomotor tone and plays an important modulating role in the here-to-fore poorly understood mechanisms of hypoxic pulmonary vasoconstriction. These themes are extended in the second section where important aspects of pulmonary vasomotor tone, hypoxia and lung disease are described. Perhaps no time interval is more pivotal for the pulmonary circulation than birth, when the pulmonary circulation progresses from a minor hypoperfused organ to become the most perfused and singly most important organ for immediate survival in the neonatal period. In the third section, classic pulmonary physiology is presented in all its technological brilliance punctuated by novel insights and pathophysiologic relationship. Clinical relevance and practical applications define the profit from these investigations. In the fourth section, the topics switch to the alveolar interface where acute lung injury plays out its most obvious battles. This linkage between the alveolar surface and the circulation marks the single most unique aspect of the pulmonary circulation and correctly is described last, along with perspectives on clinical trials in the treatment of acute lung injury and pulmonary edema.

No story about science is static, nor is this volume exhaustive in its treatment of the topics. Relevant references are given to push the reader onward. However, the publication of this work comes quickly upon its presentation, making the subject matter up-to-date as well as pertinent to both the clinical scientist and practicing physician who must address issues of pulmonary pathology every day. It is to these people that this volume is directed. Finally, the organizing committee believes that we were truly fortunate to have the opportunity to create this program and to now share it with the reader.

Michael R. Pinsky, MD
Pittsburgh, PA

17 February 1996

Abbreviations

ALI, acute lung injury
AM, alveolar macrophage
ANP, atrial natriuretic peptide
ARDS, acute respiratory distress syndrome
BAL, bronchoalveolar lavage
CDH, congenital diaphragmatic hernia
cDO_2, critical level of oxygen delivery (DO_2 crit)
CFA, cryptographic fibrosing alveolitis
COP, colloid osmotic pressure
COPD, chronic obstructive pulmonary disease
COX, cyclooxygenase
DIC, disseminated intravascular coagulopathy
ECE, endothelin-converting enzyme
ECMO, extracorporeal membrane oxygenation
EDRF, endothelium-derived (or -dependent) relaxing factor
EF, ejection fraction
ET, endothelin
FEV_1, forced expiratory volume in the first second
F_iO_2, fraction of inspired O_2
HAPE, high-altitude pulmonary edema
HFOV, high-frequency oscillatory ventilation
HPV, hypoxic pulmonary vasoconstriction
ICAM, intercellular adhesion molecule
ITP, intrathoracic pressure
L-NAME, N^{ω}-nitro-L-arginine methyl ester
LNA, L-nitroarginine
L-NNA, *N*-nitro-L-arginine
L-NMMA, *N*-monomethyl-L-arginine
MAS, meconium aspiration syndrome
MOF, multiple organ failure
O, oxymizer

OI, oxygenation index
OSAS, obstructive sleep apnea syndrome
P_{aw}, airway pressure
PAF, platelet-activating factor
PAP, pulmonary artery pressure
$Pa{O_2}$, partial pressure of arterial oxygen
PECAM-1, platelet endothelial cell adhesion molecule
PEEP, positive end-expiratory pressure
PFC, persistent fetal circulation
PFT, pulmonary function test
PVR, pulmonary vascular resistance
PVRI, pulmonary vascular resistance index (dyn s cm^{-5} m^2)
PVZ, pulmonary vascular impedance
rt-PCR, reverse transcription polymerase chain reaction
RVEF, right ventricular ejection fraction
SIRS, systemic inflammatory response syndrome
SVR, systemic vascular resistance
TR, tricuspid regurgitation
TTC, transtracheal catheter
TXA_2, thromboxane A_2
V_A/Q, ventilation/perfusion
VCAM, vascular cellular adhesion molecule

Introduction

The Pulmonary Circulation: Evolving Concepts of Control and Interaction

Michael R. Pinsky

INTRODUCTION

This chapter attempts to summarize the salient points of the following chapters as presented in the International Symposium of the same title in September 1995 which Antonio Artigas, Jean-Francois Dhainaut, and myself organized and edited for this volume. This overview is meant to serve as an executive summary only and includes statements relevant to data presented at the symposium as well as in the chapters. It should not be assumed to cover the topics of each chapter or even the salient aspects of each chapter as defined by the individual chapter's authors. I offer my apologies ahead of time to all the authors, who reflect many of the leaders in this important field.

The symposium was divided into four parts, so as to develop the pulmonary circulatory themes, although many aspects of each chapter may cross-reference with others from other sections. In the first part, issues of local and global endocrine functions are developed. In the second part, more attention is focused on the emerging aspects of nitric oxide (NO) in the regulation of local vasomotor tone and matching of ventilation to perfusion. In Part III, classic concepts of pressure–flow relations, as defined by prior workers, are applied to this complex vascular bed in an effort to understand the determinants of pulmonary blood flow from the perspective of vascular resistance and vasomotor tone. In the final part, we jump from the blood lumen through the interstitium into the alveoli and address issues of alveolar interactions as related to diseases such as acute lung injury and septic shock. In this format, the chapters cover all aspects of the pulmonary circulation and address in some fashion most of the latest and most relevant new findings in this rapidly developing field.

THE PULMONARY ENDOTHELIUM: A LOCAL AND GLOBAL ENDOCRINE ORGAN

The pulmonary vasculature represents the single largest vascular endothelial surface area in the body. It also comprises the only vascular endothelium exposed to all the blood during a single circulation. Thus, it is poised to be a major factor in regulating global function, and its local function, if abnormal, may alter global performance indirectly because of abnormalities in pulmonary blood flow and function (Figure 1). Starting first with the local effects of the vascular endothelium, Claes Frostell examined the endogenous production of NO by constitutive NO synthase species (cNOS), referred to as type III NOS or cNOS in the literature. This enzyme coverts arginine to citrulline and NO, and requires NADH, FAD and molecular oxygen. He also cautioned us about examining exhaled NO levels blindly because cNOS is also present in the nonadrenergic noncholinergic (NANC) receptors of the airway epithelium, inducing marked elevations in exhaled NO in asthmatics and other diseases associated with airway inflammation, and is produced in the gut which makes sampling of exhaled gas, if contaminated by gastric air, meaningless. Finally, he described the important and dominant role that the nasal passages play in producing NO. This auto-inhalation of NO is lost by endotracheal intubation and may play a greater role in determining pulmonary blood flow in intubated patients than we presently think. Clearly, this is a major area of active research throughout the world.

Next, Jack Reeves and Steven Abman addressed the issue of pulmonary blood flow regulation in exercise and hypoxia. Assuming that NO is tonically produced by the pulmonary vascular endothelium in response to shear stress, then if pulmonary blood flow were to increase, more NO would also be produced, inducing the commonly seen decrease in pulmonary vascular resistance during high flow states, like exercise. If this is so, then one would predict that exhaled NO levels would increase. This hypothesis has not been tested. Finally, Dr. Reeves elaborated on the important modulating effect that hypoxia has on basal NO production inducing loss of vasodilation and thus facilitating the hypoxic pulmonary vasoconstrictor response.

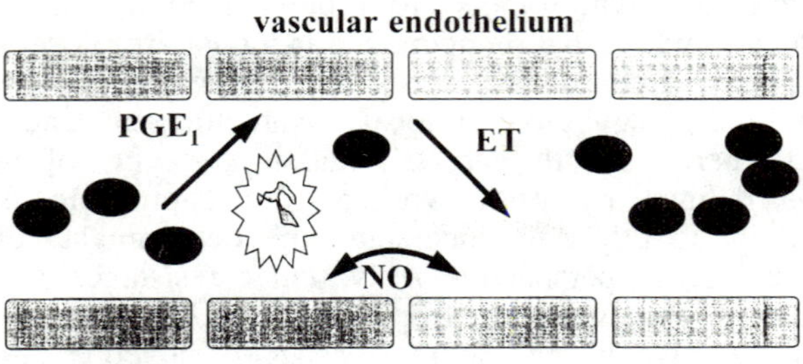

Figure 1. Diagram of the major components of the endocrine process of the pulmonary vascular endothelium. Vasodilating substances are taken up from the systemic circulation, vasoconstricting substances are enhanced and local vasodilation via NO is induced. PGE_1, prostaglandin E_1; ET, endothelin.

Next, Daniel Traber and Paul Schenarts explored the important interaction between circulating vasodilating substances and the pulmonary vascular endothelium, using sepsis models to explore these interactions. Conventional wisdom states that the pulmonary vascular endothelium takes up and metabolizes all vasodilating substances while either allowing passage of or augmenting intravascular vasoconstricting substances. Their data suggest that, during sepsis, this role may be altered, making the pulmonary vasculature less effective in defending systemic vasomotor tone. Based on their chapter, one may hypothesize that sepsis may reflect pulmonary vascular endothelial metabolic failure.

Finally, W.D. Watkins and C.S.R. Gandhi explored the evolving field of endothelin function. Endothelin is the most potent vasopressor hormone available and if present over time may induce vascular medial hypertrophy and persistent pulmonary hypertension. With the recent development of potent anti-endothelin agents, the pharmacologic study of this arm of vasomotor tone is just taking clinical trials form. Is the vascular remodeling of acute (or adult) respiratory distress syndrome (ARDS) due to imbalances in vasodilating and vasoconstricting substances? These points are discussed in their chapter, leading the reader to conclude that much of what is presently seen as end-stage lung disease may reflect a primary pulmonary vascular endothelial abnormality.

THE PULMONARY ENDOTHELIAL–SMOOTH MUSCLE INTERFACE: HYPOXIA AND VASOMOTOR TONE

Perhaps no new biological interaction has so captured the interest of the medical community as much as NO and smooth muscle tone (Figure 2). Presently, vasodilating agents are categorized as either NO-related or NO-unrelated agents. Timothy Evans and Nicholas Curzen explored the biochemistry of NO production and the effects of endotoxemia on this interaction. NOS species are of two distinct types, with various isotypes within each grouping. One group of NOS, often referred to as constitutive

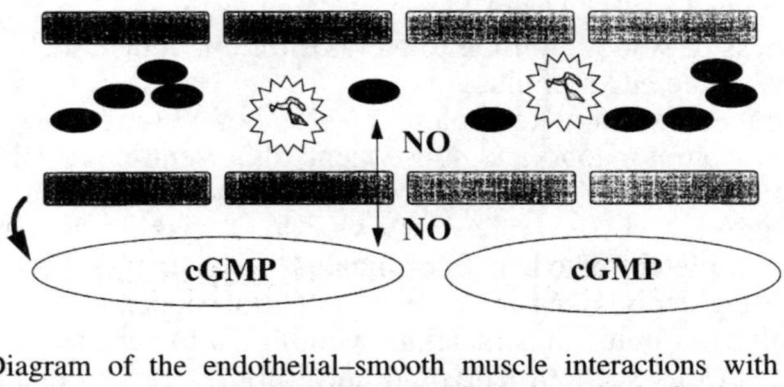

Figure 2. Diagram of the endothelial–smooth muscle interactions with NO. NO is synthesized by the vascular endothelium and released on both the lumenal and anti-lumenal sides. Lumenal NO is rapidly scavenged while that on the anti-lumenal side is taken up by vascular smooth muscle and induces vasodilation via cGMP.

NOS (cNOS) or type III NOS makes NO from arginine at a relatively slow rate, is dependent on calmodulin activation and thus is dependent on molecular oxygen. cNOS is thought to play a major role in maintaining the low basal pulmonary vasomotor tone. The other NOS species are often referred to as inducible NOS (iNOS) or type II NOS, although some iNOS exist in the native state. iNOS appears to have an activated calmodulin moiety as part of its structure, requires no molecular oxygen and can make NO at high rates thereby depleting arginine pools. Curzen and Evans presented evidence that endotoxemia decreases cNOS gene expression and augments iNOS gene expression, making NO production a function of iNOS in the vascular endothelium. Thus, the often observed loss of hypoxic pulmonary vasoconstrictor response in sepsis may reflect this imbalance in NOS activity. If cNOS is downregulated whereas iNOS is expressed, is there need for selective iNOS inhibition to reverse this process or could nonspecific NOS inhibition with arginine analogs (e.g. L-NMMA or Met-arginine) reduce this effect of sepsis? This question remains to be answered.

A.T. Dinh-Xuan, J.-C. Mercier and Steven Abman went further to explore the dynamic interaction between endothelium and NO in patients with chronic hypoxia and ARDS. Using the paradigm developed by Curzen and Evans above, they suggested that loss of endothelial function by injury or chronic hypoxia may be a primary factor determining pulmonary hypertension. Although not discussed in this chapter, in the symposium Dr. Mercier expounded on the role of both endothelin and endothelin receptor activity as well as the expression of persistent fetal circulation in the newborn. Endothelin receptor activation on endothelial cells may induce vasodilation whereas activation of endothelin receptors on the vascular smooth muscle will induce vasoconstriction. This counterbalancing interaction between endothelin and NO will continue to play out in the ensuing years as more information of these complex interactions surfaces.

Joan Barberà then proceeded to explain the role of acute inflammation on airway-exhaled NO, showing that cNOS is reduced in smokers, who are chronically exposed to high levels of NO in cigarette smoke, and increased in asthmatics. Furthermore, inhaled NO at 40 ppm or less has no measurable bronchodilating effects in normals and patients with chronic obstructive pulmonary disease (COPD), although pulmonary vasomotor tone is reduced in patients with COPD by NO levels of 40 ppm or less. Thus, the relative responsiveness of smooth muscle to NO is different depending on basal state and location of the NO stimulus.

R. Rossaint et al went on to explore the effect of NO-modulated changes in pulmonary vasomotor tone and subsequent right ventricular (RV) function. They demonstrated, not surprisingly, that pharmacologic agents that reduce pulmonary arterial pressure relieve RV workload, making the right ventricle eject more completely. The benefit of inhaled NO over systemic vasodilators, such as prostaglandin E, is that the vasodilation appears to occur only in ventilated alveolar units, thus matching ventilation to perfusion.

Finishing up this section, Christian and Enric Domingo documented the beneficial effects of long-term O_2 therapy on pulmonary vasomotor tone and Kang Lee et al demonstrated that measures of split lung VO_2 or VCO_2 can be used to accurately predict the proportion of blood flow to either lung when a tracheal divider allows such sampling.

PULMONARY BLOOD FLOW

Using classic themes of pressure–flow relations as they have been applied to the pulmonary circulation, one may identify not only the pulmonary vascular resistance, but its distension and critical closing pressure (Figure 3). Resistance is the pressure–flow relation as flow or pressure are independently varied. Distension reflects decreases in resistance at a constant perfusion pressure gradient (inflow pressure minus outflow pressure), as mean intralumenal pressure varies. Finally, downstream critical closing pressure for a vascular bed can be ascertained by determining what level of downstream pressure elevation is needed to increase upstream pressure at a constant flow. Using these constructs Robert Naeije developed the concepts of change in underlying pulmonary vascular resistance and critical closing pressure in ARDS. Furthermore, he also described the effects of positive end-expiratory pressure (PEEP) on these relations by altering only the critical closing pressure and not the pressure–flow resistance. Interestingly, vasodilator therapies may increase total blood flow up to twice as much as they decrease pulmonary artery pressure, suggesting that factors other than RV ejection pressure determine cardiac output in ARDS.

Considering the importance that pulmonary arterial pressure must play on RV function, Sadek Beloucif and Didier Payen examined the effects of combined inhaled NO and an agent that enhances hypoxic pulmonary vasomotor tone, almitrine, on gas exchange in patients with unilateral lung injury. Their data demonstrate that, although either agent alone had modest effects on gas

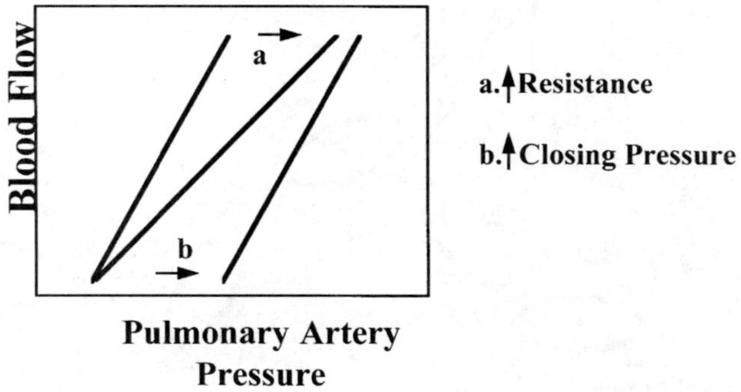

Figure 3. Plots of three pressure–flow relations for a pulmonary vascular circuit. With an increase in resistance (arrow a), the slope of this relation decreases, whereas with increases in critical closing pressure of the downstream vessels (arrow b), the zero-flow intercept point increases without a change in slope. Note that pulmonary arterial pressure for a constant flow increases in both conditions although the mechanism for the increase is different.

exchange, when combined, the benefit was impressive. These data are important because they demonstrate the importance of both vasodilation and vasoconstriction in the balance of ventilation to perfusion.

J. J. Rouby took this analysis further to examine why some patients might respond to inhaled NO whereas others with seemingly similar disease processes do not. Regrettably, the data to date show that one cannot predict who will respond and who will not based on baseline pulmonary arterial pressure, pulmonary vascular resistance, intrapulmonary shunt fraction or measures of lung compliance. Importantly, if the patient can demonstrate alveolar recruitment, then the improvement in gas exchange and pulmonary blood flow is greater than if no recruitment occurs. These data suggest that unrecruited lung may be the major site of action of NO and that ventilated alveolar units may already be fully dilated.

Francisco Baigorri et al demonstrated that, in patients with severe COPD, inhaled NO may decrease pulmonary arterial pressure but will not alter cardiac output, suggesting that RV function is not the limiting factor in chronic pulmonary hypertension complicating COPD. The chronicity of the hypertension suggests that RV adaptation allows pulmonary arterial pressure to vary without markedly altering blood flow. The implications of these data are that NO therapy may not benefit such patients even though pulmonary hypertension may be alleviated.

THE ALVEOLAR INTERFACE: DOORWAY TO THE CIRCULATION

The role of the pulmonary circulation is first and foremost to promote effective gas exchange between the blood and ambient air through the alveolar interface (Figure 4). All issues of endocrine control, pulmonary hypertension and vasomotor tone are subservient to this role. Patients with acute lung injury or ARDS present with impaired gas exchange due to loss of

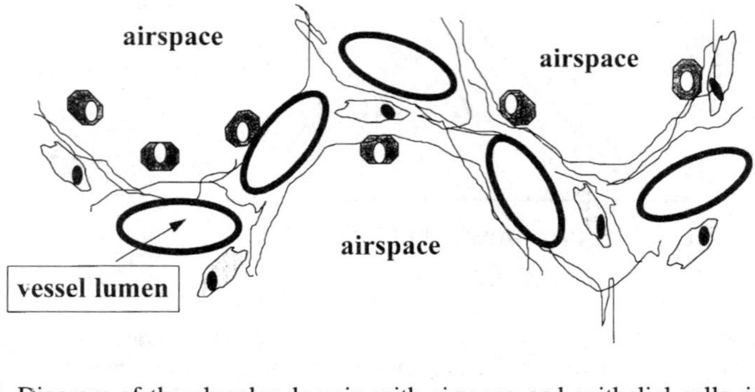

Figure 4. Diagram of the alveolar domain with airspace and epithelial cells, interstitial cells and vessel lumens. Note the complex nature of these cellular elements and the potential for compartmentalization of responses depending on which side of the airway the insult or therapeutic agent arrives.

alveolar epithelial integrity. In that light, Thomas Martin described the effect that neutrophil migration into the alveolar airspace from the vascular space has on alveolar epithelial integrity. Presumably, if neutrophil migration broke epithelial tight junctions, then alveolar disrupture would be the result of this migration and not a result of the neutrophil activation in the airspaces, *per se*. He demonstrated that neutrophil migration does not damage airway epithelial integrity, thus showing that alveolar damage, if present, represents a subsequent injury. These data are interesting for a number of reasons, not the least being that methods of neutrophil inactivation via airway-administered agents may mitigate the inflammatory response even if neutrophil accumulation does occur. Low levels of NO are anti-inflammatory and may represent such a strategy.

Alveolar epithelial injury can occur from mechanisms other than just neutrophil migration. Didier Dreyfuss and Georges Saumon described the important contribution that alveolar distension makes in the development of both alveolar injury and microvascular injury. These data, developed over a series of studies, demonstrate that repetitive hyperinflation of the lungs can induce microvascular injury, capillary leak, acute lung injury and even death, if persistent. This barotrauma, or correctly volutrauma, has a strong vascular component with an associated activation of the intravascular inflammatory cascade.

Gordon Bernard continued this theme in his report on clinical trials of ARDS therapy using anti-inflammatory agents. These data demonstrate that cyclooxygenase blockage can inhibit the immediate increase in pulmonary arterial pressure seen in experimental sepsis in sheep and may mitigate the detrimental aspects of sepsis in humans. This line of investigation reflects active ongoing large-scale clinical trials and remains a major focus of many groups including large federally funded projects and pharmaceutical industry efforts.

Finally, Luis Oppenheimer et al explored the possibility of driving back edema fluid into the interstitium and vascular space by manipulating plasma oncotic pressure. He shows that artificial increases in oncotic pressure induced by colloid loading can reduce lung water in experimental animals. Thus, it appears that we are offered a wide variety of potential agents and approaches to the treatment of acute lung injury which may be complementary in their applications. The results of ongoing and future clinical trials based on these constructs will shape our future management of the patient with, or at risk for the development of, ARDS. Such multifaceted approaches represent the logical extension of ongoing research and hopefully describe cost-effective care, since many of these novel approaches are relatively inexpensive.

The editors of this volume wish to thank all the contributing authors for their efforts in making this volume a reality. We are also grateful for the opportunity to collate these topics into one volume for the benefit of the physician who must address these very real issues of patient care on a daily basis.

Part I

The Pulmonary Endothelium: A Local and Global Endocrine Organ

1

Endogenous Nitric Oxide Production in the Respiratory System

Claes G. Frostell

INTRODUCTION

It is the bias of this presentation that endogenously produced nitric oxide (NO) has a variety of important functions in the respiratory system, many of them not yet fully determined. The literature on the biological effects of NO has exploded since 1987, when strong evidence for the identity of NO with endothelium-derived relaxing factor (EDRF) was presented.[1,2] Many aspects of endogenously formed NO have been previously reviewed,[3,4] as has the relevance of NO for the respiratory system.[5]

Endogenous NO can be synthesized from L-arginine by at least three different types of NO synthases.[6] It is usually stated that NO combines with heme in guanylate cyclase, which in turn increases production of cGMP, [3,4] resulting in biological effects. However, it is important to keep in mind that living tissue contains several other possible targets for NO in addition to heme.[7,8] One or several of the NO-producing enzymes (NO synthases of neuronal, inducible and constitutive type) can be found in abundance in several respiratory system cell types including the endothelial cells of the pulmonary vasculature.[9]

Interestingly markedly reduced expression of endothelial NO synthase in the lung vasculature has been described in patients with chronic pulmonary hypertension compared with controls.[10] Endogenously produced NO has been shown to increase ciliary beat frequency in respiratory epithelium,[11] to stimulate neurotransmitter-like activity of the inhibitory non-adrenergic non-cholinergic nerves in the human airway,[12] to modulate hypoxia-induced expression of the potent vasoconstrictor, endothelin,[13] and to contribute to unspecific immunity against viruses, mycobacteria and intracellular protozoa.[6,14] In addition, NO can influence vascular morphology. Roberts et al[15] studied rats during chronic hypoxia (10% oxygen) with or without the addition of 20 parts per million (ppm) NO. They observed decreased hypoxic pulmonary vascular structural changes and somatic growth retardation, and the increase in right ventricular weight caused by the addition of inhaled NO was prevented. These are just some examples of the diversity of functions influenced by NO in respiratory biology.

BLOCKING OF ENDOGENOUS NO PRODUCTION BY L-ARGININE ANALOGS

When acutely blocking endogenous NO production with an L-arginine analog N^{ω}-nitro-L-arginine methyl ester (L-NAME), Persson et al[16] noted profound enhancement of hypoxic pulmonary vasoconstriction and basal lung vascular tone in the normoxic anesthetized rabbit lung. This demonstrated a physiological role for endogenous pulmonary vascular NO production in rabbits. Also in humans pulmonary vascular resistance increases after administration of an arginine analog.[17] Blocking of endogenous NO production results in enhanced bronchoconstriction after provocation with aerosolized ovalbumin to immunized guinea-pigs.[18] In this context it is interesting to note that NO may be stabilized as a reduced thiol in the form of an *S*-nitrosothiol (RS-NO) in the airway-lining fluid and exert bronchodilating activity.[19] Blocking endogenous NO production with an intravenously given L-arginine analog in anesthetized pigs resulted in sharply reduced blood perfusion of a hypoxic left lower lobe studied with an ultrasonic flow probe.[20] Perfusion could be almost restored by adding exogenous NO to hypoxic gas administered to this lung region. Thus NO is also an important modulator of regional pulmonary blood flow during hypoxia in the pig.

ENDOGENOUSLY PRODUCED NO IN EXHALED AIR

Minute amounts of NO have been measured in the air exhaled from several species including humans,[21] further supporting the notion that endogenous NO production occurs somewhere in the respiratory system. NO in exhaled air was detected by chemiluminescence and also by chemical trapping with subsequent nitrate analysis.[21] With chemiluminescence, mixed expired levels of 5–20 parts per billion (ppb) of NO are typically measured.[21–23] Tracings of exhaled NO from anesthetized guinea-pigs repeatedly showed lower levels of NO during hypoxic (6%) provocation. Exhaled NO levels increased again after the inspired oxygen fraction had been restored to normal. Administration of an arginine analog sharply reduced exhaled NO, with partial recovery after administration of L-arginine.[21] Attempting single-breath analysis on exhaled gas, Persson et al[24] demonstrated a high peak of NO concentration that appeared early in a recovered tidal volume, followed by a much lower plateau level when alveolar gas was measured late in the tidal volume. A possible interpretation is that a major portion of NO in exhaled air originates from the airways, with alveolar gas being in part scavenged from NO by hemoglobin in the vasculature surrounding the alveoli. Thus the true production of NO in the pulmonary endothelium and regions close to the alveoli would always be underestimated in measurements of NO in exhaled gas. When lungs are perfused with saline instead of blood, exhaled NO concentration increases, strengthening the impression that endogenous NO is to some extent scavenged by hemoglobin.[25]

EXHALED NO FROM OTHER THAN PULMONARY ORIGIN

Recently presented data suggest that the major contribution to exhaled NO is from the nasopharynx or the nasal cavity.[22,26,27] Only minor quantities are measured after intubation of the trachea, both in healthy adults and during acute lung injury.[22,28] We may speak about 'endogenously formed inhaled NO'. More than 90% of an inhaled dose of NO is retained in the lung upon inhalation.[29] The normal nasopharyngeal excretion in adult humans can be calculated as 10–15 nmol NO per minute.[22] Curiously, patients with Kartagener's syndrome have little or no nasal production of NO.[27] Large amounts of NO are also formed in the gut. Lundberg et al[30] measured NO concentrations in the low ppm range in expelled air from the stomach. The intragastric formation of NO was seen to increase after oral intake of nitrate-containing food (lettuce) digested in an acidic environment. Obviously exhaled pulmonary NO may be contaminated with NO present in regurgitated air or with NO secreted into nasal gas.

FACTORS INFLUENCING EXHALED NO CONCENTRATION

The exhaled concentration of NO has been reported to be altered by many factors such as physiological state, disease, treatment with NO donors and antibiotic therapy.

As stated above exhaled NO is lower during hypoxia. During physical exercise, the peak level of exhaled NO has been shown to be somewhat reduced, although the exhaled amount of NO was calculated to increase more than 2-fold concomitant with exercise-induced hyperventilation.[24] Prolonged breath-holding increased peak NO levels severalfold. Ethanol intake significantly lowers exhaled levels of NO.[31] The exact nature of the interaction between the L-arginine/NO pathway and ethanol is not known. Asthmatic subjects not treated with glucocorticoids have higher peak NO concentrations than healthy normal volunteers.[32,33] Smokers exhale less NO than control subjects.[32] Massaro et al[23] studied patients presenting for emergent treatment of asthma, and found that the initial high levels of exhaled NO decreased after a few days of successful treatment of the clinical condition. The authors speculated that measurement of exhaled NO could be used to follow the clinical course of asthma, specifically evaluating its severity and treatment efficacy.

The concentration of exhaled NO rises after the intravenous administration of an NO donor such as nitroglycerin or sodium nitroprusside.[34,35] The development of nitrate tolerance is paralleled by a lower peak level of exhaled NO just after intravenous injection of the NO donor. Rovira et al[36] found a severalfold increase in exhaled NO a few hours after the start of an infusion with *Escherichia coli* endotoxin.

Gerlach et al[28] suggested that some of the NO produced in the respiratory system is caused by bacterial stimulation of inducible NO synthase. These researchers reported a lower nasopharyngeal NO level in patients on antimicrobial therapy than in controls.

As mentioned above exhaled NO in guinea-pigs is reduced during hypoxia.[21] Lundberg et al[37] found up to 20 ppm NO in gas aspirated from a paranasal sinus in healthy volunteers. Also, in newborn infants, peak nasal airway concentrations of several ppm NO have been recently measured.[38] In contrast with adults, the newborn baby has only poorly developed paranasal sinuses. We can conclude that humans inhale NO produced in the upper airways throughout life. The pathophysiological consequences of withdrawal of this NO by prolonged endotracheal intubation are as yet uncertain.

SUMMARY AND CONCLUSIONS

1. NO is continuously produced in a variety of cell types in the respiratory system, and participates in a number of biologically important activities other than relaxation of vascular smooth muscle in the vessel walls.
2. Constitutive and inducible NO synthases, producing NO from L-arginine, are present in many cell types found in the respiratory system. Expression of these enzymes is reduced throughout the lung vascular bed in patients with chronic pulmonary hypertension.
3. NO can be demonstrated in exhaled air from several species including man, and has been shown to vary with degree of physical activity, hypoxia, ethanol ingestion and airway disease.
4. In healthy humans considerable amounts of NO are produced in the gut and may be added to exhaled (or inhaled) air from either the nose or regurgitated gas from the stomach.
5. In man ppm peak levels of NO can be measured in nasal gas after timed occlusions as early as within 10 minutes of birth. The biological effects of autoinhalation of endogenously produced NO have not yet been determined, but this NO could impact upon ventilation to perfusion matching as well as host defense.
6. The state of the *pulmonary circulation* may in some clearly defined circumstances be studied by measuring exhaled NO, possibly more reliably so by using single-breath analysis. However, recent developments have made it clear that several other sources of NO add to the total exhaled NO level. These sources vary independently of the pulmonary circulation and threaten to confound any study of this circulation.
7. The *state of the airway* can to some extent be assessed by measuring exhaled NO. More specifically the degree of inflammation connected with acute asthma attacks might be clinically usefully evaluated using exhaled NO data collected intermittently over a few days.

REFERENCES

1. Palmer RMJ, Ferrige AG & Moncada S (1987) Nitric oxide release accounts for the biological activity of endothelium-derived relaxing factor. *Nature* **327:**524–526.
2. Ignarro LJ, Buga GM, Wood KS & Byrns RE (1987) Endothelium-derived relaxing factor produced and released from artery and vein is nitric oxide. *Proceedings of the National Academy of Sciences USA* **84:**9265–9269.
3. Moncada S & Higgs A (1993) The L-arginine–nitric oxide pathway. *New England Journal of Medicine* **329:**2002–2012.
4. Moncada S, Palmer RMJ & Higgs EA (1991) Nitric oxide: physiology, pathophysiology, and pharmacology. *Pharmacological Reviews* **43:**108–142.
5. Gaston B, Drazen JM, Loscalzo J & Stamler JS (1994) The biology of nitrogen oxides in the airways. *American Journal of Respiratory and Critical Care Medicine* **149:**538–551.
6. Nathan C & Xie Q (1994) Nitric oxide synthases: roles, tolls, and controls. *Cell* **78:**915–918.
7. Stamler JS, Singel DJ & Loscalzo J (1992) Biochemistry of nitric oxide and its redox-activated forms. *Science* **258:**1898–1902.
8. Stamler JS (1994) Redox signaling: nitrosylation and related target interactions of nitric oxide. *Cell* **78:**931–936.
9. Kobzik L, Bredt DS, Lowenstein CJ, Drazen J, Gaston B, Sugarbaker D & Stamler JS (1993) Nitric oxide synthase in human and rat lung: immunocytochemical and histochemical localization. *American Journal of Respiratory Cell and Molecular Biology* **9:**371–377.
10. Giaid A & Saleh D (1995) Reduced expression of endothelial nitric oxide synthase in the lungs of patients with pulmonary hypertension. *New England Journal of Medicine* **333:** 214–221.
11. Jain B, Rubinstein I, Robbins RA, Leise KL & Sisson JH (1993) Modulation of airway epithelial cell ciliary beat frequency by nitric oxide. *Biochemical and Biophysical Research Communications* **191:** 83–88.
12. Ward JK, Barnes PJ, Springall DR, Abelli L, Tadjkarimi S, Yacoub MH, Polak JM & Belvisi MG (1995) Distribution of human i-NANC bronchodilator and nitric oxide-immunoreactive nerves. *American Journal of Respiratory Cell and Molecular Biology* **13:**175–184.
13. Kourembanas S, McQuillan LP, Leung GK & Faller DV (1993) Nitric oxide regulates the expression of vasoconstrictors and growth factors by vascular endothelium under both normoxia and hypoxia. *Journal of Clinical Investigation* **92:**99–104.
14. Liew FY, Millott S, Parkinson C, Palmer RMJ & Moncada S (1990) Macrophage killing of *Leishmania* parasite *in vivo* is mediated by nitric oxide from L-arginine. *Journal of Immunology* **144:**4794–4797.
15. Roberts JD, Roberts CT, Jones RC, Zapol WM & Bloch KD (1995) Continuous nitric oxide inhalation reduces pulmonary artery structural changes, right ventricular hypertrophy, and growth retardation in the hypoxic newborn rat. *Circulation Research* **76:**215–222.
16. Persson MG, Gustafsson LE, Wiklund NP, Moncada S & Hedqvist P (1990) Endogenous nitric oxide as a probable modulator of pulmonary circulation and hypoxic pressor response *in vivo. Acta Physiologica Scandinavica* **140:**449–457.
17. Stamler JS, Loh E, Roddy MA, Currie KE & Creager MA (1994) Nitric oxide regulates basal systemic and pulmonary vascular resistance in healthy humans. *Circulation* **89:**2035–2040.
18. Persson MG, Friberg SG, Hedqvist P & Gustafsson LE (1993) Endogenous nitric oxide counteracts antigen-induced bronchoconstriction. *European Journal of Pharmacology* **249:**R7–R8.

19. Jansen A, Drazen J, Osborne JA, Brown R, Loscalzo J & Stamler JS (1992) The relaxant properties in guinea pig airways of *S*-nitrosothiols. *Journal of Pharmacology and Experimental Therapy* **261:**154–160.
20. Freden F, Wei SZ, Berglund JE, Frostell C & Hedenstierna G (1995) Nitric oxide modulates pulmonary blood flow distribution during lobar hypoxia. *Anesthesiology* **82:**1216–1225.
21. Gustafsson LE, Leone AM, Persson MG, Wiklund NP & Moncada S (1991) Endogenous nitric oxide is present in the exhaled air of rabbits, guinea pigs and humans. *Biochemical and Biophysical Research Communications* **181:**852–857.
22. Schedin U, Frostell C, Persson MG, Jacobsson J, Andersson & Gustafsson LE (1995) Contribution from upper and lower airways to exhaled endogenous nitric oxide in humans. *Acta Anaesthesiologica Scandinavica* **39:**327–332.
23. Massaro AF, Gaston B, Kita D, Fanta C, Stamler JS & Drazen JM (1995) Expired nitric oxide levels during treatment of acute asthma. *American Journal of Respiratory and Critical Care Medicine* **152:**800–803.
24. Persson M, Wiklund NP & Gustafsson LE (1993) Endogenous nitric oxide in single exhalations and the change during exercise. *American Review of Respiratory Disease* **148:**1210–1214.
25. Persson MG, Midtvedt T, Leone AM & Gustafsson LE (1994) Ca^{2+}-dependent and Ca^{2+} independent exhaled nitric oxide, presence in germfree animals, and inhibition by arginine analogues. *European Journal of Pharmacology* **264:**13–20.
26. Alving K, Weitzberg E & Lundberg JM (1993) Increased amount of nitric oxide in exhaled air of asthmatics. *European Respiratory Journal* **6:**1368–1370.
27. Lundberg JON, Weitzberg E, Nordvall SL, Kuylenstierna R, Lundberg JE & Alving K (1994) Primarily nasal origin of exhaled nitric oxide and absence in Kartagener's syndrome. *European Respiratory Journal* **7:**1501–1504.
28. Gerlach H, Rossaint R, Pappert D, Knorr M & Falke KJ (1994) Autoinhalation of nitric oxide after endogenous synthesis in nasopharynx. *Lancet* **343:**518–519.
29. Nathorst-Westfelt U, Benthin G, Lundin S, Stenqvist O & Wennmalm A (1995) Conversion of inhaled nitric oxide to nitrate in man. *British Journal of Pharmacology* **114:**1621–1624.
30. Lundberg JON, Weitzberg E, Lundberg JM & Alving K (1994) Intragastric nitric oxide production in humans: measurements in expelled air. *Gut* **35:**1543–1546.
31. Persson MG, Cederqvist B, Wiklund CU & Gustafsson LE (1994) Ethanol causes decrements in airway excretion of endogenous nitric oxide in humans. *European Journal of Pharmacology* **270:**273–278.
32. Persson MG, Zetterstrom O, Agrenius V & Gustafsson LE (1993) Single-breath nitric oxide measurements in asthmatic patients and smokers. *Lancet* **343:**146–147.
33. Kharitonov SA, Yates D, Robbins RA, Logan-Sinclair R, Shinebourne EA & Barnes PJ (1993) Increased nitric oxide in exhaled air of asthmatic patients. *Lancet* **343:**133–135.
34. Husain M, Adrie C, Ichinose F, Kavosi M & Zapol WM (1994) Exhaled nitric oxide as a marker for organic nitrate tolerance. *Circulation* **89:**2498–2502.
35. Persson MG, Agvald P & Gustafsson LE (1994) Detection of nitric oxide in exhaled air during administration of nitroglycerin *in vivo*. *British Journal of Pharmacology* **111:**825–828.
36. Rovira I, Fita G, Lopez A, Carrero E, Herrero S, Sala X & Nalda MA (1995) Increased exhaled nitric oxide in the early phase of experimental endotoxemia. *American Journal of Respiratory and Critical Care Medicine* **151:**A730. (Abstract).
37. Lundberg JON, Rinder J, Weitzberg E, Lundberg JM & Alving K (1994) Nasally exhaled nitric oxide in humans originates mainly in the paranasal sinuses. *Acta Physiologica Scandinavica* **152:**431–432.

38. Schedin U, Norman M, Frostell C & Gustafsson LE (1995) Endogenous nitric oxide in the upper airways of healthy newborn children. *British Journal of Anaesthesia* **74(Suppl 1):**101–102 (A333).

2

Nitric Oxide as the Principal Endothelium-Dependent Relaxing Factor

John T. Reeves
Steven H. Abman

INTRODUCTION

Increasing evidence supports the concept that nitric oxide (NO) is indeed the principal endothelium-dependent relaxing factor (EDRF).[1–10] It seems remarkable that so simple a molecule as nitric oxide (which by analogy with carbon monoxide, CO, might be called nitrogen monoxide) with such profound biological effects has only recently achieved the attention which it seems to deserve. NO is a remarkable molecule, for which scientists are discovering an increasing number of physiological and pathological functions. We are concerned here with the role of the endothelium in vascular control, but apart from the endothelium, NO has been implicated in neurotransmission, penile erection, bacterial killing, inhibition of platelet aggregation, and the regulation of renin secretion, to name but a few.[3,5,9,11] The present brief review looks first at the progress of scientific thought relative to our current understanding of EDRF, next at some of the evidence that EDRF is NO, and finally at selected examples of physiological function to illustrate the schema whereby endothelial L-arginine metabolism ultimately leads to vascular regulation. Because we have been concerned with the developmental evolution of the NO cascade, we will often use examples from the fetal and newborn lamb. In depth treatment of the larger issues, and particularly the physiology, pharmacology and biochemistry of the NO synthases, cGMP, and NO itself are beyond the scope of the present report and the interested reader is referred to other, more detailed reviews.[2,3,5,9,10,12]

HISTORICAL PERSPECTIVE

An historic root of NO research might justly be attributed to Brunton who in

1867 as a 23-year-old intern showed that 'nitrite of amyl' was useful therapy in a patient with angina pectoris.[13] He knew the chemical structure of the compound, and that it lowered blood pressure in dogs, and postulated that an analogous effect in man would relieve chest pain. His subsequent research into nitrogen-containing organic compounds, including nitroglycerin, suggested to him that the vasodilator effect resided with the nitrogen–oxygen moiety within the various active molecules. There was no way he could have known that amyl nitrite probably released NO in the body, for even as late as 1940, Krantz et al[14] could not identify the active principle. However, we can credit Brunton's work of more than four decades with initiating interest in the nitrovasodilators.

Two decades after Krantz's paper, there was a clue that the endothelium might be important in vascular control. In 1959 Prinzmetal et al[15] described an unusual form of angina pectoris, namely that which occurred at rest, often during the early morning hours. Reasoning from the history, physical examination, and electrocardiogram he made the remarkably prescient suggestion that the cause of the chest pain was neurally mediated vasospasm of a large coronary artery at a *locus of endothelial damage*. Further, he reported that nitroglycerin was particularly effective in such patients. Thus by 1960, there were clues in the medical literature that some combination of nitrogen and oxygen originating from certain organic compounds caused profound vasodilation, that a healthy endothelium might be necessary to avert vasoconstriction, and that the nitrovasodilators could relax constricted arteries in the presence of endothelial damage. However, there was not enough evidence to allow medical scientists to link the endothelium to the vasodilation; hindsight is ever clearer than foresight.

The next step occurred in 1977, when Arnold et al[16] showed for a number of tissues that NO stimulated guanylate cyclase. Although he did not study vascular smooth muscle, he reported that '*NO activation of guanylate cyclase appears to be a novel mechanism of enzyme regulation* . . .'. He also showed that the effect of NO could be blocked by oxidizing agents such as methylene blue and H_2O_2, and enhanced by reducing substances such as glutathione or dithiothreitol, findings that later were key in leading Furchgott[11] and Ignarro et al[4] to suspect that EDRF was NO. The 1980 report of Furchgott[17] initiated worldwide intense interest in EDRF. He found, almost by accident,[18] that acetylcholine was a vasodilator in isolated vessels, and he went on to show that it caused the vascular release of a vasodilating substance only when an intact endothelium was present (Figure 1). He called the substance endothelium-dependent relaxing factor (EDRF, where the letters RF are also the initials of Robert Furchgott).[18] His and other laboratories soon identified those substances, such as acetylcholine, bradykinin, and ATP, that were dependent on the presence of endothelium for their vasodilating effect, and other substances, such as prostacyclin, that caused vasodilation independently of the endothelium. Those dependent on endothelium required the presence of calcium for their effect. Furchgott's laboratory also showed that the effect was rapid, and that it was accompanied by the accumulation of cGMP (Figure 2). The similar time course of the cGMP accumulation and the relaxation in these vessels indicated a close relation between the two

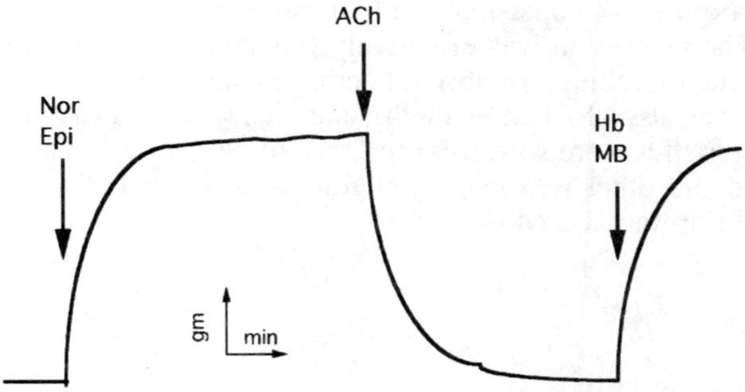

Figure 1. Inhibition by acetylcholine (ACh) of a norepinephrine-induced contraction (Nor Epi) in vascular smooth muscle with endothelium intact. Reversal of the acetylcholine effect by addition of solutions of hemoglobin (Hb) or methylene blue (MB) is shown. Redrawn and schematized from Furchgott.[11] (Time is in min and force in grams.)

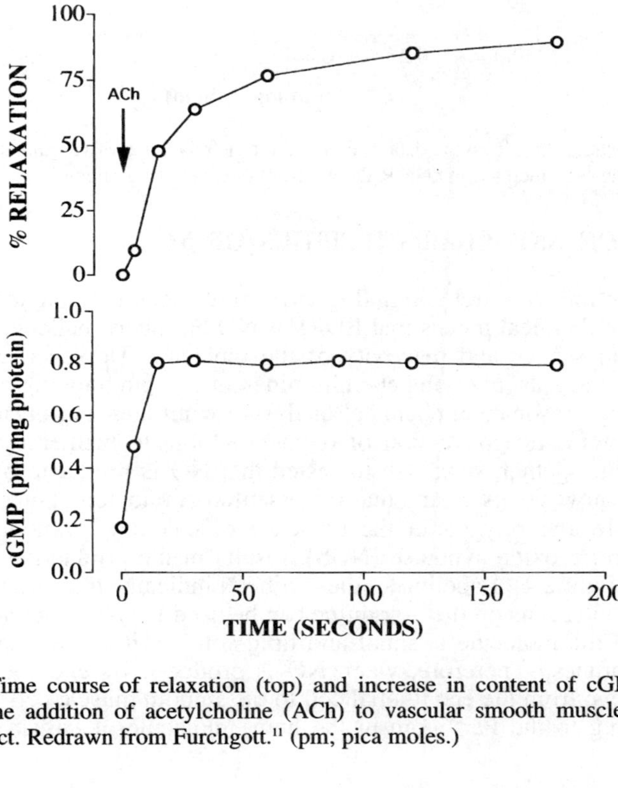

Figure 2. Time course of relaxation (top) and increase in content of cGMP (bottom) following the addition of acetylcholine (ACh) to vascular smooth muscle with endothelium intact. Redrawn from Furchgott.[11] (pm; pica moles.)

variables (Figure 3) consistent with a role for cGMP in the relaxation response. The relaxation was effectively blocked by hemoglobin (Figure 1), but not methemoglobin, probably reflecting the avid binding of NO by heme. Relaxation was also blocked by methylene blue (Figure 1) and other oxidants. The characteristics were so similar to those of NO, as noted by Arnold et al,[16] that for this and other reasons, Furchgott[11] and Ignarro et al[4] suggested that EDRF might, in fact, be NO.

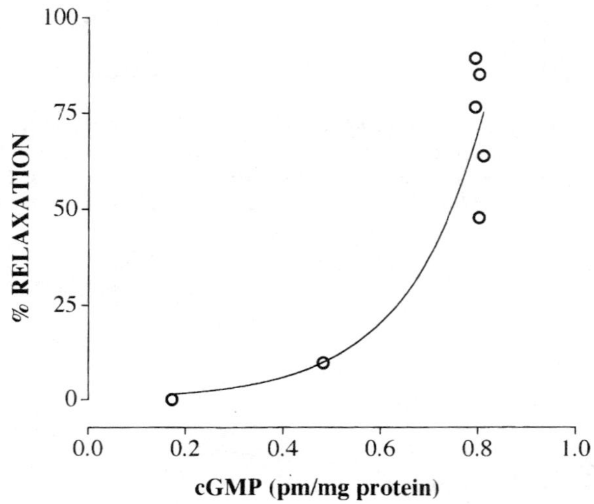

Figure 3. Relationship, from the data in Figure 2, of the relaxation of vascular smooth muscle to the simultaneous increase in cGMP. Drawn from the data of Furchgott.[11] (pm; pica moles.)

FORMATION AND CHARACTERISTICS OF NO

The suggestions of Furchgott and Ignarro were easier to make than to prove. Proving by chemical means that EDRF is NO has been challenging, because of the evanescence and reactivity of the molecule. However, as reviewed recently,[2,6] methods involving chemiluminescence, spin trapping plus electron paramagnetic resonance, chemical analysis for nitrates and nitrites, and the spectrophotometric conversion of oxyhemoglobin to methemoglobin have, when taken together, strongly suggested that NO is produced by the endothelium. It now seems clear[7,8] that the essential amino acid, L-arginine, acted on by molecular oxygen in the presence of calcium, calmodulin and an enzyme, nitric oxide synthase (NOS), results in the production of NO and citrulline (Figure 4). Labeling studies with ^{15}N indicated that either of the two guanidino nitrogens on the L-arginine can be used for NO generation.

Because the molecule is small and lipid-soluble, it moves rapidly across cell membranes.[1] Therefore, when NO is produced by endothelium it can rapidly move from the endothelial cell to the smooth muscle cell. Because of avid binding to the Fe^{2+} atom in the heme molecule, it has an affinity for

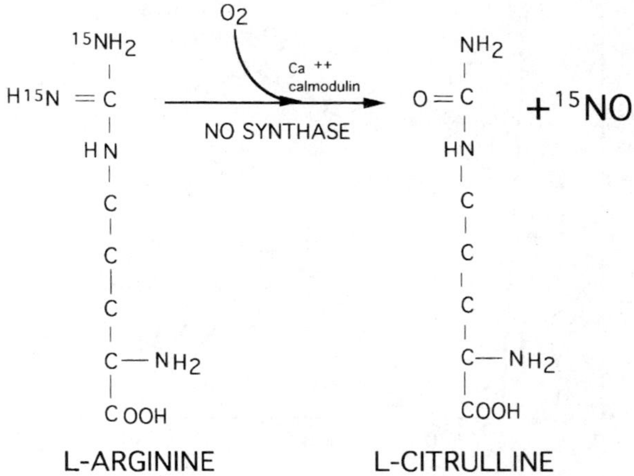

Figure 4. Schematic representation from Palmer et al[7] of the conversion of L-arginine (guanidino nitrogens labelled with ^{15}N) to L-citrulline in the presence of oxygen (O_2), free calcium (Ca^{2+}), and calmodulin, to NO where the isotopically labeled nitrogen was identified.

hemoglobin that is 10^6 times that of CO.[1] Also, because NO is a reactive species, which can be rapidly oxidized,[12] it has a half-life in the body of but a few seconds.[1] NO produced by the endothelium acts locally because that which diffuses into the vascular lumen is quickly bound to hemoglobin in the blood, and that which diffuses in the opposite direction, i.e. to the adjacent vascular smooth muscle cell, is rapidly inactivated.

Palmer et al[6] indicated that pharmacologically stimulated endothelial cells produced NO in concentrations sufficient to account for the relaxation of vessels. By combining their bioassay with their chemiluminescence data, from two separate but analogous experiments, the data suggest that NO itself, bradykinin-stimulated release of NO from endothelial cells, and the NO equivalent of nitroglycerin, all fall on a similar stimulus–response curve (Figure 5), which is compatible with the concept that NO probably is the common element.

SCHEMA FOR NO-INDUCED VASODILATION

L-Arginine

A great deal of evidence (see reviews[2,3,5,11,19]) has led to the development of a schema involving endothelium-derived NO, and leading from L-arginine to vasodilation of vascular smooth muscle (Figure 6). An examination of the evidence should begin with the overall effect, for example, whether inhibiting L-arginine metabolism along the proposed pathway does, in fact, oppose vasodilation by leading to vasoconstriction. If so, then one may consider that

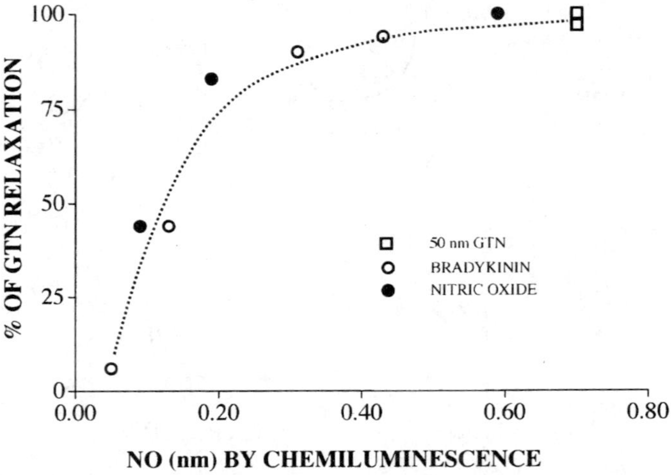

Figure 5. Correlation of measurements of relaxation in precontracted vascular smooth muscle (without endothelium) perfused from a column of endothelial cells, with analogous but non-simultaneous data of nitric oxide (NO) assay by chemiluminescence. The bradykinin relaxations occurred with NO concentrations equivalent to those from NO itself. Relaxation to nitroglycerin (GTN) and equivalent NO concentration are also shown. Drawn from the data of Palmer et al.[6]

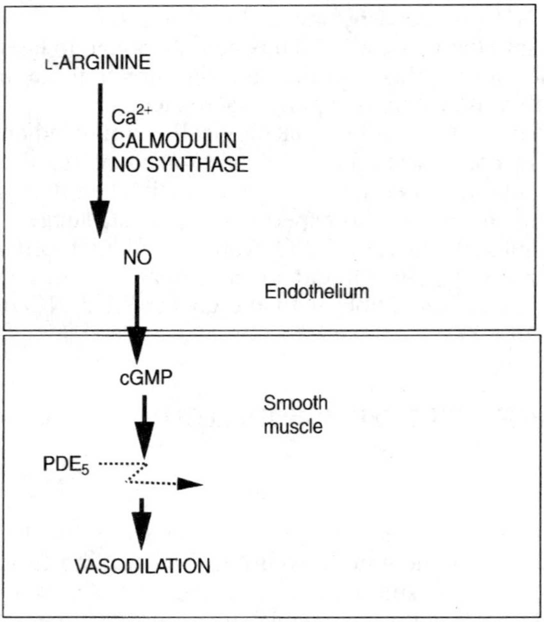

Figure 6. Schema for the metabolism of L-arginine to NO in endothelial cells and the NO-induced relaxation in vascular smooth muscle. PDE_5, phosphodiesterase.

one may be removing a mechanism that contributes to normal physiological control. Testing of the schema has been markedly facilitated by the development of numerous analogs that block NOS activity by competing with L-arginine. The most frequently used analogs involve the modification of a guanidino nitrogen (^{15}N; Figure 4) on L-arginine which probably alters the geometry of the molecule. Further, if the analog is operating by competing with L-arginine, giving L-arginine as the true substrate should reverse the vasoconstriction, unless the metabolic pathway has been damaged.

One of these competitive analogs, *N*-monomethyl-L-arginine (L-NMMA), when given as a single dose to anesthetized rabbits, raises systemic arterial pressure for many minutes (Figure 7) and the effect can be reversed by the administration of L-arginine.[20] Such data suggested that an active L-arginine pathway involving the endothelium participated in maintaining a relatively low vascular tone, and blocking the pathway allowed vascular tone to rise. If so, the pathway was involved in the acute regulation of the systemic blood pressure. This concept was supported by studies in conscious dogs by Chu et al[21] (Figure 8), in which L-NMMA acutely raised systemic arterial pressure and simultaneously caused a narrowing of a small coronary artery. If one takes their measurements in small coronary arteries as indicative of changes in systemic arterioles in general, then their results can be interpreted to show a dose-dependent response to inhibition of the L-arginine pathway, where systemic vasoconstriction increases vascular resistance and raises systemic arterial pressure. In addition, considering the constriction with L-NMMA in coronary arteries themselves supports the remarkable early suggestion of Prinzmetal et al[15] that a healthy endothelium is necessary to maintain the normal diameter of the coronary arteries. Thus in either anesthetized rabbits or conscious dogs, blocking endothelial metabolism of L-arginine increases systemic arterial tone.

Inhibition of L-arginine metabolism not only increases systemic arterial pressure acutely, but also chronic inhibition leads to chronic elevation of systemic pressure. Thus when rats were given the analog *N*-nitro-L-arginine methyl ester (L-NAME) for 4 weeks, their systemic arterial pressure as measured by tail cuff rose from a mean of 120 to 160 mmHg.[22] In addition, renal histology showed fibrinoid necrosis in the glomeruli, indicating that

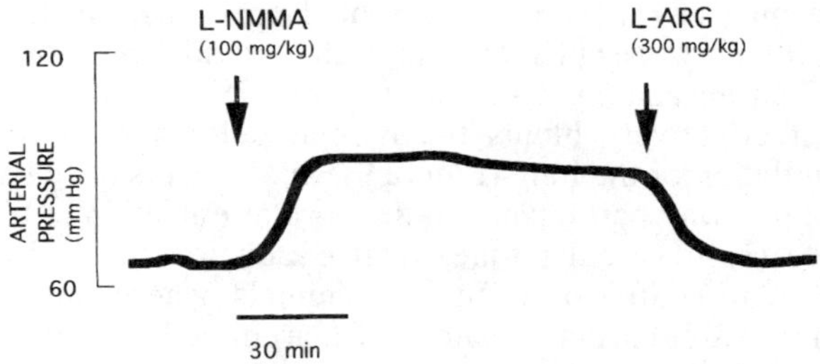

Figure 7. Pressor effect of the L-arginine analog L-NMMA on arterial pressure of the anesthetized rabbit, and return of pressure with L-arginine administration. Schematized redrawing of data presented by Rees et al.[20]

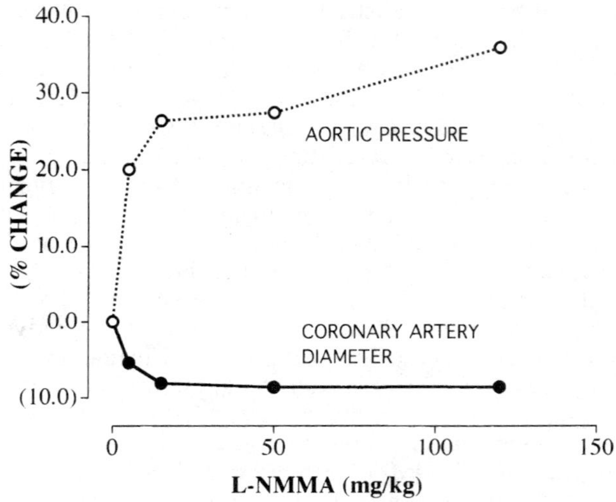

Figure 8. Decreasing coronary arterial diameter and simultaneously increasing systemic arterial pressure with increasing doses of the L-arginine analog L-NMMA. Data replotted from Chu et al.[21]

severe hypertension had been produced. After 4 weeks the hypertension could not be fully reversed by chronically administering, for 1 week, the true substrate, L-arginine. This failure to restore the pressure to normal was in contrast with the effect of L-arginine when it was given to the acutely hypertensive rabbit (Figure 7). Taken together these experiments suggest not only that the endothelial L-arginine pathway contributes to the acute and chronic regulation of arterial pressure, but also that chronic inhibition of the pathway by an L-arginine analog may damage the metabolic machinery for the endothelial production of NO.

The above studies have examined the systemic circulation where vascular tone is normally present, and one wonders whether the L-arginine pathway participates in the regulation of the pulmonary circulation, where high vascular tone may or may not be present. Experiments in the fetal lamb, where the pulmonary vascular tone is high, provide one approach to this question.[23] When an analog, *N*-nitro-L-arginine (L-NA) is given to mature fetal lambs, it effectively blunts the normal pulmonary vasodilation that occurs on ventilation of the lung (Figure 9). Such results have suggested that the L-arginine pathway participates in the normal transition at birth from the high-resistance (high vascular tone) fetal circulation to the low-resistance (low-tone) circulation after birth. In adult animals, where there is little or no basal pulmonary vascular tone, analogs of L-arginine have little acute effect, but they exaggerate the increase in tone when pulmonary vasoconstrictors are given. Thus the concept has arisen for both systemic and pulmonary circulation that, in the presence of vascular tone, the L-arginine pathway is involved in vascular control. From the above, it can be seen that, in the

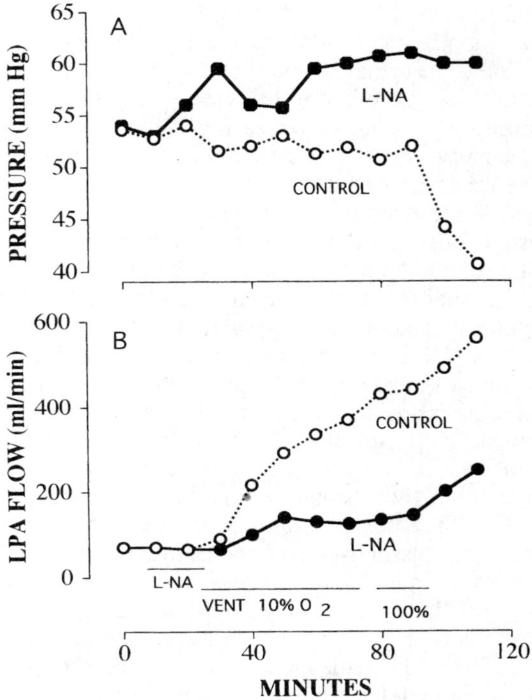

Figure 9. Measurements from the left main pulmonary artery (LPA) in mature fetal lambs. A, The L-arginine analog, L-NA, prevented the fall in pulmonary arterial pressure on ventilation of the lungs with either hypoxic gas or 100% oxygen. B, The L-arginine analog, L-NA, prevented the increase in pulmonary arterial flow on ventilation of the lungs with either hypoxic gas or 100% oxygen. Redrawn from Cornfield et al.[23]

presence of vascular tone, endothelial function seems to be a normal regulator of arterial function in a variety of animal species, in the systemic as well as the pulmonary circulation, and in the fetal, newborn, and adult mammal. Thus, the available evidence supports the overall schema shown in Figure 6.

Ca^{2+} and endothelial shear

Numerous studies (see review by Moncada et al[5]) show that acetylcholine, bradykinin, ATP, and other endothelium-dependent vasodilators require an increase in endothelial cell-free Ca^{2+} ions for the production of NO from L-arginine (Figure 6). However, we have chosen to illustrate the importance of Ca^{2+} entry into endothelial cells subjected to shear stress. Shear stress would seem to be the primary physiological endothelial cell stimulus for NO production, in part because the circulating concentrations of the endothelium-dependent vasodilators are too low to stimulate the release of NO. By contrast, endothelial cells, which line the vascular lumen, are constantly subjected to shear stresses by the flowing blood, and they have long been known to release another vasodilator, prostacyclin, even with small increments in shear force.[19] Further, throughout life, continuous NO production seems to be greatest in systemic arterioles which are subjected to the greatest shear, and least in low-pressure systems such as veins.[21] Endothelial cells may be particularly sensitive to stimulus by shear stress. High flow rates which create high shear are capable of damaging them and even stripping them from the vascular wall. If the arterial (or venous) endothelial cells sense increased shear and release a substance that increases arterial diameter, the shear stress would thereby be reduced. Further, a feedback mechanism which minimizes shear stress on the endothelium would also control arterial diameter. Since Ca^{2+} is necessary for the endothelial production of NO, then one would expect that, if increased shear is an important stimulus, it would increase Ca^{2+} entry into the endothelial cell, resulting in the production and release of NO, which would then lead to an increase in vascular diameter.

Such seems to be the case. In excised rat cremaster artery, simultaneous measurements of vessel diameter and intracellular Ca^{2+} were made from fluorescent images after the endothelium had been loaded with the Ca^{2+}-sensitive dye, fura-2.[24] When flow was increased there was a prompt and simultaneous increase in the vessel diameter and in intracellular Ca^{2+} (Figure 10A), compatible with shear-induced responses. Acetylcholine induced both the increase in Ca^{2+} and the vasodilation in the absence of flow change, and removing the endothelium prevented both the response to acetylcholine and that to increased flow. The data indicate that increased shear, like acetylcholine, increased endothelial free Ca^{2+} and arterial diameter. That shear actually increased NO production was assumed in these studies, but had previously been shown in cultured endothelial cells.[25] Further chronically increased flow in dogs with a femoral arterial–venous fistula for 6 weeks was associated with an enhanced capacity for endothelial-dependent vasodilation.[26] Although arterial and venous diameters were not reported in this study, they are known to be increased in vessels carrying a high shunt flow. The evidence is consistent with the view that increased shear increases Ca^{2+} entry into the endothelial cell, which then contributes to the activation of the L-arginine pathway to increase NO production, which then causes vasodilation, as indicated by the schema in Figure 6. Further, the shear-stress-induced mechanism appears to function both acutely and chronically.

The response to vascular shear stress has also been examined in the fetal lamb lung.[23] When the ductus arteriosus of the fetus is compressed, the pulmonary arterial pressure is increased and increasing volumes of blood are forced through the lung, thereby increasing shear stress on the pulmonary arteries. The normal acute response to the increase in pressure is pulmonary vasodilation, an increase in blood flow (Figure 10B), and a fall in pulmonary vascular resistance. However, when an analog of L-arginine is given, the flow increase is blunted. These data indicate that, in the fetal lung arterial circulation, L-arginine metabolism and the NO cascade are important for the normal vasodilation that occurs with increasing shear stress. Taking all these data together, we can say that increasing flow within vessels of many species, whether *in vitro* or *in vivo* and

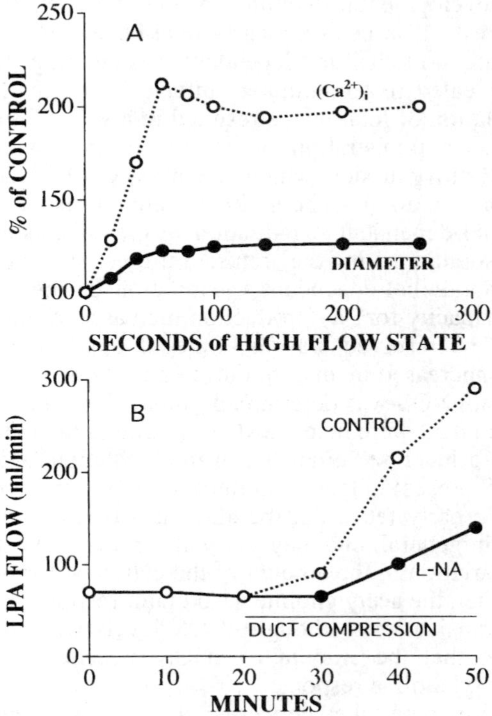

Figure 10. Measurements relating to increased shear stress in arteries. A, Time courses of the simultaneous increases in diameter and intracellular Ca^{2+} concentration in isolated arteries of the rat following an increase in flow through the artery at time 0. Removing the endothelium prevented the flow-related increases both in diameter and intracellular Ca^{2+} (data not shown). Redrawn from Falcone et al.[24] B, Time course of left pulmonary artery (LPA) flow in mature fetal lambs following the partial occlusion of the ductus arteriosus at time 20 minutes. The administration of the L-arginine analog, L-NA, inhibited the normal increase in flow seen in the control lambs following ductal compression. Redrawn from the data of Cornfield et al.[23]

whether in fetuses or adults, increases vascular diameter. Blocking endothelial metabolism of L-arginine blocks the increase in diameter. A reasonable speculation is that deformation of the endothelial cell by shear stress is the likely stimulus for Ca^{2+} entry, where increased intracellular Ca^{2+}, in turn, is the likely stimulus for NO production. If so, then endothelial-dependent vasodilation is an important mechanism for control of vascular tone and diameter.

Nitric oxide synthase (NOS) and phosphodiesterase (PDE_5)

The structure, chemistry, and function of the various isoforms of NOS have been extensively studied (see review of Griffith & Sthuer[2]). However, in our laboratory, the developmental evolution of the endothelial isoform (eNOS) has been of interest. At issue is the early fetal development and subsequent maturation of the endothelium-dependent vasodilating mechanism. The investigations revealed that continuous infusions of acetylcholine into the pulmonary circulation of fetal lambs resulted in a vasodilation that was only transient, whereas administration of endothelial-independent vasodilators (NO, 8-Br-cGMP, nitroprusside, which increases cGMP in the smooth muscle cell) gave sustained dilation[15]. The findings were consistent with the concept that the endothelial-dependent vasodilation was less robust than endothelial-independent vasodilation in the fetus. Further evidence supporting a maturation of endothelial-dependent vasodilation during fetal life was the finding that the capacity for NO production increases during gestation.[24] The first question to be resolved was the time of appearance of eNOS, and whether or not it increased in amount during gestation.

The presence of eNOS was determined immunologically, and estimates of endothelial cell content were made. eNOS was found to be present very early in fetal life and to increase somewhat in mid-gestation[27] (Figure 11A). The amounts of eNOS present in late gestation and in the newborn were similar to that present in the early fetus, but the amount was less in the adult (Figure 11A). However, in general, one may say that for the ovine species there was relatively little variation in the amount of the eNOS isoform from early fetal to adult life. Further, the acetylcholine vasodilator responses in mid- and late-gestation were transient even though eNOS levels were maximal at these times, suggesting that the amount of eNOS present did not explain the transient fetal acetylcholine response.

The next question to be asked concerned the activity of the enzyme, which can be determined by the rate of conversion of L-arginine to L-citrulline, as seen from the reaction shown in Figure 4. From preliminary findings, the activity of the enzyme increased greatly from 117 to 140 days of gestation (from 80% to 95% of the value at term which is 147 days in the lamb) and increased further after birth (Figure 11B). If the enzyme in the fetus, though present, was relatively inactive, then one might expect that a high production of NO in fetal life might not be easily sustained. However, if in the adult the enzyme is in a very active form, sustained NO production becomes possible even though less of the enzyme is present. Thus, in contrast with the presence of the enzyme, its activity appears to be more closely related to NO production and the capacity of the lung circulation to sustain a vasodilator response to acetylcholine. The factors responsible for the increase in enzyme activity in later gestation and after birth are not known, but are clearly of great importance.

Not only the production of NO, but also its rate of removal could be important in the non-sustained vasodilation with acetylcholine in the fetus. As shown in Figure 6, the breakdown of cGMP is catalyzed by the phosphodiesterase isoenzyme, PDE_5. Thus another factor that could contribute to an unsustained vasodilation in the fetus is a high activity of PDE_5, which is an important regulator of cGMP concentration within the vascular smooth muscle cell. Preliminary data suggest (Figure 11C) that the activity of this enzyme is higher in the term fetus than in the newborn, which, if confirmed,

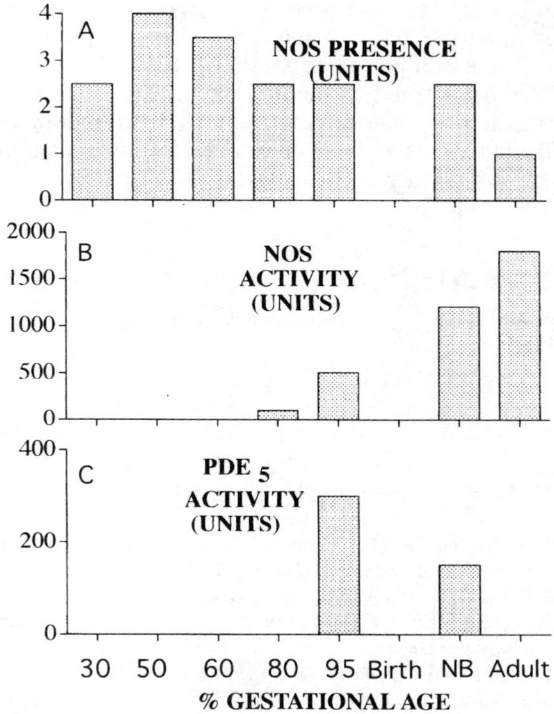

Figure 11. Measurements from pulmonary arterial tissue in lambs of varying gestational age (term is 147 days), in newborn lambs (NB; <6 days), and in adult sheep. A, The changes during development in immunologically determined NOS content of endothelium. Redrawn from Halbower et al.[27] B, Changes during development in activity of NOS in endothelium as determined from the rate of conversion of L-arginine to L-citrulline (unpublished data). C, Changes from mature fetus to the newborn in the activity of an isoenzyme of phosphodiesterase (PDE_5) (unpublished data).

could also help account for the transient nature of the acetylcholine vasodilatory response in the fetus.

SUMMARY

There seems to be ever increasing evidence that NO is the essential EDRF. Even though final chemical proof is difficult to establish because of the evanescent and reactive nature of the molecule, the multiple approaches used mutually reinforce the role for NO. Further, intense investigation from around the world has put into place considerable understanding of the reactions by which L-arginine is converted into L-citrulline with the release of NO, and the cascade of events leading from NO to the ultimate vasodilation that occurs. The physiological role for endothelial production of NO in vascular control would seem primarily to involve endothelial shear stress. The mechanisms of the NO cascade appear to be particularly important where vascular tone is high, as in fetal life for the developing lung (and probably for the developing systemic) circulation, and after birth in the systemic arterial tree. Further efforts to understand endothelium-dependent relaxation will almost certainly lead to a better understanding of vascular control in health and disease.

ACKNOWLEDGEMENTS

This work was supported in part by the National Institute of Health grants HL-01932, HL-41012, and SCOR grant HL-46481.

REFERENCES

1. Archer S (1993) Measurement of nitric oxide in biological models. *FASEB Journal* **7:**349–360.
2. Griffith OW & Sthuer DJ (1995) Nitric oxide synthases: Properties and catalytic mechanism. *Annual Reviews of Physiology* **57:**707–736.
3. Griffith TM & Edwards DH (1990) Nitric oxide in arterial networks. In Moncada S & Higgs EA (eds) *Nitric Oxide from* L*-Arginine: A Bioregulatory System*, pp 397–408. Amsterdam: Elsevier.
4. Ignarro LJ, Burns RE & Wood KS (1988) Biochemical and pharmacological properties of endothelium-derived relaxing factor and its similarity to the nitric oxide radical. In Vanhoutte PM (ed), *Vasodilation: Vascular Smooth Muscle, Peptides, Autonomic Nerves, and Endothelium*, pp 427–436. New York: Raven Press.
5. Moncada S, Palmer RMJ & Higgs EA (1991) Nitric oxide: Physiology, pathophysiology, and pharmacology. *Physiological Reviews* **43:**109–142.
6. Palmer RM, Ferrige AG & Moncada S (1987) Nitric oxide release accounts for the biological activity of endothelium-derived relaxing factor. *Nature* **327:**524–526.
7. Palmer RMJ, Ashton DS & Moncada S (1988) Vascular endothelial cells synthesize nitric oxide from L-arginine. *Nature* **333:**664–666.
8. Palmer RMJ, Reese DD, Ashton DS & Moncada S (1988) L-arginine is the physiologic precursor for the formation of nitric oxide in endothelium-dependent relaxation. *Biochemical and Biophysical Research Communications* **153:**1251–1256.
9. Umans JG & Levi R (1995) Nitric oxide in the regulation of blood flow and arterial pressure. *Annual Reviews of Physiology* **57:**771–790.
10. Vanhoutte PM (1988) *Relaxing and Contracting Factors*, Clifton, NJ: The Humana Press.
11. Furchgott RF (1988) Studies on relaxation of rabbit aorta by sodium nitrite: the basis for the proposal that the acid-activatable inhibitory factor from retractor penis is inorganic nitrite and that the endothelium-derived relaxing factor is nitric oxide. In Vanhoutte PM (ed) *Vasodilation: Vascular Smooth Muscle, Peptides, Autonomic Nerves and Endothelium*, pp 401–414. New York: Raven Press.
12. Freeman B (1994) Free radical chemistry of nitric oxide. *Chest* **105:**79S–84S.
13. Reeves JT (1995) Brunton's use of amyl nitrite in angina pectoris: an historic root of nitric oxide research. *News of Physiological Sciences* **10:**141–144.
14. Krantz JC, Carr CJ, Forman SE & Cone N (1940) Mechanism and action of organic nitrates. *Journal of Pharmacology and Experimental Therapy* **70:**323–327.

15. Prinzmetal M, Kennamer R, Merliss R, Wada T & Bor N (1959) Angina Pectoris I. A variant form of angina pectoris. *American Journal of Medicine* **27:**375–388.
16. Arnold WP, Mittal CK, Katsuki S & Murad F (1977) Nitric oxide activates guanylate cyclase and increases guanosine 3′:5′ monophosphate levels in various tissue preparations. *Proceedings of the National Academy of Sciences USA* **74:**3203–3207.
17. Furchgott RF & Zawadzki JV (1980) The obligatory role of endothelial cells in the relaxation of arterial smooth muscle by acetyl choline. *Nature* **288:**373–376.
18. Furchgott RF (1993) The discovery of endothelium-dependent relaxing factor. *Circulation* **87 (Suppl V):**V3–V8.
19. van Grondelle AS, Worthen GS, Ellis D, Mathias MM, Murphy TC, Strife RJ, Reeves JT & Voelkel NF (1984) Altering hemodynamic variables influences PGI_2 production by isolated lungs and endothelial cells. *Journal of Applied Physiology* **57:**388–395.
20. Rees DD, Palmer MJ & Moncada S (1989) Role of endothelium-derived nitric oxide in the regulation of blood pressure. *Proceedings of the National Academy of Sciences USA* **86:**3375–3378.
21. Chu A, Lin C-C, Chambers DE, Kuehl WD, Palmer RMJ, Moncada S & Cobb FR (1991) Effects of inhibition of nitric oxide formation on basal tone and endothelium-dependent responses of the coronary artery in awake dogs. *Journal of Clinical Investigation* **87:**1964–1968.
22. Ribiero MO, Antunes E, de Nucci G, Lovisolo SM & Zatz R (1992) Chronic inhibition of nitric oxide synthesis, a new model of arterial hypertension. *Hypertension* **20:**298–303.
23. Cornfield DN, Chatfield BA, McQueston JA, McMurtry IF & Abman SH (1992) Effects of birth-related stimuli on L-arginine-dependent vasodilation in the ovine fetus. *American Journal of Physiology* **262:**H1474–H1481.
24. Falcone JC, Kuo L & Meininger GA (1993) Endothelial cell calcium increases during flow-induced dilation in isolated arteries. *American Journal of Physiology* **264:**H653–H659.
25. Buga GE, Gold ME, Fukuto JM & Ignarro LJ (1991) Shear stress-induced release of nitric oxide from endothelial cells grown on beads. *Hypertension* **17:**187–193.
26. Miller VM, Aarhus LL & Vanhoutte PM (1986) Modulation of endothelium-dependent responses by chronic alterations of blood flow. *American Journal of Physiology* **251:**H520–H527.
27. Halbower AC, Tudor RM, Pollock JS, Forstermann U & Abman SH (1994) Maturation-related changes in immunolocalization of endothelial nitric oxide synthase in the developing ovine circulation. *American Journal of Physiology* **267:**L585–L591.

3

Interaction Between Vasodilating Substances and Lung Function

Paul J. Schenarts
Daniel L. Traber

INTRODUCTION

Increased vasomotor tone of the pulmonary vasculature resulting in the development of pulmonary hypertension is a typical feature of acute lung injury associated with sepsis, polytrauma, pneumonia, and critical illness. Pulmonary hypertension may also be due to idiopathic causes as in the case of primary pulmonary hypertension or may be a secondary complication of chronic disease states such as chronic obstructive pulmonary disease. This increased pulmonary vascular smooth muscle tone, particularly on the venous side of the circulation, causes an increase in pulmonary transvascular fluid flux with resultant interstitial edema and subsequent impairment of gas exchange. Pulmonary hypertension also increases the afterload on the right ventricle, which not only causes right heart failure but also shifts the interventricular septum into the left ventricular chamber, ultimately resulting in biventricular heart failure.

In response to acute lung injury and changes in ventilatory pattern, the lung is able to assert active control of its circulation by synthesizing and releasing vasodilatory substances into the pulmonary vasculature. In this way the lung is able to limit the pulmonary hypertension, edema, hypoxemia, and ventricular dysfunction associated with acute lung injury. Several of these vasodilators have also been shown to have therapeutic applications. The purpose of this chapter is to: (1) briefly describe the mechanisms that govern pulmonary vasoactivity under normal and pathologic conditions; (2) delineate the general therapeutic implications of pulmonary vasodilators; (3) discuss in detail pulmonary vasodilators the therapeutic use of which has been recently explored such as nitric oxide (NO), prostaglandin I_2, and prostaglandin E_1, and (4) briefly discuss other pulmonary vasodilatory agents, including prostaglandin E_2, atrial natriuretic peptide, and the endothelins.

NORMAL MECHANISMS OF PULMONARY VASOMOTOR CONTROL

Vasomotor control of the pulmonary circulation differs from systemic circulation in that hypoxia induces vasoconstriction in contrast with the vasodilatory response seen in the systemic circulation. This pulmonary vascular mechanism is responsible for matching ventilation with perfusion. Alteration of this mechanism results in ventilation–perfusion mismatch and impaired gas exchange.

Vasoconstriction

The principal pulmonary vasoconstrictor is hypoxia. Von Euler and Liljestrand first described the phenomenon of hypoxic pulmonary vasoconstriction (HPV) in 1946.[1] However, despite intense scientific efforts, the exact mechanisms and mediators responsible for this complex process have remained elusive. Numerous vasoconstrictive agents such as angiotensin, adrenergic agonists, histamine, serotonin, and products of arachidonic acid metabolism have been shown to contribute to or augment the process of HPV but none have qualified as the unique effector of HPV.[2] It has become increasingly likely that pulmonary vascular smooth muscle tone is regulated by pulmonary-derived endothelial factors. The endothelial cell is capable of producing vasoactive substances, such as platelet-activating factor, in response to hypoxia, which may react with pulmonary vascular smooth muscle receptors with resultant vasoconstriction.[3]

Low oxygen tension may also directly induce vasoconstriction by electromechanical coupling, changes in cellular metabolism, or alterations of plasma membrane signal transduction.[2] Alternatively, hypoxia has been shown to cause impaired release of endothelium-derived relaxing factor (nitric oxide (NO)),[4] a substance that is known to reverse HPV.[5] Potassium channels may also be sensitive to hypoxia and cause vasoconstriction by closure, which results in depolarization and opening of calcium channels.[6] Regardless of the initial mechanism, the final common pathway involves increasing the concentration of intracellular calcium in pulmonary vascular smooth muscle, which results in pulmonary vasoconstriction.

Vasodilatation

In contrast with the many different mechanisms that induce pulmonary vasoconstriction, the intracellular mechanisms responsible for pulmonary vasodilatation are mediated through one of two intracellular mediators, either cyclic adenosine monophosphate (cAMP) or cyclic guanosine monophosphate (cGMP).

Activation of adenylate cyclase via G stimulatory proteins may occur by direct β-adrenergic receptor stimulation (e.g. isoproterenol) or by production of endothelium-derived substances such as prostaglandin I_2, prostaglandin E_1, or prostaglandin E_2, each of which increases intracellular cAMP and in turn induces pulmonary vasodilatation.[7] The endothelial production of vasodilators such as prostaglandin I_2 is normally stimulated by shear forces and pulse pressure.[7] This production is known to decrease with advancing age, diabetes mellitus, and atherosclerosis.[7]

cGMP-dependent pulmonary vasorelaxation is also mediated by both endothelium-dependent and -independent mechanisms. The prototypic cGMP endothelium-dependent pulmonary vasodilator is acetylcholine, which interacts with endothelial muscarinic receptors leading to the production of NO.[8] NO activates cytoplasmic guanylate cyclase, thus increasing cGMP, which in turn promotes calcium pumping from the cell and dephosphorylation of myosin light chains, which results in pulmonary vasorelaxation.[9] Endothelial-dependent NO production can also be stimulated by ATP, ADP, bradykinin, and histamine.[7] Like prostaglandin I_2, NO can also be produced by shear stress and may act synergistically with prostaglandin I_2.[7] Endothelium-independent pathways are not dependent on an interaction with the endothelium and are commonly used therapeutic agents such as sodium nitroprusside and nitroglycerin, each of which function as NO analogs.[7] In addition to these therapeutic agents, atrial natriuretic peptide (ANP) induces production of NO by acting on the particulate membrane form of guanylate cyclase,[10] which ultimately increases intracellular cGMP by an endothelium-independent pathway.[3]

Summary

In summary, the balance between vasoconstriction and vasodilatation in the pulmonary circulation is responsible for matching ventilation with perfusion. Vasoconstriction is primarily due to hypoxia; however, the exact mechanism responsible for this remains elusive. Multiple mediators are capable of inducing pulmonary vasodilatation and do so by increasing either cAMP or cGMP, which leads to a reduction in intracellular calcium (Figure 1). These mechanisms that govern pulmonary vasomotor control may be altered in acute and chronic lung disease.

ALTERATIONS OF VASOMOTOR CONTROL IN RESPONSE TO ACUTE LUNG INJURY AND OTHER DISEASE STATES

Ventilation–perfusion matching is dependent upon the dynamic balance of pulmonary vasodilatation and vasoconstriction. In acute lung injury and other chronic disease states this balance is disrupted, thus impairing gas exchange, which ultimately leads to systemic tissue hypoxia and injury.

Using an animal model of acute lung injury induced by mesenteric ischemia–reperfusion, Fullerton et al[11] showed that cAMP-mediated pulmonary vasodilatation was dysfunctional. Therefore it appears that in the setting of acute lung injury the pulmonary vasomotor balance is tipped in favor of vasoconstriction.[11] This conclusion is further substantiated by the

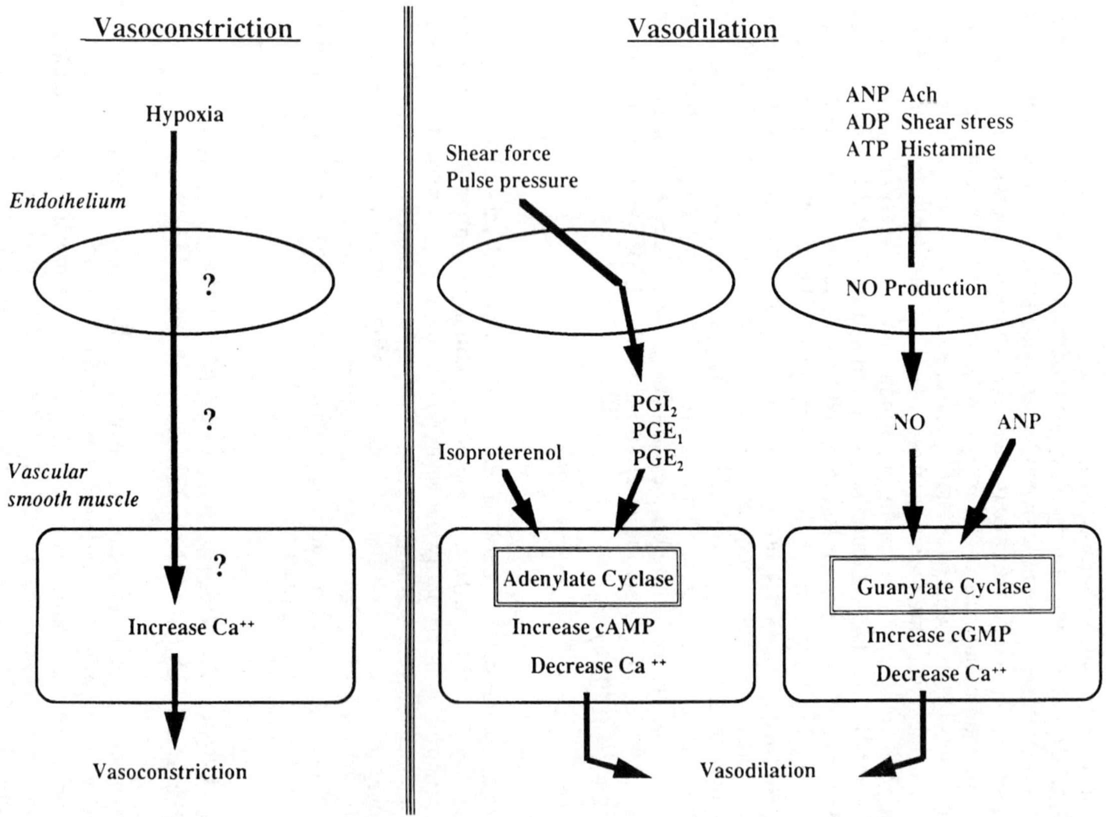

Figure 1. Summary of pulmonary vasomotor control mechanisms. PGI_2, prostaglandin I_2; PGE_1, prostaglandin E_1; PGE_2, prostaglandin E_2 Ach, acetylcholine.

finding that mesenteric ischemia–reperfusion depletes pulmonary endothelial ATP, a known pulmonary vasodilator,[7] via a humoral mechanism.[12] However, endothelium-dependent as well as endothelium-independent cGMP-mediated vasodilatation remain essentially normal.[7]

Hypoxia is also thought to play an important role in the disrupted vasomotor balance of both acute lung injury and some chronic pulmonary disease states. Hypoxia has been shown to impair β-adrenergic signal transduction, resulting in impaired cAMP mechanisms of pulmonary vasodilatation.[7] However, both endothelium-dependent and -independent mechanisms of cGMP-mediated vasodilatation appear to be intact during hypoxia.[7] Thus hypoxia not only causes pulmonary vasoconstriction, but it also inhibits pulmonary vasodilatation, thereby further tipping the balance in favor of vasoconstriction. The chronic hypoxia noted in patients with chronic obstructive pulmonary disease is thought to induce remodeling of the pulmonary vasculature, which further increases pulmonary vascular resistance.[13]

In addition to the pulmonary vasomotor dysfunction associated with acute lung injury, a number of mechanical factors, such as platelet microemboli, *in situ* thrombosis, and vascular compression from edema may further impair pulmonary blood flow and complicate gas exchange.[14,15] Additional pulmonary vasoconstriction may also occur, as a result of the release from distant injury sites, of vasoconstrictor substances such as thromboxane. These mediators may circulate to the pulmonary vasculature where they can induce further vasoconstriction.

In summary, lung injury and hypoxia favor vasoconstriction over vasodilatation, which may lead to impaired gas exchange owing to ventilation–perfusion mismatch. These dysfunctional vasomotor control mechanisms are further complicated by mechanical factors that obstruct pulmonary blood flow. These pathophysiologic mechanisms account for substantial morbidity and mortality after acute and chronic lung injury. Therefore, the use of selective pulmonary vasodilators would be therapeutically advantageous.

THERAPEUTIC IMPLICATIONS OF SELECTIVE PULMONARY VASODILATORS

There are two principal criteria that pulmonary vasodilators must meet to be therapeutically useful. The first is that it should act selectively on the pulmonary circulation and not the systemic circulation. Acute lung injury is often associated with multisystem trauma, sepsis, major surgical procedures, and critical illness; in these settings, systemic vasodilatation would lead to disastrous circulatory collapse. The second important requirement is that the selective pulmonary vasodilator should improve perfusion only to well-ventilated alveolar units. Should blood flow be restored to nonventilated areas this would lead to an increased ventilation–perfusion mismatch and would further impair oxygenation.

Several pulmonary vasodilators have been shown to be synthesized, released, and metabolized by the lung. Three of these have been examined for use in treatment of pulmonary hypertension secondary to acute lung injury as well as chronic pulmonary disease.

PULMONARY VASODILATORS WITH POTENTIAL THERAPEUTIC APPLICATION

Several vasodilatory substances are released by the lung in response to pulmonary injury. Of these, NO, prostaglandin I_2 (PGI_2), and prostaglandin E_1 (PGE_1) have been investigated in the treatment of acute and chronic lung disease. Several of these agents are, however, limited by lack of pulmonary selectivity or exacerbation of ventilation–perfusion mismatch.

Nitric oxide

Within the past decade NO has progressed from an environmental pollutant found in engine exhaust to 'molecule of the year' in 1992[16] for its integral role in normal and abnormal physiology. The role of NO in pulmonary vasodilatation under normal conditions was briefly discussed above. Additionally, NO has been shown to play an important role in the pathogenesis of a number of serious medical conditions, including hemorrhagic[17] and septic shock,[18–20] and gastrointestinal ischemia–reperfusion injury.[21] Therefore, the potential pharmacological value of NO as well as that of agents that manipulate its metabolism may prove useful in the critical care setting.

NO, previously known as endothelium-derived relaxing factor,[22] is a potent endogenous vasodilator. It is normally produced by a constitutive NO synthase (cNOS) in the endothelium from L-arginine by a metabolic pathway that requires calcium, calmodulin, and NADPH. The enzyme NOS also has an inducible form that does not require calcium for its activity. In addition to its vasodilatory properties NO is also known to regulate a number of other physiologic processes including platelet aggregation,[23] neurotransmission,[24] as well as antitumor and antimicrobial activities.[25,26] NO has also been shown to preserve microvascular permeability to protein after acute lung injury.[27]

Upon stimulation of the endothelium receptor, activation leads to increased cytosolic calcium, which activates constitutive NOS to produce NO. This small lipophilic molecule freely diffuses out of the endothelium and into vascular smooth muscle cells where it stimulates the production of cGMP; this in turn causes a decrease in the concentration of free cytosolic calcium that results in smooth muscle relaxation and vasodilatation.

Stimulation of the vascular endothelium to produce NO has also been shown to occur in response to shear forces, pulsatile pressure,[7] substances released from nerves (e.g. acetylcholine, excitatory amino acids), and substances released from platelets (e.g. thrombin, serotonin).[28] In addition, ANP also causes the release of NO.[3]

In vivo, NO is labile, with a biologic half-life of 111 and 130 ms, depending on the ambient oxygen concentration.[29] Once in the circulation, NO binds albumin[30] or is quickly inactivated by reacting with hemoglobin, resulting in the formation of nitrite, nitrate, nitrosylated protein, and methemoglobin.[30–32] Thus, the vascular endothelium normally regulates vasomotor tone locally without affecting the body as a whole.

If the inducible form of NOS is created, as in the case of sepsis, NO can be formed in such abundance as to result in systemic vasodilatation and circulatory collapse.

While this increased production of NO may appear to provide an element of pulmonary protection, by limiting the associated pulmonary hypertension, it may do so at a significant cost. In addition to pulmonary hypertension, an increased intrapulmonary shunt is also associated with sepsis. This increased intrapulmonary shunt and secondary hypoxemia are likely due to this increased production of NO, which abolishes HPV[5] and thereby increases ventilation–perfusion mismatch. Using a sepsis model induced by a continuous infusion of endotoxin, we have found that the associated increase in intrapulmonary shunt fraction was returned to normal by administration of an NOS inhibitor.[33] Further, in pulmonary vessels obtained from sheep that had been given a continuous infusion of endotoxin or bacteria, contractility to norepinephrine and potassium was depressed. This depression in contractility occurred predominately in pulmonary veins and was not reversed by the administration of NOS inhibitor (Figure 2).[34–36] However, these vessels were also found to have particularly high levels of cGMP, which was reversed by addition of an NOS inhibitor (Figure 3).[34–36] The reasons for these apparently contradictory results are unclear.

It would appear from the above discussion that NO would not be useful as a therapeutic agent for pulmonary hypertension because it is not a selective

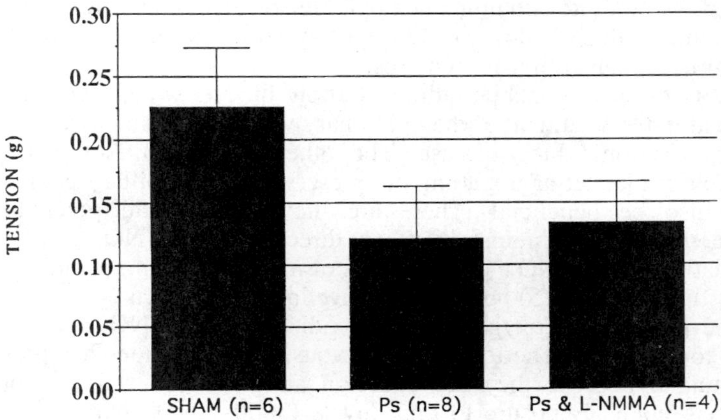

Figure 2. Maximal contractile responses (E_{max} in g) to KCl in pulmonary veins from control sheep (SHAM), sheep given a 48 h infusion of *Pseudomonas aeruginosa* (Ps), or a 48 h infusion of *Pseudomonas* and a 24 h infusion of L-N^G-monomethyl-L-arginine (100 μM; Ps & L-NMMA). The data are presented as means ± S.E.M. There was a decrease in contractility in both groups treated with *Pseudomonas* compared with the SHAM group; however, this decrease in contractility was not reversed by L-NMMA.

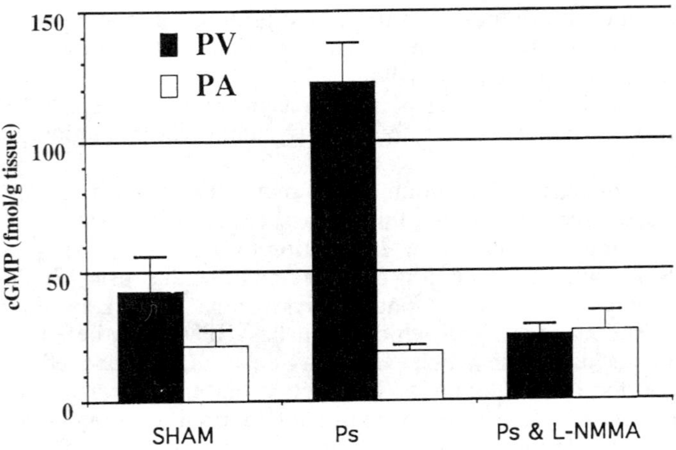

Figure 3. Pulmonary vascular levels of cGMP in pulmonary arteries (PA; open bars) and veins (PV; solid bars) from control sheep (SHAM), sheep given a 48 h infusion of *Pseudomonas aeruginosa* (Ps) or a 48 h infusion of *Pseudomonas* and a 24 h infusion of L-N^{G}-monomethyl-L-arginine (100 μM; Ps & L-NMMA). The data are presented as means ± S.E.M. There was an increase in cGMP in the PV but not PA; this was reversed by L-NMMA.

pulmonary vasodilator. However, its gaseous properties allow it to be inhaled, thereby vasodilating only those alveolar units which are adequately ventilated, thus preventing exacerbation of ventilation–perfusion mismatch. Since NO rapidly binds to albumin, hemoglobin, or is oxidized to nitrates and nitrites, the inhaled gas does not cause the systemic vasodilatation that would be harmful in many clinical scenarios.

Short-term transbronchial administration of NO would appear to be beneficial in the treatment of the pulmonary vasoconstriction associated with acute and chronic lung disease. The other actions of NO, particularly inhibition of platelet aggregation and preservation of capillary permeability, would also be beneficial. There are, however, several potential risks associated with NO administration:[9] (1) direct toxicity of NO, (2) toxicity of its oxidative product NO_2, (3) formation of methemoglobin, (4) inhibition of platelet function, and (5) possible negative inotropic effects.

In the presence of oxygen, NO is oxidized to NO_2. NO_2 and NO have known toxic effects. The toxicity of various nitrogen oxides has previously been studied because they are common air pollutants and are found in cigarette smoke.[9] Exposure to high levels (5000–20 000 ppm) of NO and NO_2 also causes the formation of HNO_3 and HNO_2, both of which cause silo filler's disease, a type of acute interstitial pneumonitis.[9] However, mice exposed to NO (10 ppm) for 6 months[37] and rabbits exposed to 43 ppm of NO (3.6 ppm NO_2) for 6 days showed no apparent lung damage.[38] Another concern, particularly in the treatment of acute lung injury, is that acute inflammation enhances the formation of toxic oxygen metabolites. NO reacts with superoxide radical ($O_2^{-\bullet}$) to form peroxynitrite, an extremely cytotoxic metabolite.[39]

As described above, NO reacts with hemoglobin to form methemoglobin. Methemoglobin is eliminated by the enzyme methemoglobin reductase found in erythrocytes. Patients with partial or complete deficiency in this enzyme may have difficulty oxygenating as the oxygen may preferentially bind to the methemoglobin in place of hemoglobin.[9] Neonatal patients are known to have an immature methemoglobin reductase and therefore may be more subject to this phenomenon.[40]

While the antiplatelet effects of NO may be desirable because NO prevents the mechanical obstruction of the pulmonary microvasculature by platelet aggregates associated with acute lung injury,[15] it may also lead to bleeding complications.[41]

Another potential limitation of NO therapy is that it may mediate negative inotropic effects on the heart.[42] In patients with severe congestive heart failure, inhalation of NO may cause a further increase in pulmonary capillary wedge pressure, resulting in worsening pulmonary edema.[43,44]

Despite these limitations the potential benefits of inhaled NO therapy for the vasoconstriction associated with acute and chronic lung disease are tremendous. Animal studies, such as the one by Frostell et al[5] which showed the ability of NO to dilate the pulmonary circulation after acute vasoconstriction induced by thromboxane or hypoxia in animal models, have rapidly advanced NO therapy from the laboratory to clinical trials.

In a recent clinical trial, inhaled NO was used to treat patients with the adult (or acute) respiratory distress syndrome (ARDS).[45] In this study pulmonary artery pressure was reduced and improved matching of ventilation and perfusion increased oxygenation. Inhaled NO has also been especially useful in the treatment of persistent pulmonary hypertension of the newborn,[46,47] in acute pulmonary vasospasm after surgical correction of congenital heart disease,[48] and chronic pulmonary hypertension after mitral valve surgery, and may be efficacious in primary pulmonary hypertension.[49] In patients with primary pulmonary hypertension, inhaled NO may also be useful as a preoperative diagnostic study to determine the reversibility of the pulmonary hypertension. If the pulmonary hypertension is reversible with vasodilators, only a heart transplant is needed. However, if the vasoconstriction is unresponsive both heart and lung transplantation are necessary.[9]

While inhaled NO has shown promise in the treatment of a number of different pulmonary diseases, it does have some significant limitations. There is strong evidence that the beneficial effects of inhaled NO are dependent on the type of lung injury. In our laboratory, using an ovine model of smoke inhalation injury, Booke et al[27] found that inhaled NO lowered pulmonary artery pressure, improved right ventricular stroke work index, and left heart function but failed to improve oxygenation or intrapulmonary shunt. In another ovine model of smoke inhalation, Ogura et al[50] found similar results. This is likely due to the pulmonary edema and cast formation associated with smoke inhalation.[51,52] The presence of pulmonary edema (a hallmark of this injury) increases the diffusion distance for NO, making it possible for it to be converted to nitrates and nitrites before vasodilatation. On the other hand,

Kikuchi et al,[53] using our chronic lung lymph model, demonstrated that the administration of NO 22 h after inhalation injury resulted in a reduction in lung lymph flow, pulmonary microvascular pressure, and wet/dry ratio. Lung tissue conjugated diene levels were elevated in the control group but not in the NO-treated animals (Figures 4 and 5).

In addition to the contradictory results in smoke inhalation, the therapeutic benefit of NO has been questioned in other models of critical illness. In a piglet model of group B streptococcal sepsis, Berger et al[54] found that inhalation of NO reduced pulmonary artery pressure but did not improve oxygenation. This lack of correlation between reduction in pulmonary hypertension and improvement in intrapulmonary shunt has also been reported by Rovira et al.[55] Failure of inhaled NO to reduce pulmonary hypertension or to improve gas exchange has also been reported in a dog model of acute lung injury induced by oleic acid, despite the fact that concentrations of 145 ppm were administered.[56] In this study the authors hypothesized that endogenous production of NO is already maximal in the ventilated areas of the lung as a result of the injury; therefore further administration of exogenous NO has no additional benefit.

In summary, NO is a potent endogenous vasodilator which also has many other important physiologic actions. NO production increases in response to sepsis, which not only causes systemic vasodilatation but also induces an increase in intrapulmonary shunt due to the ability of NO to abolish HPV. However, despite its contribution to the pathophysiology of sepsis it is capable of reducing pulmonary hypertension and improving biventricular function. While there are many potential therapeutic benefits of inhaled NO

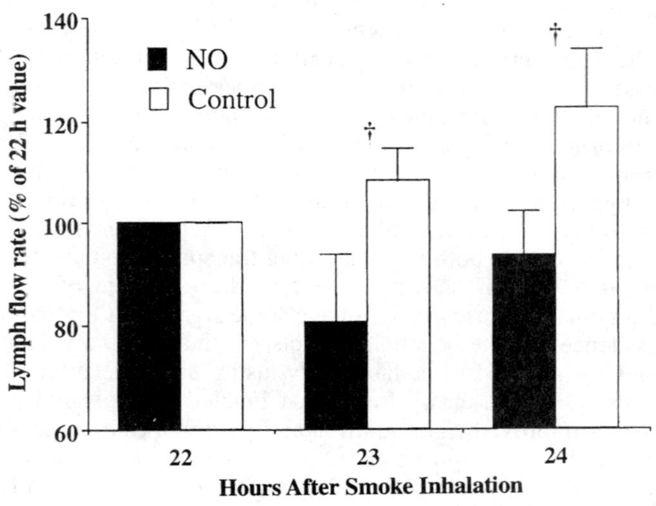

Figure 4. Comparison of lung lymph flow in sheep treated with inhaled NO versus control 22 h after smoke inhalation. Data are presented as percentage of 22 h baseline and are means ± S.E.M. †$P < 0.05$ between groups by anova with post-hoc Dunnett's test.

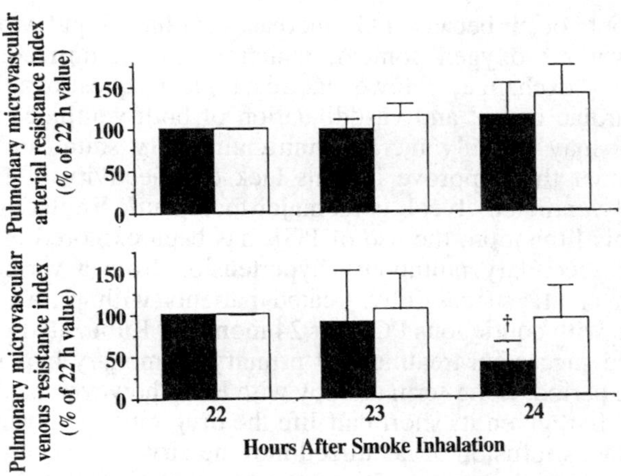

Figure 5. Comparison of pulmonary microvascular arterial and venous resistance index in sheep treated with inhaled NO (■) versus control (□) 22 h after smoke inhalation. Data are presented as percentage of 22 h baseline and are means ± S.E.M. †$P < 0.05$ between groups by anova and post-hoc Dunnett's test.

therapy, there are also a number of risks and therapeutic limitations. This is certainly an area that needs to be evaluated further.

Prostaglandin I_2

PGI_2 (prostacyclin, epoprostenol) is another potent endogenous vasodilator with potential therapeutic benefit in pulmonary hypertension. This prostanoid is mainly generated in the pulmonary vascular endothelium from arachidonic acid and prostaglandin endoperoxidases.[57] PGI_2 production by the lung has been demonstrated in both experimental animal models[57,58] and humans.[59] Ventilatory pattern appears to influence production of PGI_2 in several animal studies, where hyperventilation increased the release of PGI_2 from the lung.[57,60] However, evidence that this phenomenon occurs in humans has been inconclusive.[59,61,62] It is most likely that hyperventilation does not influence synthesis in humans.[61,62] PGI_2 induces pulmonary vasodilatation by increasing intracellular AMP.[63] It is likely that the actions of PGI_2 are more significant locally in the pulmonary circulation rather than in the systemic circulation.[61]

In addition to its potent vasodilatory properties PGI_2 has very potent antiplatelet aggregation properties.[58] Given that the pulmonary hypertension of acute lung injury is due to a combination of vasoconstriction and mechanical obstruction by microthromboemboli, PGI_2 appears to be an attractive agent with both vasodilatory and antiplatelet effects.

PGI_2 has a half-life of 1–3 min, which makes it relatively easy to titrate hemodynamic effects to achieve optimal effect.[64] However, this short half-life also necessitates continuous infusion. While it would seem likely that PGI_2 would cause an increased imbalance of ventilation–perfusion mismatch, this is thought not to occur because PGI_2 increases cardiac output, which increases the mixed venous oxygen content, which would in turn compensate for worsening gas exchange.[13] However, this logic is questionable in that an increased cardiac output and vasodilatation of both ventilated and unventilated alveoli may actually increase intrapulmonary shunt and worsen gas exchange rather than improve it. This lack of selectivity of PGI_2 in vasodilating well-ventilated alveoli is its major therapeutic limitation.

Despite this limitation, the use of PGI_2 has been explored in treatment of primary and secondary pulmonary hypertension from a variety of causes. Higinbottam et al[65] successfully treated patients with primary pulmonary hypertension with continuous PGI_2 for 24 months.[68] Rubin et al[66] also reported a randomized successful treatment of primary pulmonary hypertension over an 18-month period. Long-term therapy with PGI_2, however, has several other limitations. First, given its short half-life the drug must be given as a continuous intravenous infusion or nebulized into the airway.

The intravenous route necessitates chronic central venous access such as that provided by a Hickman catheter, which has inherent infectious complications. Second, despite the potential for in-home therapy, close monitoring of dosage is required as any sudden increase or decrease in dose may cause severe fluctuation in a patient's hemodynamic status. Finally, the cost of this therapy is extremely high, with each 500 μg vial costing $100.[67] Intravenous PGI_2 has also been used in patients with ARDS, in order to decrease pulmonary vascular pressures and thus reduce pulmonary fluid filtration and right heart afterload.[68] This treatment, however, was limited by lack of pulmonary selectivity, as vasorelaxation of both the systemic and pulmonary circulation, and within the pulmonary vasculature in both ventilated and nonventilated areas.

Recently, these limitations have been circumvented by application of aerosolized PGI_2 via the transbronchial route. This strategy provides pulmonary selectivity without systemic vasodilatation and also limits intrapulmonary shunt by acting only at well-ventilated alveolar units. Welte et al[69] showed that inhalation of aerosolized PGI_2 caused selective pulmonary vasodilatation in hypoxia-induced pulmonary hypertension in dogs. This strategy has also been found to induce pulmonary vasodilatation accompanied by improvement in intrapulmonary shunt and arterial oxygenation in patients with ARDS.[70] Additional applications of transbronchial aerosolized PGI_2 include treatment of severe pneumonia[71] and asthma.[72] In a comparison study of the effects of inhaled NO and nebulized PGI_2 on HPV in anesthetized sheep, we found that PGI_2 at a dosage of 10 μg/min reduced pulmonary artery pressure and improved the ventilation–perfusion ratio, without untoward systemic vasodilatory effects.[73] The advantages of inhaled PGI_2 include pulmonary selectivity with minimal systemic side effects and is nontoxic even given over extended periods. In addition PGI_2 does not require the sophisticated ventilators needed to administer NO in a controlled fashion. Further, the transbronchial route avoids the need for chronic venous cannulation and its associated complications.

PGI_2 has also been found to be useful as a bridge to heart–lung transplantation in the treatment of primary pulmonary hypertension,[67] and in conjunction with the single-flush technique, to enhance graft preservation at the time of tissue harvest. The rapid onset of action and short half-life of PGI_2 make it useful in testing reversibility and response to vasodilators in patients with primary and secondary pulmonary hypertension.[13]

In summary, PGI_2 is a potent vasodilator and antiplatelet agent that is potentially useful in the treatment of pulmonary hypertension. It has been successfully used intravenously for long-term treatment of primary pulmonary hypertension. Its major drawbacks include infectious risks associated with long-term vascular access, cost, increased intrapulmonary shunt, and lack of pulmonary selectivity. Recently, limitations have been circumvented by the use of aerosolized PGI_2.

Prostaglandin E_1

PGE_1 is another endogenous prostaglandin with potent vasodilatory effects that has similar properties and structure to PGI_2.[74] Like PGI_2, PGE_1 is a product of arachidonic acid metabolism and acts as a local hormone, influencing pulmonary vasorelaxation while having limited systemic circulatory effects. PGE_1 also induces vasorelaxation by activation of adenylate cyclase and has antiplatelet aggregation effects but these are less potent than PGI_2. In addition, PGE_1 may influence leukocyte trafficking in the lung.[75]

PGE_1 would be expected to have similar therapeutic benefits to PGI_1 but would also be limited by the lack of pulmonary selectivity and an increase in intrapulmonary shunt. PGE_1 has recently been examined for use in the treatment of ARDS.[76] However, in this study, while PGE_1 decreased pulmonary hypertension it did so at the expense of pulmonary gas exchange. It may be that aerosolization of PGE_1 may also circumvent these limitations.

PGE_1 has shown promise in the treatment of other pulmonary diseases. In a comparison study of PGE_1 and PGI_2 in infants after heart surgery, Kermode and associates[77] found that each were equally effective in treating pulmonary hypertension but recommended PGE_1 because it was more cost-effective. Further, PGE_1 has been demonstrated to be effective in secondary pulmonary hypertension associated with chronic obstructive pulmonary disease[78] and systemic collagen vascular disease.[79,80] PGE_1 has also been shown to be useful in the pretransplant evaluation of pulmonary vasoreactivity in patients with chronic heart failure[81] as well as in improving early graft function after lung transplant.[82,83]

In addition to the effects of PGE_1 on pulmonary vascular smooth muscle, Slotman et al[84] have shown that intravenous administration of PGE_1 improved cardiac performance, hepatic function, and leukocyte availability during clinical ARDS.[84] These effects may also be attributed to an action on the pulmonary circuit. Elevation of pulmonary arterial pressure can affect left heart function; resultant right ventricular pressure causes the ventricular septum to bulge into the left ventricle, affecting its compliance and geometry.[85] Similarly, the associated elevation in systemic pressures may affect hepatic function. Thus, by reducing pulmonary artery pressure the dilator prostaglandins would affect these functions. PGE_1 and PGI_2 may also affect leukocyte trafficking by downregulation of adherence molecules in the pulmonary endothelium.[86,87]

In summary, PGE_1 has potential therapeutic actions similar to PGI_2; however, it is also subjected to the same limitations of lack of pulmonary selectivity and increased intrapulmonary shunt.

OTHER PULMONARY VASODILATORS

In addition to NO, PGI_2 and PGE_1, a number of other vasodilators have been shown to be synthesized and released from the lung. While these vasodilators have limited therapeutic application, understanding them provides insight into how the lung actively controls its vasomotor tone.

Prostaglandin E_2

Another prostaglandin of the E series that may act as a pulmonary vasodilator is prostaglandin E_2 (PGE_2). Like PGE_1, PGE_2 is synthesized and released from the lung in response to hyperinflation, anaphylaxis, and embolization.[88–90] PGE_2 is also almost completely metabolized by a single passage through the pulmonary circulation.[91] Both PGEs act as dilators of the perinatal pulmonary circulation.[92] However, PGE_2 has been shown to be less effective than PGE_1 in counteracting hypoxic pulmonary vasoconstriction in newborn goats.[92] Data on the effects of PGE_2 in the adult pulmonary circulation are conflicting. Kadowitz et al[93] have shown that PGE_2 actually causes pulmonary vasoconstriction resulting in an increased pulmonary vascular resistance.

Atrial natriuretic peptide

ANP is a recently discovered hormone originally found by de Bold et al[94] in the cardiac atria, which is capable of inducing diuresis, natriuresis, and reduction of systemic blood pressure. Given its anatomical location, it is likely that the lung is the first target organ for ANP.[95] In addition to the cardiac atria, ANP synthesis occurs in type II alveolar cells, respiratory epithelium, and smooth muscle cells of pulmonary veins.[95] Once released, ANP migrates to the pulmonary circulation where it activates guanylate cyclase in an endothelium-independent manner.[96] This results in an increase in cGMP, which decreases intracellular calcium and induces vasorelaxation. Unlike NO, ANP acts on granular guanylate cyclase as opposed to the cytoplasmic form of the enzyme.[97,98] This granular guanylate cyclase lacks the heme group that interacts with NO and Evan's blue and consequently is unaffected by these materials.[98] ANP relaxes both the pulmonary arteries and especially the pulmonary veins. This action increases the capacitance of pulmonary vasculature. ANP is removed from the pulmonary circulation by two main mechanisms. First, it may bind to an internalized receptor and be degraded by lysosomal enzymes. Another possibility is that ANP is metabolized by endopeptidase.[95] In the pulmonary artery the vasodilatory effects of ANP are enhanced when pulmonary vascular resistance is increased secondary to acute[99] or chronic hypoxia.[100,101] The importance of ANP in counteracting the pulmonary hypertension associated with *Pseudomonas aeruginosa* sepsis has also been demonstrated.[102] In this study HS 142-1, a selective ANP inhibitor, had greater contractility effects in the pulmonary vasculature than in the mesenteric or femoral arteries. In addition to its vasodilatory effects, ANP is also thought to regulate endothelial permeability.[103–105] Hinder et al[106] have demonstrated that inhibition of ANP with HS 142-1 increased pulmonary transvascular fluid flux in an ovine model of sepsis. These changes in pulmonary vascular permeability may be of some physiological benefit. If pulmonary microvascular permeability to protein after injury is increased secondary to the margination and activation of neutrophils, ANP will reduce the permeability effects.[105] On the other hand, ANP causes an increase in permeability to small molecules (increases filtration coefficient) in the normal pulmonary microvasculature.[107] This latter action may be part of the physiological role of ANP in maintenance of vascular volume. In addition to its effects on vascular permeability, ANP has also been shown induce broncho-relaxation.[108] These ANP effects would be beneficial to patients with acute lung injury, given the ability of ANP to reduce the associated pulmonary hypertension and pulmonary edema, maintain permeability, and improve oxygenation. In the future, ANP levels may be used as a marker of pulmonary injury. Studies have shown that plasma ANP levels increase in patients with severe lung injury[109,110] as well as endotoxemia[111,112] and decline as lung injury improves (Figure 6).[109]

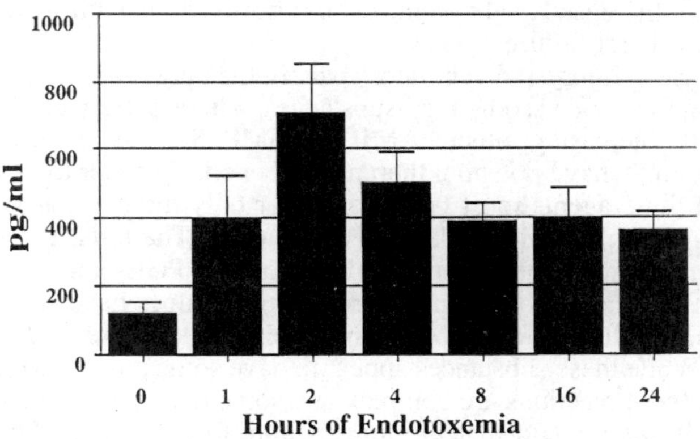

Figure 6. Plasma concentration of ANP after endotoxemia. Data are presented as means ± S.E.M.

Endothelins

The endothelins (ETs) are another group of vasoactive peptides produced by the vascular endothelial cells.[113] There are three specific peptides: ET-1, ET-2, ET-3. Plasma concentrations of ET-1 have been shown to correlate with the extent of pulmonary hypertension.[114–116] The pulmonary vascular response to ET-1 is complex and controversial. It has been demonstrated to produce a variety of vasoactive effects in the pulmonary circulation. These effects vary from sustained vasoconstriction and sustained vasodilatation to a biphasic response in which transient vasodilatation is followed by sustained vasoconstriction.[114,117–120] ET-1 has also been shown to have pulmonary vasodilatory effects which are mediated in part by endothelium-derived NO synthesis and ATP-gated potassium-channel activation.[117,121] However, the ability of ET-1 to release NO is also controversial. Whether ET-1 causes pulmonary vasoconstriction or vasodilatation appears to depend on a variety of factors, including age and the form of sepsis studied, experimental preparation, dose of ET-1, and baseline pulmonary vascular tone.[117]

ET-3 has also been shown to be a rapid, transient, yet potent vasodilator capable of complete reversal of hypoxic vasoconstriction.[122] ET-3 vasodilatory effects appear to be due to activation of ATP-gated potassium channels.[121] Like ET-1, the effects of ET-3 on pulmonary vasomotor tone are complex and controversial.

CONCLUSIONS

The lung normally maintains a balance between pulmonary vasoconstriction and vasodilatation. In the setting of acute and chronic lung injury this balance is tipped in favor of vasoconstriction. This pulmonary hypertension in turn causes increased transvascular fluid flux with resultant interstitial edema and hypoxemia. Increased right ventricular afterload also ultimately leads to biventricular heart failure.

In response to injury and ventilatory pattern the lung is able to synthesize and release a number of vasodilatory substances. These substances induce vasodilatation by increasing either cAMP or cGMP. Several of these pulmonary vasodilators may have potential therapeutic benefit. In order to be therapeutically useful these agents must be selective for only the pulmonary circulation and vasodilate only well-ventilated alveolar units. The three vasodilators that have been examined for therapeutic use are NO, PGE_1 and PGI_2. Of these, inhaled NO appears to be the most promising but does have some significant limitations. The lung is also able to synthesize and release PGE_2, ANP, ET-1 and ET-3. While these substances appear to have some pulmonary vasodilatory properties, these reactions are complex and some data are conflicting.

Overall it can be said that the lung is able to assert active control of its vasomotor tone in the setting of lung injury. With improved understanding of the mechanisms that govern the synthesis, release, and metabolism of these pulmonary vasodilators, clinicians of the future may be able to actively control these vasomotor mechanisms in the settings of both acute and chronic lung injury.

REFERENCES

1. von Euler U & Liljestrand G (1946) Observations on the pulmonary arterial blood pressure in the cat. *Acta Physiologica Scandinavica* **12:**301–320.
2. Voelkel NF, Marletta MA, Yoon PS, Iyengar R, Leaf CD & Wishnok JS (1988)

Mechanisms of hypoxic pulmonary vasoconstriction. *American Review of Respiratory Disease* **27:**8706–8711.
3. Peacock A (1993) Vasodilators in pulmonary hypertension. *Thorax* **48:**1196–1199.
4. Adnot S, Raffestin B, Eddahibi S, Braquet P & Chabrier PE (1991) Loss of endothelium-dependent relaxant activity in the pulmonary circulation of rats exposed to chronic hypoxia. *Journal of Clinical Investigation* **87:**155–162.
5. Frostell C, Fratacci MD, Wain JC, Jones R & Zapol WM (1991) Inhaled nitric oxide. A selective pulmonary vasodilator reversing hypoxic pulmonary vasoconstriction. *Circulation* **83:**2038–2047.
6. Albarwani S, Xia N & Nye PCG (1993) Excitation of small isolated pulmonary blood vessels from the rat by 4-aminopyridine and hypoxia. *Journal of Physiology* **467:**46.
7. McIntyre RC, Jr, Harken AH & Fullerton DA (1994) Mechanisms of pulmonary vascular control in normal and injured lungs. *Surgery* **115:**273–275.
8. Furchgott RF & Zawadzki JV (1980) The obligatory role of endothelial cells in the relaxation of arterial smooth muscle by acetylcholine. *Nature* **288:**373–376.
9. Lunn RJ (1995) Inhaled nitric oxide therapy. *Mayo Clinic Proceedings* **70:**247–255.
10. Gerzer R, Heim JM, Schutte B & Weil J (1987) Cellular mechanisms of action of atrial natriuretic factor. *Klinische Wochenschrift* **65(Suppl 8):**109–114.
11. Fullerton DA, Hahn AR, Koike K, Banerjee A & Harken AH (1993) Intracellular mechanisms of pulmonary vasomotor dysfunction in acute lung injury caused by mesenteric ischemia–reperfusion. *Surgery* **114:**360–366.
12. Gerkin TM, Oldham KT, Guice KS, Hinshaw DB & Ryan US (1993) Intestinal ischemia–reperfusion injury causes pulmonary endothelial cell ATP depletion. *Annals of Surgery* **217:**48–56.
13. Jones K, Higenbottam T & Wallwork J (1989) Pulmonary vasodilation with prostacyclin in primary and secondary pulmonary hypertension. *Chest* **96:**784–789.
14. Zapol WM & Snider MT (1977) Pulmonary hypertension in severe acute respiratory failure. *New England Journal of Medicine* **296:**476–480.
15. Tomashefski JF, Davies P, Boggis C, Greene R, Zapol WM & Reid LM (1983) The pulmonary vascular lesions of the adult respiratory distress syndrome. *American Journal of Pathology* **112:**112–126.
16. Culotta E & Koshland DE, Jr (1992) NO news is good news. *Science* **258:**1862–1865.
17. Thiemermann C, Szabo C, Mitchell JA & Vane JR (1993) Vascular hyporeactivity to vasoconstrictor agents and hemodynamic decompensation in hemorrhagic shock is mediated by nitric oxide. *Proceedings of the National Academy of Sciences USA* **90:**267–271.
18. Julou Schaeffer G, Gray GA, Fleming I, Schott C, Parratt JR & Stoclet JC (1990) Loss of vascular responsiveness induced by endotoxin involves L-arginine pathway. *American Journal of Physiology* **259:**H1038–H1043.
19. Evans T, Carpenter A, Kinderman H & Cohen J (1993) Evidence of increased nitric oxide production in patients with the sepsis syndrome. *Circulation Shock* **41:**77–81.
20. Ochoa JB, Udekwu AO, Billiar TR et al (1991) Nitrogen oxide levels in patients after trauma and during sepsis. *Annals of Surgery* **214:**621–626.
21. Payne D & Kubes P (1993) Nitric oxide donors reduce the rise in reperfusion-induced intestinal mucosal permeability. *American Journal of Physiology* **265:**G189–G195.
22. Palmer RM, Ferrige AG & Moncada S (1987) Nitric oxide release accounts for the biological activity of endothelium-derived relaxing factor. *Nature* **327:**524–526.
23. Radomski MW, Palmer RM & Moncada S (1990) An L-arginine/nitric oxide pathway present in human platelets regulates aggregation. *Proceedings of the National Academy of Sciences USA* **87:**5193–5197.

24. Garthwaite J, Charles SL & Chess-Williams R (1988) Endothelium-derived relaxing factor release on activation of NMDA receptors suggests role as intercellular messenger in the brain. *Nature* **336:**385–388.
25. Marletta MA, Yoon PS, Iyengar R, Leaf CD & Wishnok JS (1988) Macrophage oxidation of L-arginine to nitrite and nitrate: nitric oxide is an intermediate. *Biochemistry* **27:**8706–8711.
26. Stuehr DJ & Nathan CF (1989) Nitric oxide. A macrophage product responsible for cytostasis and respiratory inhibition in tumor target cells. *Journal of Experimental Medicine* **169:**1543–1555.
27. Booke M, Bradford DW, Hinder F et al (1995) Inhaled nitric oxide selectively reduces pulmonary hypertension after ovine smoke inhalation but does not improve oxygenation. *Critical Care Medicine*. In Press.
28. Anggard E (1994) Nitric oxide: mediator, murderer, and medicine. *Lancet* **343:**1199–1206.
29. Kelm M & Schrader J (1990) Control of coronary vascular tone by nitric oxide. *Circulation Research* **66:**1561–1575.
30. Stamler JS, Jaraki O, Osborne J et al (1992) Nitric oxide circulates in mammalian plasma primarily as an S-nitroso adduct of serum albumin. *Proceedings of the National Academy of Sciences USA* **89:**7674–7677.
31. Rimar S & Gills CN (1993) Selective pulmonary vasodilation by inhaled nitric oxide is due to hemoglobin inactivation. *Circulation* **88:**2884–2887.
32. Yoshida K & Kasama K (1987) Biotransformation of nitric oxide. *Environmental Health Perspectives* **73:**201–205.
33. Meyer J, Lentz CW, Stothert JC, Traber LD, Herndon DN & Traber DL (1994) Effects of nitric oxide synthesis inhibition in hyperdynamic endotoxemia. *Critical Care Medicine* **22:**306–312.
34. Nelson SH, Ehardt JS, Lingnau W, Traber L & Traber D (1994) Influence of sepsis and nitric oxide synthase (NOS) inhibition in pulmonary artery and vein. *Shock* **1:**60.
35. Lingnau W, Nelson SH, Ehardt JS, Traber LD & Traber DL (1994) c-GMP levels of pulmonary vessels after nitric oxide inhibition in ovine bacteremia. *FASEB Journal* **8:**A367.
36. Nelson SH, Ehardt JS, Lingnau W, Dehring DJ & Traber D (1995) Influence of sepsis and nitric oxide synthase inhibitors on pulmonary arteries and veins. *Journal of Cardiovascular Pharmacology*. In Press.
37. Oda H, Kusumoto S & Nakajima T (1975) Nitrosyl-hemoglobin formation in the blood of animals exposed to nitric oxide. *Archives of Environmental Health* **30:**453–456.
38. Hugod C (1979) Effect of exposure to 43 ppm nitric oxide and 3.6 ppm nitrogen dioxide on rabbit lung. A light and electron microscopic study. *International Archives of Occupational Environmental Health* **42:**159–167.
39. Koppenol WH, Moreno JJ, Pryor WA, Ischiropoulos H & Beckman JS (1992) Peroxynitrite, a cloaked oxidant formed by nitric oxide and superoxide. *Chemical Research Toxicology* **5:**834–842.
40. Ross JD (1963) Deficient activity of DPH-dependent methemoglobin diaphorase in cord blood erythrocytes. *Blood* **21:**51–62.
41. Hogman M, Frostell C, Arnberg H & Hedenstierna G (1993) Bleeding time prolongation and NO inhalation. *Lancet* **341:**1664–1665.
42. Finkel MS, Oddis CV, Jacob TD, Watkins SC, Hattler BG & Simmons RL (1992) Negative inotropic effects of cytokines on the heart mediated by nitric oxide. *Science* **257:**387–389.
43. Semigran MJ, Cockrill BA, Kacmarek R, Thompson BT, Zapol WM & Dec GW (1994) Hemodynamic effects of inhaled nitric oxide in heart failure. *Journal of the American College of Cardiology* **24:**982–988.

44. Bocchi EA, Bacal F, Auler Junior JO, Carmone MJ, Bellotti G & Pileggi F (1994) Inhaled nitric oxide leading to pulmonary edema in stable severe heart failure. *American Journal of Cardiology* **74:**70–72.
45. Rossaint R, Falke KJ, Lopez F, Slama K, Pison U & Zapol WM (1993) Inhaled nitric oxide for the adult respiratory distress syndrome. *New England Journal of Medicine* **328:**399–405.
46. Kinsella JP & Abman SH (1994) Efficacy of inhalational nitric oxide therapy in the clinical management of persistent pulmonary hypertension of the newborn. *Chest* **105:**92S–94S.
47. Kinsella JP & Abman SH (1993) Inhalational nitric oxide therapy for persistent pulmonary hypertension of the newborn. *Pediatrics* **91:**997–998.
48. Journois D, Pouard P, Mauriat P, Malhere T, Vouhe P & Safran D (1994) Inhaled nitric oxide as a therapy for pulmonary hypertension after operations for congenital heart defects. *Journal of Thoracic Cardiovascular Surgery* **107:**1129–1135.
49. Pepke-Zaba J, Higenbottam TW, Dinh-Xuan AT, Stone D & Wallwork J (1991) Inhaled nitric oxide as a cause of selective pulmonary vasodilation in pulmonary hypertension. *Lancet* **338:**1173–1174.
50. Ogura H, Cioffi WG, Jordan BS et al (1994) The effect of inhaled nitric oxide on smoke inhalation injury in an ovine model. *Journal of Trauma* **37:**294–301.
51. Herndon DN, Traber DL, Niehaus GD, Linares HA & Traber LD (1984) The pathophysiology of smoke inhalation injury in a sheep model. *Journal of Trauma* **24:**1044–1051.
52. Traber DL, Schlag G, Redl H & Traber LD (1985) Pulmonary edema and compliance changes following smoke inhalation. *Journal of Burn Care Rehabilitation* **6:**490–494.
53. Kikuchi Y, Nishida K, Hinder F, Traber L, Herndon D & Traber D (1995) Treatment of smoke-induced pulmonary injury with nitric oxide (NO) inhalation in sheep. *Journal of Applied Physiology*. In Press.
54. Berger JI, Gibson RL, Redding GJ, Standaert TA, Clarke WR & Truog WE (1993) Effect of inhaled nitric oxide during group B streptococcal sepsis in piglets. *American Review of Respiratory Disease* **147:**1080–1086.
55. Rovira I, Chen TY, Winkler M, Kawai N, Bloch KD & Zapol WM (1994) Effects of inhaled nitric oxide on pulmonary hemodynamics and gas exchange in an ovine model of ARDS. *Journal of Applied Physiology* **76:**345–355.
56. Romand JA, Pinsky MR, Firestone L, Zar HA & Lancaster JR (1994) Inhaled nitric oxide partially reverses hypoxic pulmonary vasoconstriction in the dog. *Journal of Applied Physiology* **76:**1350–1355.
57. Gryglewski RJ, Korbut R & Ocetkiewicz A (1978) Generation of prostacyclin by lungs *in vivo* and its release into the arterial circulation. *Nature* **273:**765–767.
58. Moncada S, Vane JR, Gryglewski RJ et al (1978) Pharmacology and endogenous roles of prostaglandin endoperoxides, thromboxane A2, and prostacyclin. *Archives of Pharmacology* **304:**45–50.
59. Edlund A, Bomfim W, Kaijser L et al (1981) Pulmonary formation of prostacyclin in man. *Prostaglandins* **22:**323–332.
60. Korbut R, Boyd J & Eling T (1981) Respiratory movements alter the generation of prostacyclin and thromboxane A_2 in isolated rat lungs: the influence of arachidonic acid-pathway inhibitors on the ratio between pulmonary prostacyclin and thromboxane A_2. *Prostaglandins* **21:**491–503.
61. Christ-Hazelhof E & Nugteren DH (1981) Prostacyclin is not a circulating hormone. *Prostaglandins* **22:**739–746.
62. du Toit HJ, Erasmus FR, MacFarlane CM et al (1984) The effect of ventilatory patterns on prostacyclin (PGI_2) synthesis in the lung. *South African Medical Journal* **65:**135–136.

63. MacDermot J & Barnes PJ (1980) Activation of guinea pig pulmonary adenylate cyclase by prostacyclin. *European Journal of Pharmacology* **67:**419–425.
64. Szczeklik J, Szczeklik A & Nizankowski R (1980) Haemodynamic changes induced by prostacyclin in man. *British Heart Journal* **44:**254–258.
65. Higenbottam T, Wheeldon D, Wells F & Wallwork J (1984) Long-term treatment of primary pulmonary hypertension with continuous intravenous epoprostenol (prostacyclin). *Lancet* **1:**1046–1047.
66. Rubin LJ, Mendoza J, Hood M et al (1990) Treatment of primary pulmonary hypertension with continuous intravenous prostacyclin (epoprostenol). Results of a randomized trial. *Annuals of Internal Medicine* **112:**485–491.
67. Kramer MR, Fucks S, Simon Z & Berkman N (1993) Continuous therapy with intravenous prostacyclin for primary pulmonary hypertension: a bridge to heart–lung transplantation. *Israel Journal of Medical Sciences* **29:**613–616.
68. Radermacher P, Santak B, Wüst HJ, Tarnow J & Falke KJ (1990) Prostacyclin and right ventricular function in patients with pulmonary hypertension associated with ARDS. *Intensive Care Medicine* **16:**227–232.
69. Welte M, Zwissler B, Habazettl H & Messmer K (1993) PGI_2 aerosol versus nitric oxide for selective pulmonary vasodilation in hypoxic pulmonary vasoconstriction. *European Surgical Research* **25:**329–340.
70. Walmrath D, Schneider T, Pilch J, Grimminger F & Seeger W (1993) Aerosolised prostacyclin in adult respiratory distress syndrome. *Lancet* **342:**961–962.
71. Walmrath D, Schneider T, Pilch J, Schermuly R, Grimminger F & Seeger W (1995) Effects of aerosolized prostacyclin in severe pneumonia. Impact of fibrosis. *American Journal of Respiratory and Critical Care Medicine* **151:**724–730.
72. Hardy CC, Bradding P, Robinson C & Holgate ST (1988) Bronchoconstrictor and antibronchoconstrictor properties of inhaled prostacyclin in asthma. *Journal of Applied Physiology* **64:**1567–1574.
73. Booke M, Bradford DW, Hinder F et al (1995) Effects of inhaled nitric oxide and nebulized prostacyclin on hypoxic pulmonary vasoconstriction in anesthetized sheep. *Critical Care Medicine*. In Press.
74. Moncada S, Flower R & Vane J (1985) Prostaglandins, prostacyclin, thromboxane A_2, and leukotrienes. In *Pharmacological Basis for Therapeutic Interventions*. New York: Macmillan.
75. Grant MM, Burnett CM & Fein AM (1991) Effect of prostaglandin E_1 infusion on leukocyte traffic and fibrosis in acute lung injury induced by belomycin in hamsters. *Critical Care Medicine* **19:**211–217.
76. Melot C, Lejeune P, Leeman M, Moraine JJ & Naeije R (1989) Prostaglandin E1 in the adult respiratory distress syndrome. Benefit for pulmonary hypertension and cost for pulmonary gas exchange. *American Review of Respiratory Disease* **139:**106–110.
77. Kermode J, Butt W & Shann F (1991) Comparison between prostaglandin E_1 and epoprostenol (prostacyclin) in infants after heart surgery. *British Heart Journal* **66:**175–178.
78. Naeije R, Melot C, Mols P & Hallemans R (1982) Reduction in pulmonary hypertension by prostaglandin E_1 in decompensated chronic obstructive pulmonary disease. *American Review of Respiratory Disease* **125:**1–5.
79. Kawahara R, Takezawa J, Mike N et al (1987) Prostaglandin E_1 in pulmonary hypertension of collagen disease. *Critical Care Medicine* **15:**884–885.
80. Ignaszewski AP, Percy JS & Humen DP (1993) Successful treatment of pulmonary hypertension associated with systemic lupus erythematosus with prostaglandin I_2 and prostaglandin E_1. *Journal of Rheumatology* **20:**595–596.
81. Murali S, Uretsky BF, Armitage JM et al (1992) Utility of prostaglandin E_1 in the pretransplantation evaluation of heart failure patients with significant pulmonary hypertension. *Journal of Heart and Lung Transplantation* **11:**716–723.

82. Aoe M, Trachiotis GD, Okabayashi K et al (1994) Administration of prostaglandin E_1 after lung transplantation improves early graft function. *Annals of Thoracic Surgery* **58:**655–661.
83. Matsuzaki Y, Waddell TK, Puskas JD, Hirai T, Nakajima S & Slutsky AS (1993) Amelioration of post-ischemic lung reperfusion injury by prostaglandin E_1. *American Review of Respiratory Disease* **148:**882–889.
84. Slotman GJ, Kerstein MD, Bone RC et al (1992) The effects of prostaglandin E_1 on non-pulmonary organ function during clinical acute respiratory failure. The Prostaglandin E_1 Study Group. *Journal of Trauma* **32:**480–488.
85. Sugi K, Newald J, Traber LD et al (1991) Cardiac dysfunction after acute endotoxin administration in conscious sheep. *American Journal of Physiology* **260:**H1474–H1481.
86. Gee MH, Tahamont MV, Flynn JT, Cox JW, Pullen RH & Andreadis NA (1987) Prostaglandin E_1 prevents increased lung microvascular permeability during intravascular complement activation in sheep. *Circulation Research* **61:**420–428.
87. Most J, Schwaeble W, Drach J et al (1991) Regulation of the expression of ICAM-1 on human monocytes and monocytic tumor cell lines, effects of recombinant tumor necrosis factor-alpha on cultured pulmonary artery and lung microvascular endothelial monolayers. *Journal of Immunology and American Journal of Pathology* **138:**93–101.
88. Lindsey HE & Wyllie JH (1970) Release of prostaglandins from embolized lungs. *British Journal of Surgery* **57:**738–741.
89. Piper PJ & Vane JR (1969) Release of additional factors in anaphylaxis and its antagonism by anti-inflammatory drugs. *Nature* **223:**29–35.
90. Berry EM, Edmonds JF & Wyllie H (1971) Release of prostaglandin E_2 and unidentified factors from ventilated lungs. *British Journal of Surgery* **58:**189–192.
91. Piper PJ, Vane JR & Wyllie JH (1970) Inactivation of prostaglandins by the lungs. *Nature* **225:**600–604.
92. Tyler T, Leffler C, Wallis R & Cassin S (1975) Effects of prostaglandins of the E-series on pulmonary and systemic circulations of newborn goats during normoxia and hypoxia. *Prostaglandins* **10:**963–970.
93. Kadowitz PJ, Joiner PD & Hyman AL (1975) Effect of prostaglandin E_2 on pulmonary vascular resistance in intact dog, swine and lamb. *European Journal of Pharmacology* **31:**72–80.
94. de Bold AJ, Borenstein HB, Veress AT & Sonnenberg H (1981) A rapid and potent natriuretic response to intravenous injection of atrial myocardial extract in rats. *Life Sciences* **28:**89–94.
95. Perreault T & Gutkowska J (1995) Role of atrial natriuretic factor in lung physiology and pathology. *American Journal of Respiratory and Critical Care Medicine* **151:**226–242.
96. Ignarro LJ, Wood KS, Harbison RG & Kadowitz PJ (1986) Atriopeptin II relaxes and elevates cGMP in bovine pulmonary artery but not vein. *Journal of Applied Physiology* **60:**1128–1133.
97. Cherner JA, Singh G & Naik L (1990) Atrial natriuretic factor activates membrane-bound guanylate cyclase of chief cells. *Life Sciences* **47:**669–677.
98. Garbers DL (1990) The guanylyl cyclase receptor family. *New Biology* **2:**499–504.
99. Adnot S, Chabrier PE, Brun-Buisson C, Viossat I & Braquet P (1988) Atrial natriuretic factor attenuates the pulmonary pressor response to hypoxia. *Journal of Applied Physiology* **65:**1975–1983.
100. Jin HK, Yang RH, Thornton RM, Chen YF, Jackson R & Oparil S (1988) Atrial natriuretic peptide lowers pulmonary arterial pressure in hypoxia-adapted rats. *Journal of Applied Physiology* **65:**1729–1735.

101. Rogers TK, Stewart AG & Morice AH (1992) Effect of chronic hypoxia on rat pulmonary resistance vessels: vasodilatation by atrial natriuretic peptide. *Clinical Sciences* **83:**723–729.
102. Ehardt JS, Nelson SH, Hinder F, Booke M, Traber LD & Traber DL (1995) Effects of an atrial naturetic peptide (ANP) inhibitor, HS 142-1 in isolated blood vessels from septic sheep. *FASEB Journal* **9:**5153.
103. Lofton CE, Newman WH & Currie MG (1990) Atrial natriuretic peptide regulation of endothelial permeability is mediated by cGMP. *Biochemical and Biophysical Research Communications* **172:**793–799.
104. Baron DA, Lofton CE, Newman WH & Currie MG (1989) Atriopeptin inhibition of thrombin-mediated changes in the morphology and permeability of endothelial monolayers. *Proceedings of the National Academy of Sciences USA* **86:**3394–3398.
105. Westendorp RG, Draijer R, Meinders AE & van Hinsbergh VW (1994) Cyclic-GMP-mediated decrease in permeability of human umbilical and pulmonary artery endothelial cell monolayers. *Journal of Vascular Research* **31:**42–51.
106. Hinder F, Booke M, McGuire RW, Traber LD & Traber DL (1995) Blockage of the receptor for atrial natriuretic peptide during ovine sepsis increases pulmonary transvascular fluid flux without evidence of high-protein edema. *Anesthesiology* **81(3A):**A335.
107. Myers PR, Wright TF, Tanner MA & Adams HR (1992) EDRF and nitric oxide production in cultured endothelial cells: direct inhibition by *E. coli* endotoxin. *American Journal of Physiology* **262:**H710–H718.
108. Potvin W & Varma DR (1989) Bronchodilator activity of atrial natriuretic peptide in guinea pigs. *Canadian Journal of Physiology and Pharmacology* **67:**1213–1218.
109. Mitaka C, Hirata Y, Nagura T, Sakanishi N, Tsunoda Y & Amaha K (1992) Plasma alpha-human atrial natriuretic peptide concentration in patients with acute lung injury. *American Review of Respiratory Disease* **146:**43–46.
110. Eison HB, Rosen MJ, Phillips RA & Krakoff LR (1988) Determinants of atrial natriuretic factor in the adult respiratory distress syndrome. *Chest* **94:**1040–1045.
111. Lübbesmeyer HJ, Woodson L, Traber LD, Flynn JT, Herndon DN & Traber DL (1988) Immunoreactive atrial natriuretic factor is increased in ovine model of endotoxemia. *American Journal of Physiology* **254:**R567–R571.
112. Redl G, Woodson L, Traber LD et al (1992) Mechanism of immunoreactive atrial natriuretic factor release in an ovine model of endotoxemia. *Circulatory Shock* **38:**34–41.
113. Yanagisawa M & Masaki T (1989) Molecular biology and biochemistry of the endothelins. *Trends in Pharmacological Sciences* **10:**374–378.
114. Traber DL, Booke M, Hinder F, McGuire R, Gandhi CR & Traber LD (1994) Endothelin-1 and pulmonary hemodynamics during ovine sepsis. *Pathophysiology* **1(Suppl):**410.
115. Cody RJ, Haas GJ, Binkley PF, Capers Q & Kelley R (1992) Plasma endothelin correlates with the extent of pulmonary hypertension in patients with chronic congestive heart failure. *Circulation* **85:**504–509.
116. Stewart DJ, Levy RD, Cernacek P & Langleben D (1991) Increased plasma endothelin-1 in pulmonary hypertension: marker or mediator of disease? *Annuals of Internal Medicine* **114:**464–469.
117. Wong J, Vanderford PA, Fineman JR, Chang R & Soifer SJ (1993) Endothelin-1 produces pulmonary vasodilation in the intact newborn lamb. *American Journal of Physiology* **265:**H1318–H1325.
118. Barnard JW, Barman SA, Adkins WK, Longenecker GL & Taylor AE (1991) Sustained effects of endothelin-1 on rabbit, dog, and rat pulmonary circulations. *American Journal of Physiology* **261:**H479–H486.
119. Mann J, Farrukh IS & Michael JR (1991) Mechanisms by which endothelin 1 induces

pulmonary vasoconstriction in the rabbit. *Journal of Applied Physiology* **71:**410–416.

120. Perreault T & De Marte J (1991) Endothelin-1 has a dilator effect on neonatal pig pulmonary vasculature. *Journal of Cardiovascular Pharmacology* **18:**43–50.
121. Lippton HL, Cohen GA, McMurtry IF & Hyman AL (1991) Pulmonary vasodilation to endothelin isopeptides in vivo is mediated by potassium channel activation. *Journal of Applied Physiology* **70:**947–952.
122. Crawley DE, Liu SF, Barnes PJ & Evans TW (1992) Endothelin-3 is a potent pulmonary vasodilator in the rat. *Journal of Applied Physiology* **72:**1425–1431.

4

Mediators of Vasoconstriction: Endothelin and Other Endogenous Compounds

C. Shekhar R. Gandhi
W. David Watkins

INTRODUCTION

Not long ago the vascular endothelium was considered a passive lining which permitted selective passage of circulating substances with properties influencing the underlying smooth muscle cells. An active involvement of the endothelium in the regulation of physiologic vascular tone was recognized during the 1980s when endothelial cells were discovered to process more fully a number of products with constrictor or dilator properties.[1,2] This led to the concomitant identification of endothelin-1 (ET-1) and nitric oxide (NO)[3–5] which are among the most powerful vasoconstrictors and vasodilators respectively yet identified. ET-1 and NO are produced constitutively by endothelial cells, and it is likely that a balance in the synthesis, actions, and clearance of these two mediators contributes towards the maintenance of physiologic vascular tone (Figure 1).

Endothelins are a family of four related 21-amino acid peptides: ET-1, ET-2, ET-3 and ET-β (Figure 2). They are highly vasoactive and, depending on the conditions, can produce both contraction and relaxation of blood vessels. ET-1 and ET-3 are synthesized predominantly in mammalian systems: endothelial cells in all vascular regions synthesize ET-1 and not ET-3, while nonvascular cells such as neuronal cells and macrophages synthesize both of these isopeptides. ET-1 is synthesized as a precursor protein (approximately 200 amino acid residues) that is hydrolyzed first to big ET-1 (about 40 amino acid residues); big ET-1 is then converted to mature ET-1 by a phosphoramidon-sensitive neutral endopeptidase called endothelin-converting enzyme (ECE) (Figure 3). A similar sequence of events has been predicted in the formation of other ET isopeptides by related ET-converting enzymes.

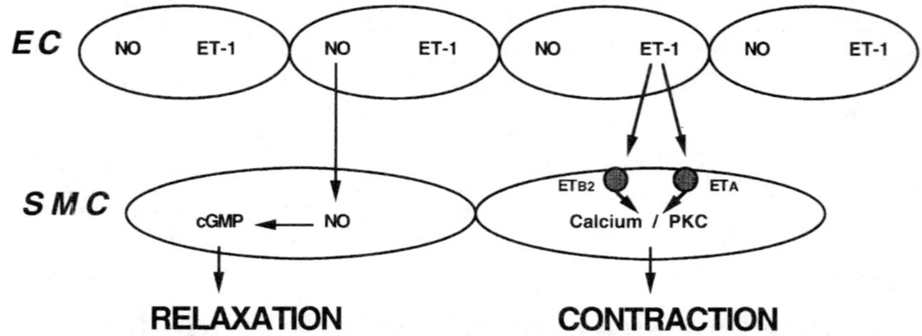

Figure 1. Regulation of vascular tone by endothelium-derived NO and ET-1. Vascular endothelial cells (EC) constitutively synthesize NO and ET-1. ET-1 binds to ET_A and ET_{B2} receptors on vascular smooth muscle cells (VSMC) and elicits vasoconstriction. NO, on the other hand, produces vasodilatation independently of a membrane receptor. While elevation of cytosolic calcium and activation of protein kinase C (PKC) are second messengers of ET-1 action, effects of NO are mediated via cGMP.

Recent years have seen an exponential growth in ET-1 and NO research, and led to the revelation that many substances associated with cardiovascular disorders influence synthesis of these mediators. Thus, altered circulating levels of ET-1 and NO have been correlated with various cardiovascular and cardiopulmonary pathologies. Current mechanisms of pulmonary pathophysiology related to NO are described elsewhere in this volume. In this review, we will describe the mechanisms with which ET-1 participates in the physiology and pathophysiology of the cardiopulmonary system, and will evaluate some related pharmacologic strategies in the treatment of pulmonary diseases with endothelin inhibitors and antagonists. For a review of biochemistry and molecular biology of endothelins, the reader is referred to previously published articles.[6–9]

SYNTHESIS AND CLEARANCE OF ET-1 IN THE PULMONARY SYSTEM

ET-1 is synthesized by endothelial cells of the pulmonary arteries, veins and microvasculature, as well as by bronchiolar and alveolar epithelial cells and macrophages in mammals, including humans.[10–14] The locally produced ET-1 acts in a paracrine way to cause vaso- or broncho-constriction. Being a regulatory step in the synthesis of ET-1, ECE has been investigated in the pulmonary system. It was shown to be a neutral endopeptidase, and therefore phosphoramidon, an inhibitor of this enzyme activity, has been used to detect the presence of ECE in biological systems. ECE purified from rat lung microsomes was found to be phosphoramidon-sensitive and preferred big ET-1 over big ET-2 and big ET-3 as a substrate.[15] Guinea-pig and porcine lung membranes also contain phosphoramidon-sensitive distinct ECE activities with varying molecular masses.[16,17] The molecular masses of these protein

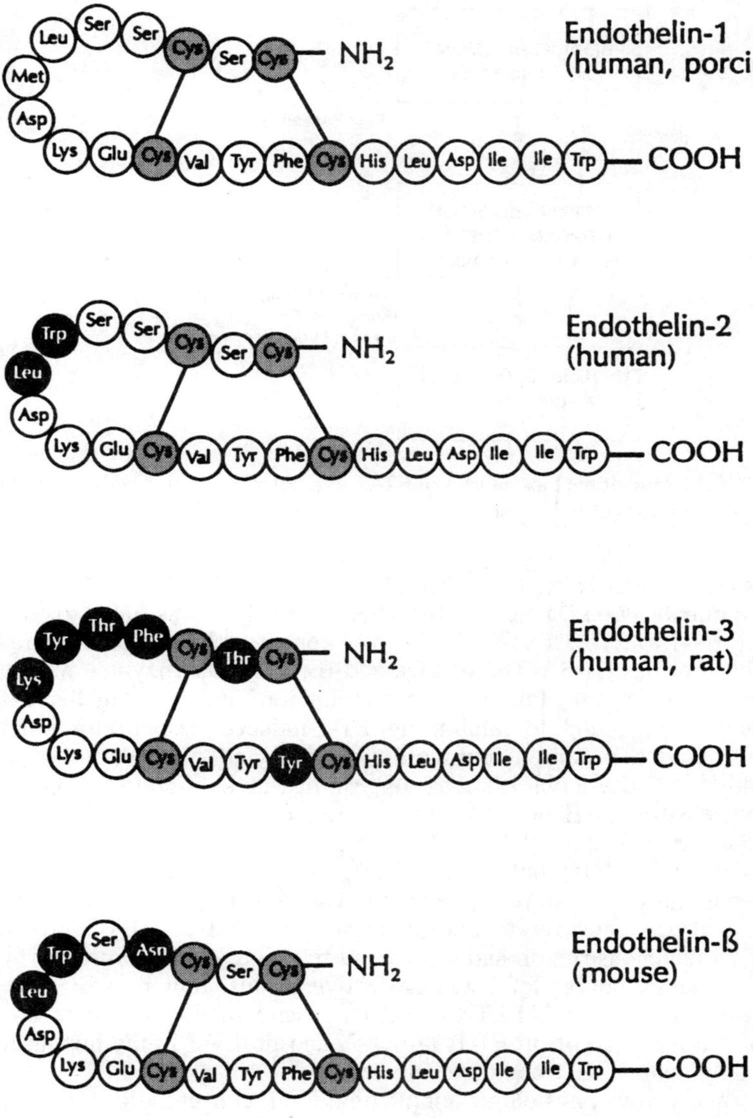

Figure 2. Amino acid sequence of the four isopeptides of the ET family. Filled circles show amino acids that differ from the ET-1 sequence. Reproduced with permission from Gandhi et al.[6]

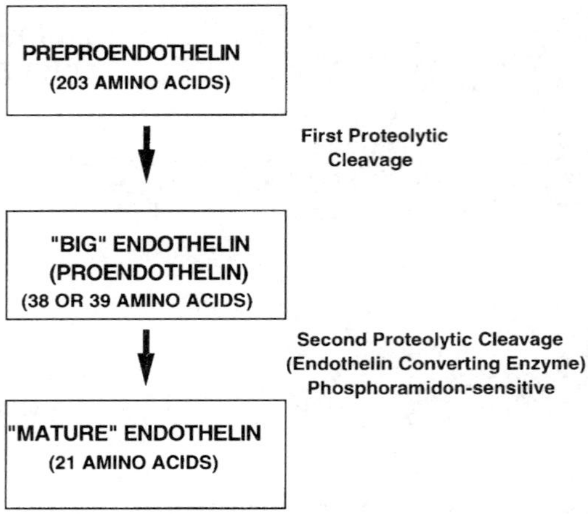

Figure 3. Schematic of the biosynthesis of ET-1 in vascular endothelial cells. Reproduced with permission from Gandhi et al.[6]

species are 108 and 162 kDa (guinea-pig lung), and 65 and 300 kDa (porcine lung). While the 300 kDa enzyme from the porcine lung was found to convert only big ET-1 to ET-1, the 65 kDa enzyme converted both big ET-1 and big ET-2, but not big ET-3.[16] The 65 kDa and the 108 kDa enzymes were also inhibited by thiorphan. Further, phosphoramidon, and to a smaller extent thiorphan, were found to inhibit big ET-1-induced vasoconstriction and bronchoconstriction and eicosanoid synthesis in the perfused lung preparations.[18,19] These observations suggest that, in addition to the phosphoramidon-sensitive ECE, non-selective enzymatic processes are also involved in the conversion of big ET-1 to ET-1 in the lung.

Infusion of big ET-1 but not big ET-3, *in vivo* and in perfused rat and guinea-pig lung preparations, elicited vasoconstrictor and prostanoid-releasing effects sensitive to phosphoramidon.[20] ET-1 and ET-2 produced similar bronchoconstriction and eicosanoid-releasing effects in the perfused guinea-pig lungs, but big ET-2 was ineffective.[19] Thus pulmonary ECE seems to discriminate between big ET-1 and other proendothelins. In this regard, in spite of the presence of proET-1, proET-2, and proET-3 in the human lung tissue, only mature ET-1 could be detected.[12]

A normally low physiologic circulating ET-1 concentration (1–5 pM), despite its constitutive synthesis, suggests a rapid and efficient mechanism of clearance at the site of synthesis. Radiolabeled ET-1 systemically administered to rats, *in vivo*, was shown to clear very rapidly ($t_{1/2} < 1$ min). The lung, kidney, liver, and heart, in that order, were found to be the principal sites of ET-1 clearance.[21,22] In anesthetized dogs also the lung was found to be a major site of ET-1 uptake.[23] Consistent with these observations, although ^{125}I-labeled ET-1 was rapidly removed from the perfusate by isolated rat lung, analysis of the radioactive material revealed that ET-1 metabolism was less than 15% in both the lung and the perfusate.[24] These results suggest that circulating ET-1 is readily taken up in the lungs, but slowly metabolized. Our experiments with tissue homogenates also indicated that, compared with other major organs, lung is ineffective in metabolizing ET-1 (Figure 4). Although it was recently demonstrated that the aortic smooth muscle cells possess a novel enzyme system on plasma membranes that rapidly metabolizes ET-1,[25] the inability of the lung to effectively metabolize ET-1 suggests the absence of such a mechanism in the pulmonary vasculature. This differential metabolism may augment the actions of elevated endogenous ET-1 in the pulmonary system.

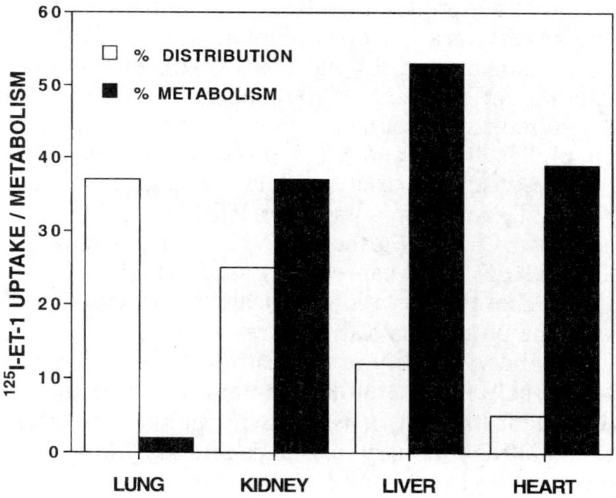

Figure 4. ET-1 clearance and ET-1-metabolizing capacity of major organs. Open bars show percentage distribution of ^{125}I-labeled ET-1 in lung, kidney, liver, and heart following its administration to the rat. These data are generated from the results described by Anggard et al[21] and Shiba et al.[22] Filled bars illustrate metabolism of ^{125}I-labeled ET-1 by these organs. In this experiment, 10% homogenates were made from rat lung, liver, kidney, and heart in Hanks' balanced salt solution containing 0.1% bovine serum albumin. After centrifugation at 1000 ***g*** (10 min; 4°C) and 10 000 ***g*** (30 min; 4°C), the pellet was suspended in the same volume of buffer as was used to prepare the homogenate. Aliquots of the suspension 1 ml each were incubated with 20 pM [^{125}I]-ET-1 for 30 min at 37°C. The reaction was terminated by the addition of 10% trichloroacetic acid, and after centrifugation radioactivity in the supernatant ([^{125}I]-ET-1 metabolites)[25] was determined.

PULMONARY ENDOTHELIN RECEPTORS AND THEIR FUNCTIONS

ET-binding sites are distributed throughout the adult human lung tissue, with maximum receptor density in parenchyma followed by airway smooth muscle and airway epithelia.[12] Endothelin receptors belong to the G-protein-linked superfamily, and are classified into three major subtypes: ET_A (specific for ET-1), ET_{B1} and ET_{B2} (nonspecific with respect to ET peptides), and ET_C

(specific for ET-3) (Table 1). Vascular smooth muscle cells contain predominantly ET_A and a small number of ET_{B2} receptors; binding of ET peptides to these receptors causes vasoconstriction. Endothelial cells contain ET_{B1} receptor, activation of which stimulates synthesis of NO and prostacyclin (PGI_2), and subsequent vasodilatation. Recent evidence suggests the presence of ET_C receptor on certain cells; however, the function of this receptor is not known. ET peptides exert a variety of biologic actions on many nonvascular cells which possess ET_A and ET_B receptors in varying proportions. ET_A and ET_B receptors were cloned from bovine[26] and rat[27] lung cDNA libraries respectively.

ET-1 was found to act predominantly as a vasodilator at lower concentration (50–100 ng/kg) and as a vasoconstrictor at higher concentration (e.g. 500 ng/kg) in lamb pulmonary arteries and veins.[28] This effect is possibly due to preferential binding of low and high concentrations of ET-1 to distinct receptors in the pulmonary vasculature. In isolated perfused lung preparations from newborn piglets, ET-1 and ET-3 produced an early-onset dilatation followed by a late-onset constriction. The ET-induced vasodilatation was inhibited by the ET_B receptor antagonist RES-701-1 but not by the ET_A receptor antagonist BQ-123. Further, BQ-123 did not alter the constrictor action of ET-3, and RES-701-1 caused only partial inhibition of ET-1-induced vasoconstriction.[29] These observations indicate the presence of ET_A, ET_{B1} and ET_{B2} receptors in the pulmonary vasculature.

There appears to be variability in the distribution of ET receptors coupled to the same functional response in the pulmonary vasculature. For example, ET-1-induced vasoconstriction in isolated rat pulmonary artery rings (2–3 mm diameter) and intrapulmonary resistance arteries (100–150 μm diameter) is mediated principally via ET_A and ET_B receptors respectively.[30] Differences were also observed between the sensitivity of large and small vessels to ET-1, with an EC_{50} of approximately 9 nM for the artery and 33 nM for the smaller vessels.[31]

In human pulmonary arteries ET-1-induced contraction is mediated via ET_A receptor, whereas ET_B receptor activation is responsible for bronchoconstriction.[32] ET_B-receptor-mediated bronchoconstriction was also observed in guinea-pig lung.[19] However, the presence of ET_A binding sites, in addition to the ET_B receptors, in tracheal smooth muscle, alveoli and small airways of ovine lung[33] and the porcine bronchus[34] indicate that both ET_A and ET_B receptors participate in airway smooth muscle contraction in response to ET peptides.

Lippton et al[35] demonstrated that, in cat, repeated intralobar arterial bolus injections of ET-1 and ET-2, but not ET-3, reversed pulmonary vasodilatation

Table 1. Endothelin receptors: their distribution and functions.

Type	Specificity	Site	Function
ET_A	ET-1>>>ET-3	Vascular smooth muscle cell	Contraction, growth
ET_{B2}	ET-1=ET-3	Vascular smooth muscle cell	Contraction
ET_{B1}	ET-1=ET-3	Endothelial cells	Relaxation (NO, PGI_2)
ET_C	ET-3>>>ET-1	?	?

to vasoconstriction. Further, repeated injections of ET-1, ET-2, or ET-3 also caused the loss of pulmonary vasodilatation to subsequent doses of ET-1, ET-2, or Sarafotoxin S6b (ET_A-selective agonist) but not to ET-3. These data suggested that the pulmonary vasodilator responses to ET-1 and ET-2, but not ET-3, undergo tachyphylaxis and cross-tachyphylaxis, and also provided a functional correlate for the existence of ET_A and ET_C receptors in the adult pulmonary vascular bed.

During the developmental stages in pig from birth to adulthood, dense ET-1-binding sites were localized over the pulmonary and bronchial arteries and veins, bronchial smooth muscle, and the parenchymal region. Muscular pulmonary arteries and pulmonary veins had a higher density of binding than elastic arteries. While between birth and adulthood, ET-binding density decreased in extrapulmonary and bronchial arteries, a transient increase in the receptor density was observed at 2–3 days and 10 days of age in the elastic and muscular intrapulmonary arteries respectively. Both ET_A and ET_B receptors were found on the medial smooth muscle cells at all ages, whereas the majority (75–92%) of binding sites in the pulmonary arteries were ET_A.[36]

SECONDARY MEDIATORS OF ET-1 ACTIONS IN THE PULMONARY SYSTEM

ET peptides have been shown to stimulate synthesis of mediators such as eicosanoids and platelet-activating factor (PAF). Eicosanoids and PAF play important roles in pulmonary pathophysiology. Interactions between ET-1, thromboxane A_2 (TXA_2) and PAF in the vasculature are apparent as ET-1-induced synthesis of TXA_2 in cultured rat vascular smooth muscle cells is inhibited by a specific PAF receptor antagonist CV-6209.[37] The ferret pulmonary circulation has been shown to be most sensitive to the TXA_2 analog U46619 and least sensitive to PAF; while U46619 and ET-1 were found to predominantly constrict veins, PAF predominantly constricted arteries.[38] D'Orleans-Juste et al[39,40] noted that activation of ET_A and ET_B receptors stimulates synthesis of the vasodilator prostanoid PGI_2 and the vasoconstrictor eicosanoid TXA_2 respectively in perfused guinea-pig lung preparation. Thus arachidonic acid metabolites and PAF appear to act as secondary mediators of bronchovascular actions of ET-1.

It was observed that inhibition of the cyclooxygenase pathway converted ET-1-induced pulmonary vasodilatation to vasoconstriction.[28] However, the mechanism of ET-1 action in pulmonary arteries and veins preconstricted with indomethacin and U46619 appears to be different. In this situation, low concentrations (50–100 ng/kg) of ET-1 converted vasoconstriction to vasodilatation, suggesting that this effect may be mediated by NO synthesis in the endothelial cells and not via cyclooxygenase metabolites.[28] Conversely, in a similar experiment, Eddahibi et al[41] observed that ET-1- and ET-3-dependent vasodilatation was potentiated upon inhibition of cyclooxygenase or thromboxane synthetase, attenuated by K^+ channel blockers, but was unaffected by inhibitors of NO synthase or guanylate cyclase. In the larger pulmonary arteries, however, potentiation of ET-1-induced constriction by the NO synthase inhibitor L-N^{ω} nitroarginine methyl ester (L-NAME), and its reversal by the ET_A antagonist FR 139317, suggest that the ET_A-receptor-mediated responses to ET-1 are suppressed by endothelium-derived NO.[30]

In guinea-pig isolated trachea, ET-1 has been shown to stimulate synthesis of a number of arachidonic acid metabolites, which include PGD_2, PGE_2, PGI_2, TXB_2, $PGF_{2\alpha}$, in the absence of epithelium and smooth muscle.[42] Attenuation of ET-1-induced contraction of isolated guinea-pig airways upon inhibition of TXA_2 synthesis suggests that the bronchopulmonary action of ET-1 is mediated, in part, by the release of TXA_2.[43,44] Further, TXA_2 receptor antagonist BM 13505 significantly potentiated the relaxant response to ET-1 in tracheal strips precontracted with carbachol. Removal of the epithelium or treatment with methylene blue, oxyhemoglobin or *N*-monomethyl-L-arginine (L-NMMA) changed the response of precontracted tracheal preparations to ET-1 from relaxation to sustained contraction. These observations and the inability of indomethacin to reverse the dilatory effect of ET-1 suggested involvement of NO and not PGI_2 in ET-1 actions in the airways.[45] Conversely, in tracheal strips under passive tension, ET-1 (1–100 nM) elicited dose-dependent contraction, which was enhanced by removal of the epithelium, but not by preincubation with methylene blue, oxyhemoglobin or L-NMMA. A concentration-dependent increase in the release of TXA_2 but not of PGE_2 and PGI_2 from intact tracheal strips following stimulation with ET-1 suggested that TXA_2 may act as a secondary mediator of ET-1-induced tracheal contraction.[44] Inhibition of TXA_2 synthesis was also found to attenuate ET-1-induced increase in lung weight and tracheal effusion without altering the vasoconstriction in rat and guinea-pig lungs; iloprost, a stable analog of PGI_2, antagonized the effects of ET-1 on perfusion pressure and lung weight without reducing tracheal effusion.[46]

A role for PAF as a secondary mediator of bronchopulmonary actions of ET-1 has been suggested, as ET-1-induced contraction of guinea-pig trachea and upper bronchi can be inhibited by the PAF receptor antagonists BN52021 and WEB 2086.[47,48] However, other investigators found that lipoxygenase inhibitors and PAF receptor antagonists did not influence the ET-1-induced increase in pulmonary inflation pressure of anesthetized and ventilated guinea-pigs and suggested that PAF and TXB_2 release cannot be the only mechanism of the bronchopulmonary effects of ET-1 in guinea pigs *in vivo*.[42,49] Conversely, unlike in guinea-pig and rat, the bronchopulmonary effects of ET-1 are not mediated via TXA_2 or PAF in humans.[50]

Leukotriene D_4 (LTD_4) and histamine are known to be potent and effective bronchoconstrictors. However, ET-1 seems to act independently of these mediators in the airways, as it does not stimulate the release of histamine or peptidoleukotrienes, and ET-1-induced bronchoconstriction is not affected by antagonists of leukotrienes and H1-histamine receptors.[42,50]

Bradykinin (BK), a powerful vasodilating peptide, regulates vascular contractility mainly through its action on the endothelium. BK appears to modulate ET-1 synthesis by enhancing endothelial synthesis of NO. In canine coronary, renal and femoral arteries, ET-1-induced contraction was inhibited by BK only in the presence of endothelium. Blockade of B2 and not B1 receptor inhibited the effect of BK on the ET-1-induced contraction.

The suppression of the ET-1-induced vasoconstriction by BK was partly reversed by inhibitors of NO synthase, guanylate cyclase and cyclo-oxygenase, and the reversing effects of methylene blue and indomethacin were additive.[51,52] Momose et al[53] also demonstrated that BK inhibition of ET-1 secretion by endothelial cells was reversed by the NO synthase inhibitor N^G-nitro-L-arginine. They observed that blockade of B1 receptors did not affect BK-induced NO production but enhanced the inhibition of ET-1 secretion by BK; B1 receptor stimulation, in contrast, enhanced ET-1 secretion by endothelial cells. These authors suggested that accumulation of endogenous BK in endothelial cells causes inhibition of ET-1 secretion primarily via B2 receptors and NO synthesis.[53] Although these observations suggest that a relationship between ET-1 and BK may be important in pulmonary pathophysiology, the mechanisms of such interactions remain to be elucidated.

It is known that elevation of cytosolic Ca^{2+} concentration is a primary step in receptor-mediated vasoconstriction. In rat, although ET-1-stimulated contraction is predominantly dependent on extracellular Ca^{2+}, nearly 35% of this effect in the pulmonary artery and 19% in the resistance vessel could be obtained in Ca^{2+}-free solution.[31] In contrast, ET-1-induced contraction of human isolated bronchus and pulmonary artery was found to be independent of the presence of Ca^{2+} in the perfusate solution.[54]

ENDOTHELIN AS A MEDIATOR OF PULMONARY PATHOLOGY

The pulmonary vasculature as well as the airways are extremely sensitive to the constrictor action of ET-1. ET-1 is also believed to play a part in fibrosis and collagen production. Further, ET-1 is a potent mitogen for vascular smooth muscle cells and fibroblasts, and its synthesis is stimulated by a number of mediators found in various pathologic conditions. As in the endothelial cells, ET-1 synthesis in alveolar epithelial cells is also stimulated by lipopolysaccharide, tumor necrosis factor α, interleukin 1, and transforming growth factor β, whereas interferon Γ and platelet-derived growth factor inhibit it.[55] These observations and the inefficiency of the lungs in degrading ET-1 suggest that, under conditions in which endogenous ET-1 is elevated, this peptide can be causal in the pathogenesis and/or complications of pulmonary disorders. In this section, we will review the findings that implicate ET-1 in some pulmonary pathologies.

Pulmonary hypertension

Pulmonary hypertension is characterized by extensive remodeling of the pulmonary vasculature, with consequent hypertrophic changes in the right ventricle. Higher plasma ET-1 concentration in patients with pulmonary hypertension than in normal subjects indicated the possibility that ET-1 may play a role in pulmonary hypertension in humans.[56] Interestingly, the arterial to venous ET-1 ratio was greater than unity in patients with primary pulmonary hypertension and near unity in patients with secondary pulmonary hypertension as against 0.6 in control subjects. A follow-up investigation demonstrated very high levels of ET-1-like immunoreactivity and expression of preproET-1 mRNA, predominantly in endothelial cells of pulmonary arteries with medial thickening and intimal fibrosis, in the lungs of patients with pulmonary hypertension.[57] These authors also observed a strong correlation between the intensity of ET-1-like immunoreactivity and pulmonary vascular resistance in patients with plexogenic pulmonary arteriopathy, but not in those with secondary pulmonary hypertension.[58] Plasma ET-1 was found to be elevated even in children with pulmonary hypertension, and the basal ET-1 correlated strongly with the degree of elevation of mean pulmonary arterial pressure during acute hypoxia. However, arterial/venous ET-1 ratios in the pulmonary hypertension group were not different from those in the control group.[59]

Increased expression of ET-1 was observed in the lung tissue from patients with interstitial lung fibrosis, which included patients with cryptographic fibrosing alveolitis (CFA), with and without pulmonary hypertension. Immunostains for ET-1 and big ET-1 and expression of preproET-1 mRNA were most prominent in airway epithelium and type II pneumocytes, particularly those lining areas of young granulation tissue. ET-1-like immunoreactivity and mRNA were also present in pulmonary vascular endothelial cells, particularly in specimens from patients with pulmonary hypertension. By contrast, lung tissue from normal subjects and patients with focal fibrosis expressed very little ET-1.[58] These findings suggest a possible role for cell-specific expression of ET-1 in the pathogenesis of CFA and associated pulmonary hypertension.

Animal models of hypoxia-induced pulmonary hypertension have been used to understand the role of ET-1 in this disorder. A positive correlation between elevated plasma ET-1 levels and increased pulmonary arterial pressure was observed in a rat model of hypoxia-induced pulmonary hypertension.[60] Further, selectively enhanced ET-1 levels and ET_A gene expression in the pulmonary vasculature, and the reversal of the pulmonary vasoconstrictor response to acute (0–90 min) and chronic (2 weeks) hypoxia by the ET_A-selective antagonist BQ-123 suggested that the intrapulmonary ET-1 acting on ET_A receptors in the pulmonary vasculature mediates hypoxia-induced pulmonary vasoconstriction and hypertension.[61] In fawn-hooded rats, a strain that develops idiopathic pulmonary hypertension, although serum ET-1 levels were not different from those of normal Sprague–Dawley rats, two- to three-fold increases in the ET-1 levels and the expression of preproET-1 mRNA were observed in the whole lung homogenate.[62]

In rats with monocrotaline-induced pulmonary hypertension, the venous plasma ET-1 concentration progressively increased before the development of pulmonary hypertension.[63,64] These effects were accompanied by concomitant increase in right ventricular systolic pressure, right ventricular hypertrophy, and increased expression of preproET-1 mRNA in the heart. However, unlike in hypoxia-induced pulmonary hypertension, expression of preproET-1 mRNA as well as immunoreactive ET-1 gradually decreased in the lungs of monocrotaline-treated rats. Pulmonary expression of ET_B

receptor mRNA was also decreased in these rats.[64] Continuous infusion of BQ-123, a selective ET_A receptor antagonist, significantly inhibited the progression of both pulmonary hypertension and right ventricular hypertrophy, and prevented pulmonary arterial medial thickening.[63] Although endogenous ET-1 does not seem to be responsible, elevated circulating ET-1 and inhibition of ET-1-induced NO synthesis due to the loss of ET_B receptors in the pulmonary vasculature may be responsible factors in monocrotalin-induced pulmonary hypertension.

Acute respiratory distress syndrome (ARDS)

Hyperdynamic circulatory state with increased cardiac output and depressed total vascular resistance and simultaneous pulmonary hypertension are common characteristics of ARDS. Studies with animal models and human patients with ARDS indicate that ET-1 may play an important role in the pathogenesis of this disorder. Reduced clearance and increased release of ET-1 by the lung caused an increase in plasma ET-1 concentration in patients with ARDS.[65,66] With clinical improvement, the mean plasma ET-1 levels, arterial/venous ET-1 ratio, and pulmonary arterial pressure fell significantly towards normal.[66] Rats injected intravenously with oleic acid is an established animal model of ARDS. After oleic acid injection into rats, plasma ET-1 was found to increase as early as within 15 min, peaked at 45 min, and reached basal levels again after 240 min. In contrast, much larger amounts of ET-1 were found in the bronchoalveolar lavage fluid, with a peak at 120 min preceding the maximum hypoxia observed at 180 min.[67] These observations were confirmed by Zhang et al,[68] and they further demonstrated that pre-administration of ET antiserum to rat with respiratory distress syndrome significantly improved hypoxemia, pulmonary edema, and histologic injury, and inhibited the leakage of protein and intracellular enzymes from alveoli.

Asthma

Increased ET-1 levels in the bronchoalveolar lavage fluid (BAL)[69,70] and plasma[71] were observed in patients with asthma. Plasma ET-1 was found to correlate with the severity of asthma, and there was significant negative correlation between ET-1 levels in plasma and BAL and the pulmonary function.[69–71] Immunohistochemical analysis of the biopsy specimens showed ET-1 in the airway epithelium of asthmatic patients and not in the control specimens.[72] Vittori et al[73] found that cultured bronchial epithelial cells from asthmatic patients but not normal subjects expressed preproET-1 mRNA and also released high amounts of immunoreactive ET-1. Interestingly, the addition of hydrocortisone to the cell culture inhibited the release of ET-1 from epithelial cells of asthmatic patients, but did not have any effect on the expression of preproET-1 mRNA.[73] In view of the powerful bronchoconstrictor property of ET-1, and its ability to stimulate fibroblast proliferation and fibrosis, the observations described above suggest that ET-1 may be an important mediator in the pathophysiology of asthma.

ENDOTHELIN ANTAGONISTS AND INHIBITORS: POTENTIAL IN THE TREATMENT OF PULMONARY DISORDERS

In recent years various pulmonary disorders have been treated by NO inhalation.[74] However, in patients with primary pulmonary hypertension, this treatment is minimally successful. NO has been shown to inhibit ET-1 synthesis in endothelial cells,[75] displace ET-1 from its receptor and inhibit the post-receptor ET-1-induced signaling pathway.[76] A recent investigation demonstrated deficiency of NO synthase in patients with pulmonary hypertension.[77] Thus, the internal control of NO over the synthesis of ET-1 and its actions appears to be compromised in these patients. This suggestion is supported by the strong increase in both ET-1 and expression of preproET-1 mRNA in the lungs of patients with pulmonary hypertension.[57,58] Treatment of pulmonary vasculature *in vivo* and *in vitro* with inhibitors of ET-1 synthesis and ET receptor antagonists has been shown to produce antagonism of ET-1 action. Further, ET receptor antagonists were found to exert beneficial effects in animal models of pulmonary hypertension. Therefore, inhibitors of ET-1 synthesis and/or ET receptor antagonists seem to offer promise in the treatment of pulmonary disorders. Attempts to design appropriate inhibitors of ET synthesis that may have clinical applicability have been unsuccessful. Hence, we will focus the discussion of this section on ET receptor antagonists.

Substitution of amino acids in ET was the initial approach toward the development of ET receptor antagonists. Of these [Dpr^1, Asp^{15}]ET-1 was found to inhibit ET-1-induced bronchoconstriction in sheep.[78] The major breakthrough in the development of ET receptor antagonists came with the discovery of the cyclic pentapeptides BE-18257A (cyclo(-D-Glu-L-Ala-D-Val-L-Leu-D-Trp)) and BE-18257B (cyclo(-D-Glu-L-Ala-*allo*-D-Ile-L-Leu-D-Trp)), which were isolated from the fermentation products of *Streptomyces misakiensis*.[79,80] These cyclic pentapeptides bind ET_A receptors in a competitive manner, and inhibit ET-1-induced vasoconstriction in isolated blood vessels and pressor responses in intact animals.[79] Chemical modification of BE-18257B to BQ-123 (cyclo(-D-Asp-L-Pro-D-Val-L-Leu-D-Trp)) and BQ-153 (cyclo(-D-Sal-L-Pro-D-Val-L-Leu-D-Trp)) improved the potency of these antagonists in inhibiting ET-1 binding to the ET_A receptor.[80] In addition to ET-1-induced contractile effects, these ET_A receptor antagonists were also shown to inhibit other cellular responses to ET-1, such as phosphoinositide metabolism and mitogenesis.[81,82]

The discovery of cyclic pentapeptide ET antagonists was followed by the development of a linear tripeptide FR 139317 ([*N*-(hexahydro-1-azepinyl)carbonyl]-Leu-D-(1-Me)Trp-D-2-pyridylalanine).[83] FR 139317, an ET_A-specific antagonist, was found to inhibit ET-1-induced vasoconstriction of guinea-pig pulmonary artery, but not the contraction of tracheal smooth muscle.[84] Another tripeptide BQ-788 (*N-cis*-2,6-dimethylpiperidinocarbonyl-L-Γ-MeLeu-D-Trp(1-CO_2Me)-D-Nle) is an ET_B-specific antagonist, which competitively inhibits binding of ET-1 to ET_B receptor and the ET-1-induced vasodepressor response without affecting its pressor effect.[85]

Peptide antagonists nonselective with respect to ET_A and ET_B were also designed, notable among them being PD 142893 (Ac-D-Dip-Leu-Asp-Ile-Ile-Trp-OH) and a more potent PD 145065 (Ac-D-Bhg-Leu-Asp-Ile-Ile-Trp-OH).

These antagonists were found to inhibit binding of ET-1 to both ET_A and ET_B receptors and to suppress ET_A- and ET_B-mediated vasoactive effects. The potency of PD 145065 was reported to be greater than that of a nonpeptide ET receptor antagonist Ro 46-2005 (see the following discussion) in inhibiting the actions of ET-1 in guinea-pig airway preparations.[86]

Although the peptide antagonists of ET receptors are useful in binding and functional assays *in vitro*, their effects *in vivo* may be limited because of their vulnerability to degradation by peptidases. Further, these substances cannot be given orally or intraperitoneally and must be administered intravenously. Therefore, attempts were made to develop orally active nonpeptide antagonists. Prominent among the antagonists that have been designed so far are SB 209670 and Ro 46-2005. SB 209670 exhibits higher affinity toward the ET_A than the ET_B receptor, and has been shown to be effective in animal models of hypertension,[87] acute renal failure,[88] and restenosis.[89] However, SB 209670 is much more effective if administered intravenously than orally. Later, a structurally similar substance, SB 217242, which is also more selective for the ET_A receptor, was found to have greater bioavailability when administered orally. The effectiveness of SB compounds in pulmonary disorders remains to be determined.

Ro 46-2005, also known as bosentan, is a low molecular-weight nonpeptide antagonist of the ET_A and ET_B receptors, and was chemically derived from a class of compounds identified by systematic screening of chemicals.[90] In binding experiments, Ro 46-2005 was found to be equipotent for inhibition of [^{125}I]-ET-1 binding on the ET_A and ET_B receptors.[91] *In vivo*, Ro 46-2005 was found to inhibit the depressor and, only at high doses (100 mg/kg intravenously) the pressor effect of ET-1. However, much lower doses (1–10 mg/kg intravenously) were sufficient to inhibit the pressor effect of the precursor big ET-1.[92] In lungs from normoxic rats, Ro 46-2005 abolished the vasodilator responses to ET-1 and the ET_B-selective agonist IRL-1620, and attenuated the vasoconstrictor responses to ET-1. In lungs from chronically hypoxic rats, the pressor response to ET-1 was abolished by Ro 46-2005 and partially reduced by the ET_A antagonist BQ-123. In conscious rats previously exposed to hypoxia for 15 days, a 3-day pretreatment with Ro 46-2005 by gavage attenuated the increase in systemic arterial pressures and the concomitant decrease in cardiac output in response to an intravenous bolus of ET-1. In rats exposed to hypoxia for 15 days and simultaneously treated with Ro 46-2005, pulmonary arterial pressure was lower and right ventricular hypertrophy was less severe than in hypoxic rats treated with vehicle.[93] These effects of Ro 46-2005 appear to be very encouraging in the treatment of pulmonary hypertension. In this regard, beneficial effects of Ro 46-2005 were reported in patients with congestive heart failure (M. Clozel, Fourth International conference on Endothelins, London, April 23–26, 1995).

CONCLUSIONS AND SUMMARY

Vascular endothelium synthesizes multiple peptides and lipids which mediate vasoconstriction. Of these mediators, ET-1 has been of particular interest because: (a) it is among the most potent vasoconstrictors yet discovered; (b) it is produced constitutively by the endothelial cells and its synthesis is stimulated by a variety of chemical and mechanical factors; (c) systemic concentrations of ET-1 appear to correlate with a variety of cardiovascular pathologies; (d) ET-1 is capable of stimulating synthesis of several vasoactive mediators, including eicosanoids and NO; and (e) in addition to its vasoconstrictor properties, ET-1 elicits actions on many mammalian cell types that are known to contribute to clinically important pathophysiologic processes.

ET-1 is a potent constrictor of the pulmonary vasculature and bronchiolar smooth muscle. Basal synthesis of ET-1 by vascular endothelial cells and bronchial epithelial cells may reflect a role in maintaining physiologic vascular and airway tone in the lung. The correlation between increased circulating ET-1 levels in acute as well as chronic pulmonary disorders is consistent with its involvement in these pathologies. Specifically, plasma ET-1 concentrations are increased in patients with primary and secondary pulmonary hypertension. Under these conditions the ratio of arterial to venous ET-1 at unity, or greater, indicates its enhanced pulmonary synthesis and/or reduced clearance in these disorders. Further, immunohistochemical and *in situ* hybridization analyses revealed elevated ET-1 levels and enhanced expression of ET-1 mRNA in pulmonary arterial and venous and bronchial vessels of patients with pulmonary hypertension. Enhanced ET-1 synthesis in the lungs of patients with pulmonary hypertension is accompanied by reduced synthesis of NO, which tends to serve as a physiologic antagonist to the vascular actions of ET-1. Increased expression of ET-1 predominantly in airway epithelium of patients with CFA and in alveolar epithelial cells close to the fibrous areas in the lungs of primary pulmonary hypertension patients suggests that ET-1 may be involved in pulmonary fibrosis. Finally, increased ET-1 in plasma and BAL from patients with ARDS and asthma suggests a role for this peptide mediator in the pathogenesis of these complex clinical conditions.

The practice of treating pulmonary diseases, including pulmonary hypertension, with inhaled NO, has helped to identify specific diseases and conditions of particular therapeutic advantage. The influence of NO seems to be dependent on continued exposure to this drug, since its effects are reversed soon after the administration is discontinued. Considering that pulmonary vascular pathologies may reflect a skewed balance between vasoconstrictor and vasodilator influences, a strategy of vasodilator agonist (NO) and vasoconstrictor antagonist (ET-1 receptor, synthesis) may be promising. The development of specific inhibitors of ET-1 synthesis with clinical applicability has not been achieved to date. However, a number of ET receptor antagonists have shown promising cardiovascular results in experimental animals and early human clinical trials. Considering the apparent role of ET-1 in multiple hemodynamic, airway and structural abnormalities associated with cardiopulmonary disorders, ET receptor antagonists and inhibitors of ET-1 synthesis may provide a novel therapeutic avenue. Additionally, the growing understanding of this relatively recent member of the important class of endogenous substances known to mediate vasoconstriction emphasizes the complex relationships that must exist for physiologic control to be maintained.

REFERENCES

1. Furchgott RF & Zawadzki JV (1980) The obligatory role of endothelial cells in the relaxation of arterial smooth muscle by acetylcholine. *Nature* **288:**373–376.
2. Demay JG & Vanhoutte PM (1982) Heterogeneous behavior of canine arterial and venous wall: importance of endothelium. *Circulation Research* **51:**439–447.
3. Ignaro LJ, Buga GM, Wood KS, Byrns RE & Chaudhuri G (1987) Endothelium-derived relaxing factor produced and released from artery and vein is nitric oxide. *Proceedings of the National Academy of Sciences USA* **84:**9295–9269.
4. Palmer RMJ, Ashton DS & Moncada S (1988) Vascular endothelial cells synthesize nitric oxide from L-arginine. *Nature* **333:**664–666.
5. Yanagisawa M, Kurihara H, Kimura S, Tomobe Y, Kobayashi M, Mitsui Y, Yazaki Y, Goto K & Masaki T (1988) A novel potent vasoconstrictor peptide produced by vascular endothelial cells. *Nature* **332:**411–415.
6. Gandhi CR, Berkowitz DE & Watkins WD (1994) Endothelins: biochemistry and pathophysiologic actions. *Anesthesiology* **80:**892–905.
7. Yanagisawa M & Masaki T. (1989) Molecular biology and biochemistry of endothelins. *Trends in Pharmacological Sciences* **10:**374–378.
8. Simonson MS & Dunn MJ (1990) Cellular signaling by peptides of the endothelin gene family. *FASEB Journal* **4:**2989–3000.
9. Anggard EE, Botting RM & Vane JR (1990) Endothelins. *Blood Vessels* **2:**269–281.
10. Black PM, Ghatei MA, Takahashi K, Bretherton-Watt D, Krausz T, Dollery CT & Bloom SR (1989) Formation of endothelin by cultured airway epithelial cells. *FEBS Letters* **255:**129–132.
11. MacCumber MW, Ross CA, Glaser BM & Snyder SH (1989) Endothelin: Visualization of mRNAs by *in situ* hybridization provides evidence for local action. *Proceedings of the National Academy of Sciences USA* **86:**7285–7289.
12. Marciniak SJ, Plumpton C, Barker PJ, Huskisson NS & Davenport AP (1992) Localization of immunoreactive endothelin and proendothelin in the human lung. *Pulmonary Pharmacology* **5:**175–182.
13. Mattoli S, Mezzetti M, Riva G, Allegra L & Fasoli A. Specific binding of endothelin on human bronchial smooth muscle cells in culture and secretion of endothelin-like material from bronchial epithelial cells. *American Journal of Respiratory Cell and Molecular Biology* **3:**145–151.
14. Ninomiya H., Uchida Y, Ishii Y, Nomura A, Kameyama M, Saotome M, Endo T & Hasegawa S (1991) Endotoxin stimulates endothelin release from cultured epithelial cells of guinea-pig trachea. *European Journal of Pharmacology* **203:**299–302.
15. Takahashi M, Matsushita Y, Iijima Y & Tanzawa K (1993) Purification and characterization of endothelin-converting enzyme from rat lung. *Journal of Biological Chemistry* **268:**21394–21398.
16. Sawamura T, Shinmi O, Kishi N, Sugita Y, Yanagisawa M, Goto K, Masaki T & Kimura S (1993) Characterization of phosphoramidon-sensitive metalloproteinases with endothelin-converting enzyme activity in porcine lung membrane. *Biochimica et Biophysica Acta* **1161:**295–302.
17. Shima H, Kawashima Y, Ohmori K, Sugiura M & Kawashima K (1994) Endothelin converting enzymes in guinea-pig lung membrane fractions: purifications and characterizations. *Biochemistry and Molecular Biology International* **34:**1227–1234.

18. Battistini B, Brown M & Vane JR (1995) Selective proteolitic activation and degradation of ETs and big ETs in parenchymal strips of the guinea-pig lung. *Biochemical and Biophysical Research Communications* **207:**675–681.
19. Gratton JP, Rae GA, Claing A, Telemaque S & D'Orleans-Juste P (1995) Different pressor and bronchoconstrictor properties of human big-endothelin-1, 2 (1–38) and 3 in ketamine/xylazine-anaesthetized guinea-pigs. *British Journal of Pharmacology* **114:**720–726.
20. Telemaque S, Gratton JP, Claing A & D'Orleans-Juste P (1993) Pharmacologic evidence for the specificity of the phosphoramidon-sensitive endothelin-converting enzyme for big endothelin-1. *Journal of Cardiovascular Pharmacology* **22 (Suppl. 8)**:S85–S89.
21. Anggard E, Galton S, Rae G, Thomas R, McLonghlin L, de Nucci G & Vane JR (1989) The fate of radiolabeled endothelin-1 and endothelin-3 in the rat. *Journal of Cardiovascular Pharmacology* **13 (suppl 5):**S46–S49.
22. Shiba R, Yanagisawa M, Miyauchi T, Ishii Y, Kimura S, Uchiyama Y, Masaki T & Goto K (1989) Elimination of intravenously injected endothelin-1 from the circulation of the rat. *Journal of Cardiovascular Pharmacology* **13 (Suppl. 5):**S98–S101.
23. Dupuis J, Goresky CA & Stewart DJ (1994) Pulmonary removal and production of endothelin in the anesthetized dog. *Journal of Applied Physiology* **76:**694–700.
24. Westcott JY, Henson J, McMurtry IF & O'Brien RF (1990) Uptake and metabolism of endothelin in the isolated perfused rat lung. *Experimental Lung Research* **16:**521–532.
25. Gandhi CR (1995) Vascular smooth muscle cells metabolize endothelin-1 in the absence of a functional receptor. *Biochimica et Biophysica Acta*, **1269:**290–298.
26. Arai H, Hori S, Aramori I, Ohkubo H & Nakanishi S (1990) Cloning and expression of a cDNA encoding an endothelin receptor. *Nature* **348:**730–732.
27. Sakurai T, Yanagisawa M, Takuwa Y, Miyazaki H, Kimura S, Goto K & Masaki T (1990) Cloning of a cDNA encoding a non-isopeptide-selective subtype of the endothelin receptor. *Nature* **348:**732–735.
28. Toga H, Usha Raj J, Hillyard R, Ku B & Anderson J (1991) Endothelin effects in isolated, perfused lamb lungs: role of cyclooxygenase inhibition and vasomotor tone. *American Journal of Physiology* **261:**H443–H450.
29. Perreault T & Baribeau J (1995) Characterization of endothelin receptors in newborn piglet lung. *American Journal of Physiology* **268:**L607–L614.
30. MacLean MR, McCulloch KM & Baird M (1994) Endothelin ET_A- and ET_B-receptor-mediated vasoconstriction in rat pulmonary arteries and arterioles. *Journal of Cardiovascular Pharmacology* **23:**838–845.
31. Leach RM, Twort CH, Cameron IR & Ward JP (1990) The mechanism of action of endothelin-1 on small pulmonary arterial vessels. *Pulmonary Pharmacology* **3:**103–109.
32. Hay DW, Luttmann MA, Hubbard WC & Undem BJ (1993) Endothelin receptor subtypes in human and guinea-pig pulmonary tissues. *British Journal of Pharmacology* **110:**1175–1783.
33. Goldie RG, Grayson PS, Knott PG, Self GJ & Henry PJ (1994) Predominance of endothelinA (ETA) receptors in ovine airway smooth muscle and their mediation of ET-1-induced contraction. *British Journal of Pharmacology* **112:**749–756.
34. Nakamichi K, Ihara M, Kobayashi M, Saeki T, Ishikawa K & Yano M (1992) Different distribution of endothelin receptor subtypes in pulmonary tissues revealed by the novel selective ligands BQ-123 and [Ala1,3,11,15]ET-1. *Biochemical and Biophysical Research Communications* **182:**144–150.
35. Lippton HL, Hauth TA, Cohen GA & Hyman AL (1993) Functional evidence for different endothelin receptors in the lung. *Journal of Applied Physiology* **75:**38–48.

36. Hislop AA, Zhao YD, Springall DR, Polak JM & Haworth SG (1995) Postnatal changes in endothelin-1 binding in porcine pulmonary vessels and airways. *American Journal of Respiratory Cell and Molecular Biology* **12:**557–566.
37. Takayasu-Okishio M, Terashita Z & Kondo K (1990) Endothelin-1 and platelet activating factor stimulate thromboxane A_2 biosynthesis in rat vascular smooth muscle cells. *Biochemical Pharmacology* **40:**2713–2717.
38. Raj JU, Toga H, Ibe BO & Anderson J (1992) Effects of endothelin, platelet activating factor and thromboxane A_2 in ferret lungs. *Respiration Physiology* **88:**129–140.
39. D'Orleans-Juste P, Telemaque S, Claing A, Ihara M & Yano M (1992) Human big-endothelin-1 and endothelin-1 release prostacyclin via the activation of ET1 receptors in the rat perfused lung. *British Journal of Pharmacology* **105:**773–775.
40. D'Orleans-Juste P, Claing A, Telemaque S, Maurice MC, Yano M & Gratton JP (1994) Block of endothelin-1-induced release of thromboxane A_2 from the guinea pig lung and nitric oxide from the rabbit kidney by a selective ET_B receptor antagonist, BQ-788. *British Journal of Pharmacology* **113:**1257–1262.
41. Eddahibi S, Springall D, Mannan M, Carville C, Chabrier PE, Levame M, Raffestin B, Polak J & Adnot S (1993) Dilator effect of endothelins in pulmonary circulation: changes associated with chronic hypoxia. *American Journal of Physiology* **265:**L571–L580.
42. Hay DW, Hubbard WC & Undem BJ (1993) Relative contributions of direct and indirect mechanisms mediating endothelin-induced contraction of guinea-pig trachea. *British Journal of Pharmacology* **110:**955–962.
43. Filep JG, Battistini B & Sirois P (1990) Endothelin induces thromboxane release and contraction of isolated guinea-pig airways. *Life Sciences* **47:**1845–1850.
44. Filep JG, Battistini B & Sirois P (1991) Pharmacological modulation of endothelin-induced contraction of guinea-pig isolated airways and thromboxane release. *British Journal of Pharmacology* **103:**1633–1640.
45. Filep JG, Battistini B & Sirois P (1993) Induction by endothelin-1 of epithelium-dependent relaxation of guinea-pig trachea in vitro: role for nitric oxide. *British Journal of Pharmacology* **109:**637–644.
46. Ercan ZS, Kilinc M, Yazar O, Korkusuz P & Turker RK (1993) Endothelin-1-induced oedema in rat and guinea-pig isolated perfused lungs. *Archives Internationales de Pharmacodynamie et de Therapie* **323:**74–84.
47. Battistini B, Sirois P, Braquet P & Filep JG (1990) Endothelin-induced constriction of guinea pig airways: role of platelet-activating factor. *European Journal of Pharmacology* **186:**307–310.
48. Filep JG, Sirois MG, Rousseau A, Fournier A & Sirois P (1991) Effects of endothelin-1 on vascular permeability in the conscious rat: interactions with platelet-activating factor. *British Journal of Pharmacology* **104:**797–804.
49. Lueddeckens G, Becker K, Rappold R & Forster W (1991) Influence of aminophylline and ketotifen in comparison to the lipoxygenase inhibitors NDGA and esculetin and the PAF antagonists WEB 2170 [correction of 2107] and BN 52021 on endothelin-1 induced vaso- and bronchoconstriction. *Prostaglandins, Leukotrienes and Essential Fatty Acids* **44:**155–158.
50. Hay DW, Hubbard WC & Undem BJ (1993) Endothelin-induced contraction and mediator release in human bronchus. *British Journal of Pharmacology* **110:**392–398.
51. Ohde H, Morimoto S & Ogihara T (1991) Bradykinin suppresses endothelin-induced contraction of coronary artery through its B2-receptor on the endothelium. *Biochemical International* **23:**1127–1132.
52. Ohde H, Morimoto S, Ohnishi K, Yamaoka E, Fukuo K, Yasuda O & Ogihara T (1992) Bradykinin suppresses endothelin-induced contraction of coronary, renal and femoral arteries through its B2-receptor on the endothelium. *Agents and Actions* **38:**14–22.

53. Momose N, Fukuo K, Morimoto S & Ogihara T (1993) Captopril inhibits endothelin-1 secretion from endothelial cells through bradykinin. *Hypertension* **21:**921–924.
54. McKay KO, Black JL & Armour CL (1991) The mechanism of action of endothelin in human lung. *British Journal of Pharmacology* **102:**422–428.
55. Markewitz BA, Kohan DE & Michael JR (1995) Endothelin-1 synthesis, receptors, and signal transduction in alveolar epithelium: evidence for an autocrine role. *American Journal of Physiology* **268:**L192–L200.
56. Stewart DJ, Levy RD, Cernacek P & Langleben D (1991) Increased plasma endothelin-1 in pulmonary hypertension: Marker or mediator of disease? *Annals of Internal Medicine* **114:**464–469.
57. Giaid A, Yanagisawa M, Langleben D, Michel RP, Levy R, Shennib H, Kimura S, Masaki T, Duguid WP & Stewart DJ (1993) Expression of endothelin-1 in the lungs of patients with pulmonary hypertension. *New England Journal of Medicine* **328:**1732–1739.
58. Giaid A, Michel RP, Stewart DJ, Sheppard M, Corrin B & Hamid Q (1993) Expression of endothelin-1 in lungs of patients with cryptogenic fibrosing alveolitis. *Lancet* **341:**1550–1554.
59. Allen SW, Chatfield BA, Koppenhafer SA, Schaffer MS, Wolfe RR & Abman SH (1993) Circulating immunoreactive endothelin-1 in children with pulmonary hypertension. Association with acute hypoxic pulmonary vasoreactivity. *American Review of Respiratory Disease* **148:**519–522.
60. Chen X (1993) Changes of endothelin in rats with normobaric hypoxia-induced pulmonary hypertension. *Chinese Medical Journal* **73:**400–402.
61. Chen YF, Li H, Elton TS, Yang RH, Jin H, & Oparil S (1994) The role of atrial natriuretic peptide and endothelin in hypoxia induced pulmonary hypertension. *Chinese Journal of Physiology* **37:**165–183.
62. Stelzner TJ, O'Brien RF, Yanagisawa M, Sakurai T, Sato K, Webb S, Zamora M, McMurtry IF & Fisher JH (1992) Increased lung endothelin-1 production in rats with idiopathic pulmonary hypertension. *American Journal of Physiology* **262:**L614–L620.
63. Miyauchi T, Yorikane R, Sakai S, Sakurai T, Okada M, Nishikibe M, Yano M, Yamaguchi I, Sugishita Y & Goto K (1993) Contribution of endogenous endothelin-1 to the progression of cardiopulmonary alterations in rats with monocrotaline-induced pulmonary hypertension. *Circulation Research* **73:**887–897.
64. Yorikane R, Miyauchi T, Sakai S, Sakurai T, Yamaguchi I, Sugishita Y & Goto K (1993) Altered expression of ETB-receptor mRNA in the lung of rats with pulmonary hypertension. *Journal of Cardiovascular Pharmacology* **22 (Suppl. 8):**S336–S338.
65. Druml W, Steltzer H, Waldhausl W, Lenz K, Hammerle A, Vierhapper H, Gasic S & Wagner OF (1993) Endothelin-1 in adult respiratory distress syndrome. *American Review of Respiratory Disease* **148:**1169–1173.
66. Langleben D, DeMarchie M, Laporta D, Spanier AH, Schlesinger RD & Stewart DJ (1993) Endothelin-1 in acute lung injury and the adult respiratory distress syndrome. *American Review of Respiratory Disease* **148:**1646–1650.
67. Simmet T, Pritze S, Thelen KI & Peskar BA (1992) Release of endothelin in the oleic acid-induced respiratory distress syndrome in rats. *European Journal of Pharmacology* **211:**319–322.
68. Zhang L, Yang J & Xu QH (1993) Protective effect of endothelin-antiserum on oleic acid-induced respiratory distress syndrome (RDS). *Chinese Journal of Tuberculosis and Respiratory Diseases* **16:**8–10.
69. Sofia M, Mormile M, Faraone S, Alifano M, Zofra S, Romano L & Carratu L (1993) Increased endothelin-like immunoreactive material on bronchoalveolar lavage fluid from patients with bronchial asthma and patients with interstitial lung disease. *Respiration* **60:**89–95.

70. Redington AE, Springall DR, Ghatei MA, Lau LC, Bloom SR, Holgate ST, Polak JM & Howarth PH (1995) Endothelin in bronchoalveolar lavage fluid and its relation to airflow obstruction in asthma. *American Journal of Respiratory Critical Care Medicine* **151:**1034–1039.
71. Aoki T, Kojima T, Ono A, Unishi G, Yoshijima S, Kaneda-Hayashi N, Yamamoto C, Hirata Y & Kobayashi Y (1994) Circulating endothelin-1 levels in patients with bronchial asthma. *Annals of Allergy* **73:**365–369.
72. Springall DR, Howarth PH, Counihan H, Djukanovic R, Holgate ST & Polak JM (1991) Endothelin immunoreactivity of airway epithelium in asthmatic patients. *Lancet* **337:**697–701.
73. Vittori E, Marini M, Fasoli A, De Franchis R & Mattoli S (1992) Increased expression of endothelin in bronchial epithelial cells of asthmatic patients and effect of corticosteroids. *American Review of Respiratory Disease* **146:**1320–1325.
74. Lunn R (1995) Inhaled nitric oxide therapy. *Mayo Clinic Proceedings* **70:**247–255.
75. Cao WB, Zeng ZP, Zhu YJ, Luo WC & Cai BQ (1994) Inhibition of nitric oxide synthesis increases the secretion of endothelin-1 *in vivo* and in cultured endothelial cells. *Chinese Medical Journal* **107:**822–826.
76. Goligorsky MS, Tsukahara H, Magazine H, Andersen TT, Malik AB & Bahou WF (1994) Termination of endothelin signaling: role of nitric oxide. *Journal of Cellular Physiology* **158:**485–494.
77. Giaid A & Saleh D (1995) Reduced expression of endothelial nitric oxide synthase in the lungs of patients with pulmonary hypertension. *New England Journal of Medicine* **333:**214–221.
78. Abraham WM, Ahmed A, Cortes A, Spinella MJ, Malik AB & Anderson TT (1993) A specific endothelin-1 antagonist blocks inhaled endothelin-1-induced bronchoconstriction in sheep. *Journal of Applied Physiology* **74:**2537–2542.
79. Ihara M, Fukuroda T, Saeki T, Nishikibe M, Kojiri K, Suda H & Yano M (1991) An endothelin receptor (ET_A) antagonist isolated from *Streptomyces misakiensis*. *Biochemical and Biophysical Research Communications* **178:**132–137.
80. Ihara M, Noguchi K, Saeki T, Fukuroda T, Tsuchida S, Kimura S, Fukami T, Ishikawa K, Nishikibe M & Yano M (1992) Biological profiles of highly potent novel endothelin antagonists selective for ET_A receptor. *Life Sciences* **50:**257–255.
81. Ohlstein EH, Arleth A, Bryan H, Elliott JD & Po Sung C (1992) The selective endothelin ET_A receptor antagonist BQ123 antagonizes endothelin-1-mediated mitogenesis. *European Journal of Pharmacology* **225:**347–350.
82. Eguchi S, Hirata Y, Ihara M, Yano M & Marumo F (1992) A novel ET_A antagonist (BQ-123) inhibits endothelin-1-induced phosphoinositide breakdown and DNA synthesis in rat vascular smooth muscle cells. *FEBS Letters* **302:**243–246.
83. Aramori I, Nirei H, Shoubo M, Sogabe K, Nakamura K, Kojo H, Notsu Y, Ono T & Nakakishi S (1993) Subtype selectivity of a novel endothelin antagonist, FR 139317, for the two endothelin receptors in transfected Chinese hamster overy cells. *Molecular Pharmacology* **43:**127–131.
84. Cardell LO, Uddaman R & Edvinson L (1993) A novel ET_A-receptor antagonist, FR 139317, inhibits endothelin-induced contraction of guinea-pig pulmonary arteries, but not trachea. *British Journal of Pharmacology* **108:**448–452.
85. Ishikawa K, Ihara M, Noguchi K, Mase T, Mino N, Saeki T, Furukoda T, Fukami T, Ozaki S, Nagase T, Nishikibe M & Yano M (1994) Biochemical and pharmacological profile of a potent and selective endothelin B-receptor antagonist, BQ-788. *Proceedings of the National Academy of Sciences USA* **91:**4892–4896.
86. Battistini B, Warner TD, Fournier A & Vane JR (1994) Comparison of PD 145065 and Ro 46-2005 as antagonists of contractions of guinea-pig airways induced by endothelin-1 or IRL 1620. *European Journal of Pharmacology* **252:**341–345.

87. Ohlstein EH, Nambi P, Douglas SA, Edwards RM, Gellai M, Lago A, Leber JD, Cousins RD, Gao A, Peishoff CE, Bean JW, Eggleston D, Elshourbagy N, Kumar C, Lee JA, Brooks DP, Ruffalo RR Jr, Feuerstein G, Weinstock J, Gleason JG & Elliott JD (1994) SB 209670, a rationally designed potent nonpeptide endothelin receptor antagonist. *Proceedings of the National Academy of Sciences USA* **91:**8052–8056.
88. Gellai M, Jugus M, Fletcher T, DeWolf R & Nambi P (1994) Reversal of post-ischemic acute renal failure with a selective endothelinA receptor antagonist in rat. *Journal of Clinical Investigation* **93:**900–906.
89. Douglas SA, Louden C, Vickery-Clark LM, Storer BL, Hart T, Feuerstein GZ, Elliott JD & Ohlstein EH (1994) A role for endogenous endothelin-1 in neointimal formation after rat carotid artery baloon angioplasty. *Circulation Research* **75:**190–197.
90. Clozel M, Breu V, Burri K, Cassal JM, Fischli W, Gray GA, Hirth G, Loffler BM, Muller M, Neidhart W & Ramuz H (1993) Pathophysiological role of endothelin revealed by the first orally active endothelin receptor antagonist. *Nature* **365:**759–761.
91. Breu V, Loffler BM & Clozel M (1993) *In vitro* characterization of Ro 46-2005, a novel synthetic non-peptide endothelin antagonist of ET_A and ET_B receptors. *FEBS Letters* **334:**210–214.
92. Clozel M, Breu V, Gray GA & Loffler BM (1993) *In vivo* pharmacology of Ro 46-2005, the first synthetic nonpeptide endothelin receptor antagonist: implications for endothelin physiology. *Journal of Cardiovascular Pharmacology* **22 (Suppl. 8):**S377–S379.
93. Eddahibi S, Raffestin B, Clozel M, Levame M & Adnot S (1995) Protection from pulmonary hypertension with an orally active endothelin receptor antagonist in hypoxic rats. *American Journal of Physiology* **268:**H828–H835.

Part II

The Pulmonary Endothelium – Smooth Muscle Interface: Hypoxia and Vasomotor Tone

5

Modulation of Pulmonary Vascular Tone in ARDS: The Role of the Endothelium

Nicholas P. Curzen
Timothy W. Evans

INTRODUCTION

Lung injury, acute (or adult) respiratory distress syndrome (ARDS) and 'sepsis syndromes'

Lung injury can occur in association with a variety of pulmonary and extra-pulmonary pathologies, and can be the response to an acute or chronic insult (Figure 1). Acute lung injury produces a spectrum of clinical severity, even though the pulmonary pathophysiological response is stereotyped. At the extreme end of this spectrum is ARDS, first described in adults in 1967 as the association of respiratory failure with non-cardiogenic pulmonary oedema.[1,2] Lung injury is common: 35% of a population with sepsis had mild to moderate lung injury, whilst 25% had severe lung injury or fully developed ARDS,[3] with a mortality of between 50 and 75%. Lung injury rarely occurs in isolation, and ARDS is now considered to be a multisystem vascular disorder[4,5] characterized not only by impaired pulmonary gas exchange, but also by a failure of oxygen uptake in the periphery, leading ultimately to multiple organ failure (MOF)[6] (Table 1). In one study respiratory failure accounted for only 16% of deaths, with the majority being attributable to MOF.[7] This is therefore consistent with the hypothesis that lung injury represents only the pulmonary manifestation of a diverse systemic insult which also produces other overlapping clinical syndromes (Figure 2, Table 2). In fact, it appears that the associated clinical conditions or risk factors and co-existing organ failures are the major determinants of survival.[5,8] Of importance is the finding that sepsis occurs up to six times more commonly in patients with ARDS compared with other critically ill patients.[7,9] As established sepsis and the systemic inflammatory response syndrome (SIRS)

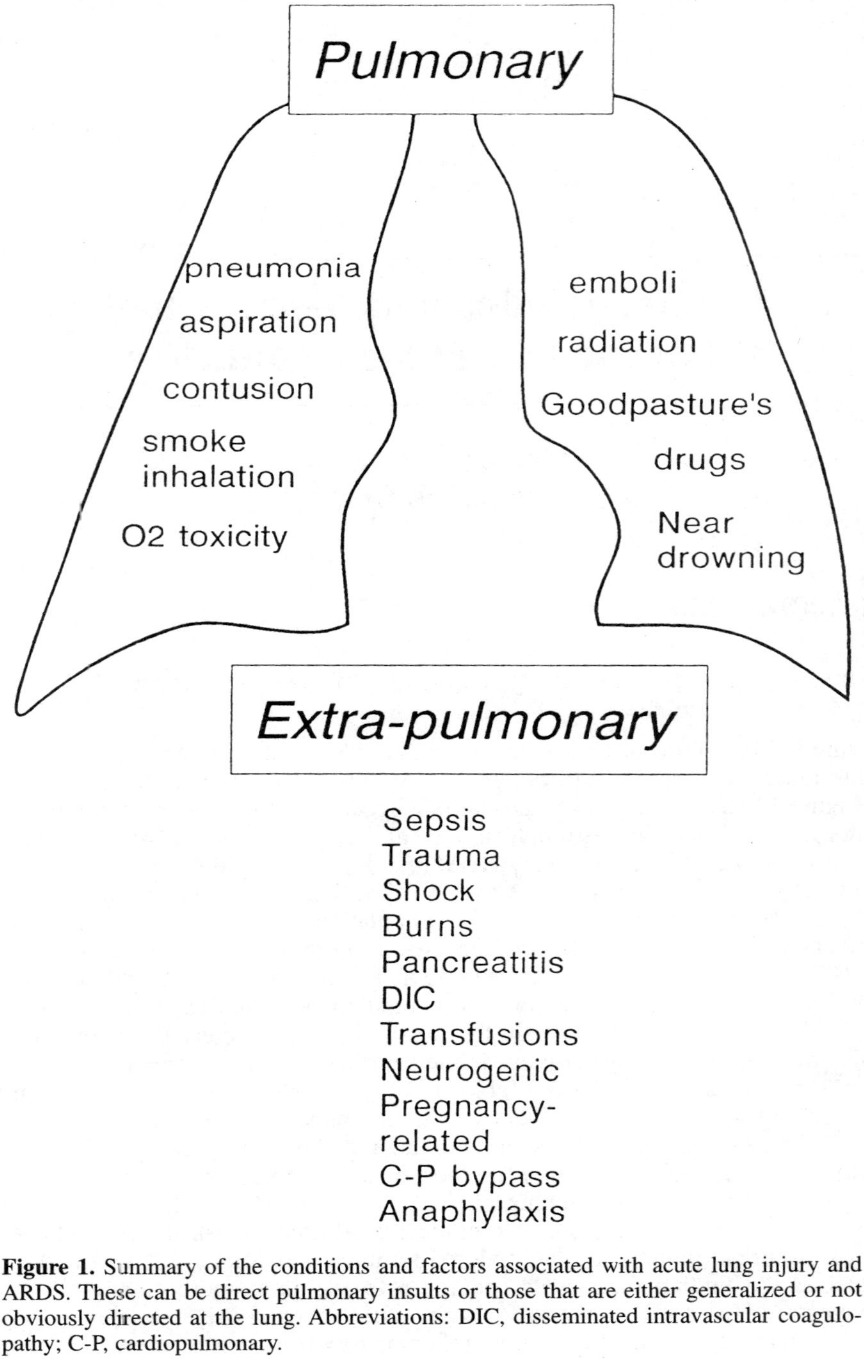

Figure 1. Summary of the conditions and factors associated with acute lung injury and ARDS. These can be direct pulmonary insults or those that are either generalized or not obviously directed at the lung. Abbreviations: DIC, disseminated intravascular coagulopathy; C-P, cardiopulmonary.

Table 1. Cardiovascular physiology of sepsis.

Site	Pathophysiology	Clinical result
Resistance & capacitance vessels	Reduced tone & hypo-responsiveness to vasoconstrictors	Hypotension with low systemic vascular resistance (SVR)
Heart	Reduced contractility	Relatively low cardiac output & O_2 delivery (although masked in early stages by low SVR & hyper-dynamic circulation)
Microvasculature	Increased capillary permeability	Non-hydrostatic oedema
	Shunting	Inefficient O_2 delivery & uptake relationship
	Coagulation abnormality: microembolism thrombosis	Microinfarction/disseminated intravascular coagulation

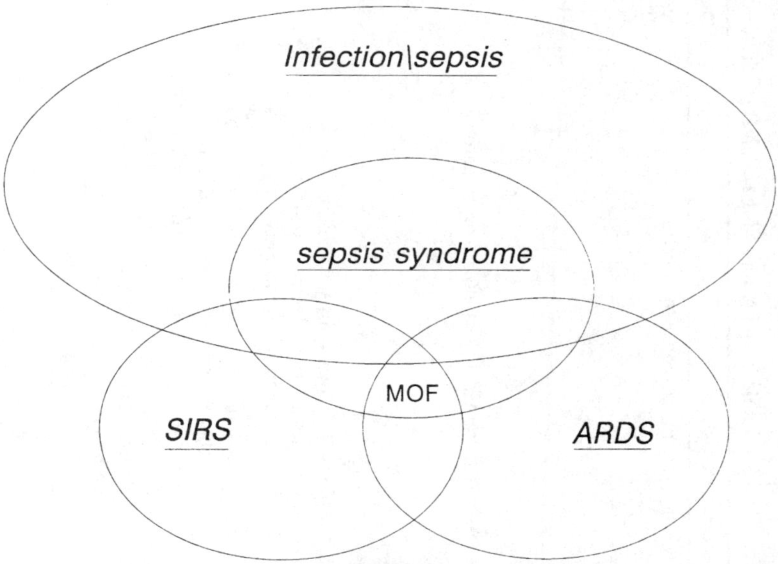

Figure 2. Diagrammatic representation of the inter-relationship between the clinical syndromes associated with the label 'sepsis'. All the clinical syndromes can be associated with an organism-positive infection, but, conversely, at least as frequently they can occur in culture-negative circumstances. Endotoxaemia is probably the commonest initiating factor in most cases, regardless of the presence of identifiable infection. The diagram also illustrates the potential relationship between lung injury and the other syndromes, with which it can overlap. Common to all the syndromes is the widespread inflammatory response that appears to focus around the endothelium.

Table 2. Definitions of the clinical syndromes associated with sepsis.

Syndrome	Definition	Comments
Sepsis	'The systemic response to infection.'	Includes two or more of the following: Temperature >38 °C or <36 °C Heart rate >90 beats/min Respiratory rate >20/min or $Pa\text{CO}_2$ <4.3 kPa White cell count >12 000/mm^3, <4000/mm^3, or >10% band (immature) forms
Sepsis syndrome	'Sepsis with evidence of altered organ perfusion.'	Altered organ perfusion includes one or more of the following: $Pa\text{O}_2/F_i\text{O}_2$ ≤280 (without other cardiopulmonary disease) Elevated lactate level (> upper limit of normal for the lab.) Oliguria <0.5 ml/kg body weight
Systemic inflammatory response syndrome	'Response to a variety of severe clinical insults (not necessarily infective), which is indistinguishable from sepsis.'	
Septic shock	'Sepsis with hypotension (sustained decrease in systolic blood pressure <90 mmHg, or drop >40 mmHg, for at least 1 h) despite adequate fluid resuscitation, in the presence of perfusion abnormalities that may include, but are not limited to lactic acidosis, oliguria or an acute alteration in mental status.'	Patients who are on inotropic or vasopressor agents may not be hypotensive at the time that perfusion abnormalities are measured

represent the biggest cause of mortality in the critically ill,[10] it is not surprising that up to 25% of such cases are complicated by ARDS. The clinical syndromes associated with sepsis represent a potentially devastating systemic inflammatory response estimated to occur in around 1% of hospitalized patients of whom 10–20% die. The mortality in those patients with septic shock is between 60 and 90%. It is important to emphasize that these clinical syndromes are associated with the positive identification of an infecting causative organism in less than 50% of cases. To avoid the requirement for an identifiable infection, as well as confusion over the term 'sepsis', the label SIRS is now used to define the resulting clinical state. Sepsis-induced *endothelium-mediated* circulatory failure is also increasingly recognized in the pathophysiology of MOF, which has an especially poor prognosis.

We can therefore present a scenario in which lung injury and ARDS are clinically recognizable sequelae of a complex inflammatory reaction to variable insults, most of which cause widespread endothelial activation and

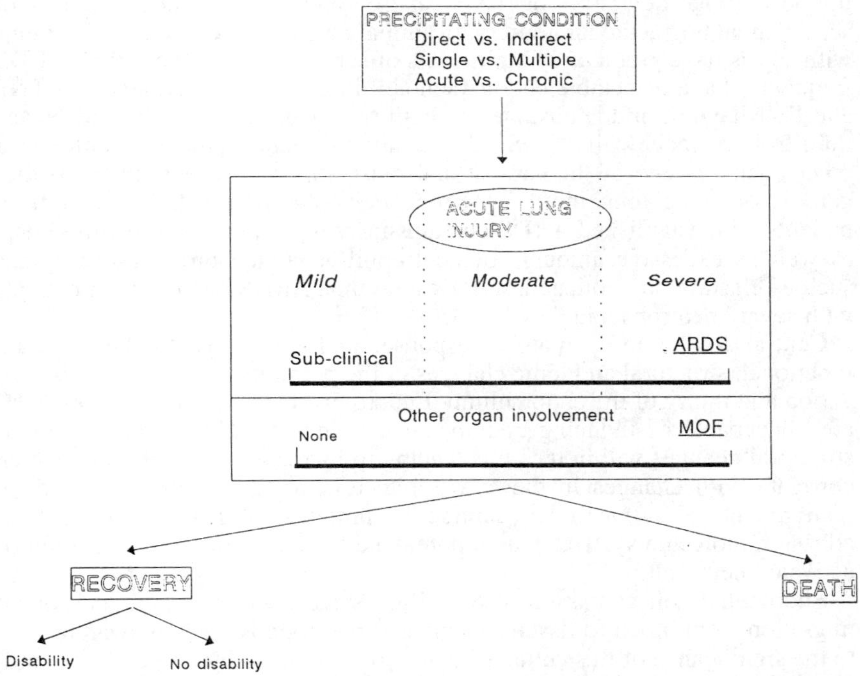

Figure 3. Lung injury can occur in response to a wide variety of insults. The response of an individual is unpredictable and the subsequent injury may present with characteristic clinical sequelae, the most severe form of which is full-blown ARDS, or it may be subclinical. Other organs may also be affected to a variable extent, in which case the most severe clinical end of this spectrum would be MOF. Currently the ability to predict those patients who are at high risk of developing significant lung injury (and other organ damage), as well as those with established ARDS who will survive, is seen as a research priority.

dysfunction, so that very frequently other organs are involved in the clinical pathology (Figure 3). The importance of this hypothesis is that the endothelium represents the fulcrum over which this inflammatory response balances between clinical and subclinical importance.

PATHOGENESIS OF LUNG INJURY

Pulmonary injury is the end result of an acute inflammatory response to a variety of local or systemic insults. In the critically ill patient, sepsis is probably the commonest and most devastating of these,[11] and is most frequently initiated by endotoxin, a lipopolysaccharide component of the cell wall of Gram-negative bacteria, and the consequent generation and release of a cascade of inflammatory mediators such as tumour necrosis factor (TNF), interleukins (IL)-1, -8, and -6 and platelet-activating factor (PAF) from neutrophils, macrophages, platelets, and endothelium[12] (Figure 4). Infusion of lipopolysaccharide (LPS) or TNF can reproduce the clinical features of sepsis, including acute lung injury, in animal models.[13–15] Critically ill patients with sepsis have predictably high levels of serum LPS and those with ARDS frequently have detectable endotoxaemia.[16] In addition, raised levels of TNF and IL-1 have been demonstrated in both serum and bronchoalveolar lavage fluid from patients with ARDS.[17,18] Activation of neutrophils by endotoxin or other agents is one of the earliest and most important events in the pathogenesis of acute lung injury.[19,20] Bronchoalveolar lavage fluid taken from patients with established ARDS contains increased numbers of neutrophils,[21] as well as excessive amounts of neutrophil-generated proteinase enzymes such as elastase and collagenase.[22] Despite this, ARDS can occur in patients with severe neutropaenia.[23]

Central to the inflammatory response, and especially to the resultant functional, structural and tonic changes of the pulmonary vasculature, is activation and injury of the endothelium. Endotoxin, TNF and other cytokines[24,25] are all capable of inducing endothelial cell injury.[26] This stimulates ultrastructural changes within the cells leading to increased permeability,[27] which correlate with changes in the cytoarchitecture of these cells produced by realignment of intracellular contractile proteins, and the activation of adhesion molecule systems which potentiate the adherence and migration of activated neutrophils.[28,29]

Endothelial cell activation also facilitates the adherence and subsequent migration from blood to tissue of activated neutrophils, and an awareness as to the significance of this cellular interaction, mediated by a steadily expanding group of 'adhesion molecules', is rapidly increasing. This adhesion molecule 'cascade' provides the machinery for the neutrophil–endothelial cell interaction that results in neutrophil migration, and as such represents an attractive set of targets for guided immunotherapy. The majority of this migration occurs in post-capillary venules. Initially there is slowing of the white cells with margination, when they can be seen under light microscopy rolling along the vessel wall as a result of loose tethering to the underlying endothelial cells. Subsequently, the neutrophils become more adherent and

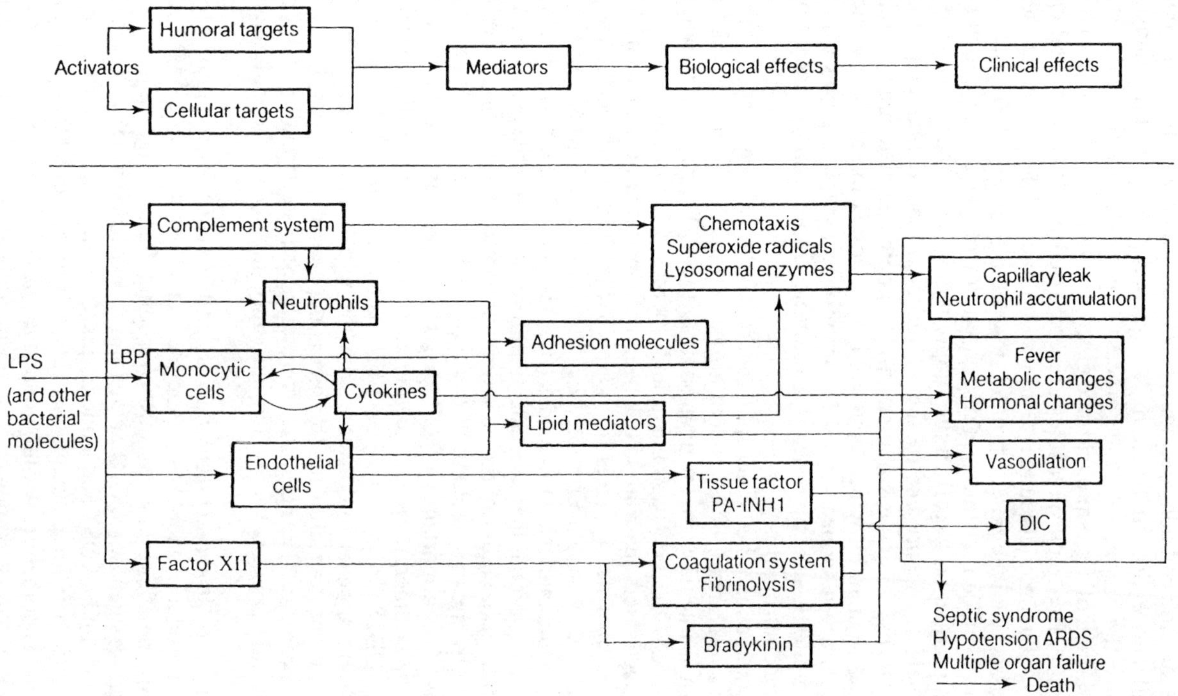

Figure 4. Interaction pathway for mediators involved in the inflammatory response to sepsis. The full complexity of this system is still being unearthed (especially in the field of the adhesion molecules), but the diagram illustrates the central role of the vascular endothelium in this response. Abbreviation: LBP, lipopolysaccharide-binding protein. Reproduced, with permission, from Glauser et al (1991) *Lancet* **338**:732–733.

they change from spherical to a flatter shape. This facilitates their slow migration between endothelial cells and then through the basement membrane into the interstitium. This process is now known to be mediated by interaction of specific cell adhesion molecules (CAM) on the surface of both the neutrophil and endothelial cell in a sequence known as the adhesion cascade.[30] Thus, the first phase of the process (slowing and rolling) depends upon the expression of a group of surface glycoprotein molecules collectively called selectins.[31] Two such molecules are expressed on the endothelial cell for this process: endothelial leukocyte adhesion molecule-1 (E-selectin), and granulocyte-associated membrane protein (P-selectin). Endothelial E-selectin expression has been demonstrated in response to cytokines and LPS, and the kinetics of its production in cell culture imply that it is dependent on protein synthesis. P-selectin is present in the granules of endothelial cells (and platelets), and its expression is stimulated by thrombin and histamine, thereby providing a mechanism by which neutrophil adhesion is initiated very early in the inflammatory response – even before protein synthetic pathways are active. Meanwhile, L-selectin is expressed on neutrophils and is shed from their cell surface during this phase.

The next stage in the neutrophil–endothelial cell interaction (firm adherence and migration) is dependent on the expression of another set of CAMs, known as integrins, on the neutrophil surface.[32] The most important of these are the CD11/CD18 complex, and increased expression of these molecules on activated neutrophils has been demonstrated in animal models both *in vivo* and *in vitro*. Ligands for these CAMs are present on the endothelial surface, and binding is promoted by cytokines including TNF, PAF and ILs. The intercellular adhesion molecules (ICAM-1 and -2) are also expressed constitutively by the endothelium, and therefore are available early on for neutrophil binding. In addition, the vascular cell adhesion molecule, VCAM-1, is expressed by the endothelium in response to the presence of endotoxin and cytokines. The importance of CD11/CD18 molecules in patients with sepsis is gradually emerging; and recently an increase in the resting expression of CD11/CD18 on granulocytes from patients with ARDS has been demonstrated and appears to correlate with the hyperadhesiveness of these cells.[33] The actual migration of neutrophils is dependent upon a chemotactic gradient, and probably also upon the expression of platelet endothelial cell adhesion molecule (PECAM-1) which is mainly situated at the endothelial cell junctions.[34]

The endothelium has other facets of its inflammatory activation. Most important of these are endotoxin-inducible genes other than CAMs, and these result in the expression of mRNA coding for a range of proteins, including cyclooxygenase (COX), constitutive and inducible nitric oxide synthase (cNOS and iNOS) and endothelins (*vide infra*). It is, to a great extent, the release of these potent vasoactive and inflammatory mediators that allows the endothelium to modulate the vascular response to sepsis. When the inflammatory response is widespread and severe, intense activation of the endothelium in some areas and destruction of it in others helps to precipitate the overwhelming and devastating clinical syndromes described above.

PATHOPHYSIOLOGY OF ACUTE LUNG INJURY

ARDS is principally a clinical diagnosis, the criteria for which differ between centres.[35] Pulmonary endothelial damage can lead to mild respiratory impairment or the overwhelming alveolar oedema that is characteristic of ARDS. A clinical scoring system is now commonly used to categorize patients according to their underlying condition and to quantify the degree of lung damage according to radiographic appearances, hypoxaemia, the requirement for positive end-expiratory pressure (PEEP), and thoracic compliance[36] (Table 3). Such scoring systems, which allow the severity of the injury to be reliably estimated, have greatly increased the utility of clinical studies. Thus, using such scoring techniques, a multicentre study was able to identify patients with milder forms of lung injury who went on to develop full-blown ARDS.[37]

Table 3. Diagnostic criteria for ARDS.

Essential	Non-essential
Antecedent history suggesting associated conditions	Normal pulmonary artery occlusion pressure (e.g. < 18 mmHg) and plasma oncotic pressure
Refractory hypoxaemia ($Pa\text{O}_2$ < 8.0 kPa on 40% $F\text{IO}_2$)	Low total respiratory system compliance
Radiological evidence of evolving bilateral pulmonary infiltrates compatible with pulmonary oedema	Evidence of raised permeability of the alveolar capillary membrane

Clinical studies have emphasized the universal finding of elevated pulmonary vascular resistance (PVR) in patient groups with respiratory failure.[38] In ARDS, PVR is increased, even after correction for arterial hypoxaemia, probably through a combination of increased vascular tone and structural factors such as extrinsic compression (i.e. oedema fluid, PEEP ventilation), thromboemboli or later remodelling of the vessel wall as part of the inflammatory response.[39,40] In ARDS, pulmonary hypertension contributes to pulmonary oedema formation,[5] and impaired right ventricular performance[41] and is associated with increased mortality.[42]

In some patients with ARDS and sepsis, an abnormal relationship between oxygen delivery (DO_2) and peripheral oxygen uptake (VO_2) has been identified.[43,44] Provided it is maintained above a critical level (cDO_2), VO_2 is normally independent of DO_2 at rest. In ARDS, however, VO_2 becomes DO_2-dependent above this threshold, so that the oxygen extraction ratio remains constant. Critically ill patients who manifest this pathological 'supply-dependency' have a higher mortality rate than those who do not.[45] This tendency, and the apparent inability of the peripheral tissues to extract oxygen, has not yet been clearly explained, but has led a number of investigators to advocate active manipulation of DO_2 to achieve predetermined target levels of VO_2. It has subsequently been shown[46,47] that critically ill patients in whom supraphysiological targets for cardiac output, DO_2 and VO_2 are attained have a lower incidence of MOF and mortality,[48] although this is an area surrounded by controversy, and is the focus of intensive research.

The microcirculation is disrupted both within the lung, thus reducing DO_2, and in the periphery, leading to suboptimal VO_2. Pathophysiological mechanisms that may account for impaired peripheral oxygen uptake in these patients include: loss of microvascular control with shunting, tissue oedema, compression of capillaries and microembolization. These changes can be largely explained by the degree of endothelial injury involved in these inflammatory conditions.

HYPOXIC PULMONARY VASOCONSTRICTION (HPV)

The phenomenon of HPV was first described in 1946[49] and is a physiological response through which blood flow is diverted away from hypoxic alveoli, with the *beneficial* result that perfusion (*Q*) and ventilation (*V*) remain 'matched'. If normal subjects breathe gas mixtures of low oxygen tension, increases in pulmonary artery pressure ensue.[50] There is conflicting evidence regarding the primary site of HPV. Although pulmonary venoconstriction has been demonstrated during hypoxia,[51,52] animal experiments using rapid-freezing histological assessment,[53,54] pulmonary angiography,[55] and direct micropuncture techniques[56] suggest that small pulmonary arteries are in fact the major site of action. Nor has the mechanism by which hypoxia elicits local vasoconstriction been fully elucidated. Autonomic innervation is not necessary for this pressor response, since HPV persists in isolated lung preparations[57,58] and in human transplanted lungs.[59] Furthermore, pharmacological intervention using adrenergic receptor blockade,[60] catecholamine depletion[61] and sympathectomy[62] does not modulate the response. This implies that HPV must be mediated via intrinsic mechanism(s). Most evidence (*vide infra*) suggests that this is an endothelium-dependent phenomenon, although interestingly cultured pulmonary artery vascular smooth muscle cells exhibit a contractile response to hypoxia that is independent of any other cell type.[63]

HPV in acute lung injury

HPV represents a beneficial homoeostatic control mechanism which is disrupted in acute lung injury.[64] This is of great clinical significance in ARDS, because the alveolar oedema and atelectasis that occur can induce enormous increases in physiological dead space. Investigations using the multiple inert gas technique[65] have demonstrated that the degree of intrapulmonary shunting is large enough to account for the observed alveolar/arterial $P\text{O}_2$ gradient, even without invoking a reduction in diffusion capacity.

The endothelium in HPV

The endothelium can modulate HPV in several ways. In some, but not all species, there is a requirement for an intact endothelium in order that hypoxia can elicit a contractile pulmonary response.[66] In the dog or rat, hypoxia-induced contractions of pulmonary arteries are reduced by endothelial removal.[67,68] Endothelial injury can enhance HPV,[69,70] and in the longer term, structural alterations in pulmonary endothelial cells may also contribute to the development of hypoxic pulmonary hypertension.[71] Theoretically, the endothelial modulation of HPV could occur via several mechanisms. The endothelium removes circulating vasoconstrictor substances,[72,73] which may become more significant in hypoxic conditions. More importantly, it releases a range of vasoactive agents locally, and a change in the dynamic balance of these factors under the influence of hypoxia could modulate the vascular tonic response.

ENDOTHELIAL MODULATION OF VASCULAR TONE

Nitric oxide

Background

It was in 1980 that the vascular relaxation induced by acetylcholine was shown to be dependent on the presence of intact endothelium and to be mediated via the release of a non-prostanoid labile vasodilator termed endothelium-derived relaxing factor (EDRF). Overwhelming evidence has since accumulated that the chemical and pharmacological properties of EDRF are shared by nitric oxide (NO). NO is synthesized *in vitro* from the semi-essential amino acid, L-arginine, by the membrane-bound enzyme NOS, a process that can be inhibited by L-arginine analogues such as N^G-monomethyl-L-arginine (L-NMMA).[74] Several distinct NOS genes have been identified, and two forms of NOS exist in the blood vessel wall: a constitutive calcium- and calmodulin-dependent enzyme, and an inducible calcium- and calmodulin-independent enzyme (Table 4). Both forms exist in the vascular endothelium.[75]

NO works by activating soluble guanylate cyclase after binding to its haem moiety, which in turn causes an increase in intracellular cyclic guanosine monophosphate (cGMP) resulting in vascular smooth muscle relaxation. This mechanism can be demonstrated experimentally. Thus, L-arginine administration has been shown to produce vasodilatation in lambs, and this effect can be blocked by the guanylate cyclase inhibitor methylene blue or by L-NMMA.[76,77] This vasodilatation can, however, be augmented by a cGMP phosphodiesterase inhibitor, whose ability to raise intracellular cGMP levels has also been shown to produce vasodilatation in other models. The measurement of cGMP levels in tissue can be used as an indicator of the degree of NOS activity, and this has become a useful tool in experimental studies of sepsis. In addition, the administration of NOS inhibitors has been shown to produce increases in mean arterial blood pressure and decreases in regional blood flow in both animals and man,[78] implying that there is a continuous basal release of NO contributing to vascular tone. The size of the

Table 4. Characteristics of the vascular isoforms of NOS.

NOS isoforms	Response in sepsis	Location	Regulation	Activation	Non-selective inhibitors	Selective inhibitors
Type II	Constitutive; immediate increase in NO activity	Endothelial cell, membrane-bound	–	Ca^{2+}-dependent	L-Arginine analogues (e.g. L-NMMA)	None known
Type III	Synthesis induced by LPS & cytokines; massive NO production after 2–6 h	Mainly smooth muscle, cytosolic	Induction prevented by corticosteroids & inhibitors of protein synthesis	Ca^{2+}-independent	L-Arginine analogues (e.g. L-NMMA)	Aminoguanidine, L-canavanine, diphenyleneiodonium

Type II: constitutive, endothelially sited; Type III: inducible, sited in smooth muscle and endothelium.

pressor response induced by intravenous L-NMMA in animal models seems to be dependent on basal vascular tone.

NO in sepsis

Suprabasal release of NO is known to occur in response to a diverse range of stimuli including endotoxin, cytokines, hypoxia, histamine, thrombin, bradykinin, calcium ionophore, endothelin and substance P (Figure 5). As a result, an increase in NO release during the inflammatory response to sepsis is inevitable. Patients and animals with septic shock lose peripheral vascular tone, and the responsiveness of systemic vessels to constrictor agents such as catecholamines is diminished, both *in vitro* and *in vivo*. The incubation of bovine aortic endothelial cells with LPS causes rapid release of an NO-like factor. Furthermore, the levels of NO metabolites are significantly elevated in patients with septic shock,[79] and the administration of NOS inhibitors in these patients,[80] or in animal models of sepsis,[81] can produce reproducible elevations in systemic vascular resistance where other vasoconstrictors are ineffective. In fact, huge quantities of NO are produced in sepsis. Endotoxin leads to the induction of the calcium-independent NOS (iNOS) in both the

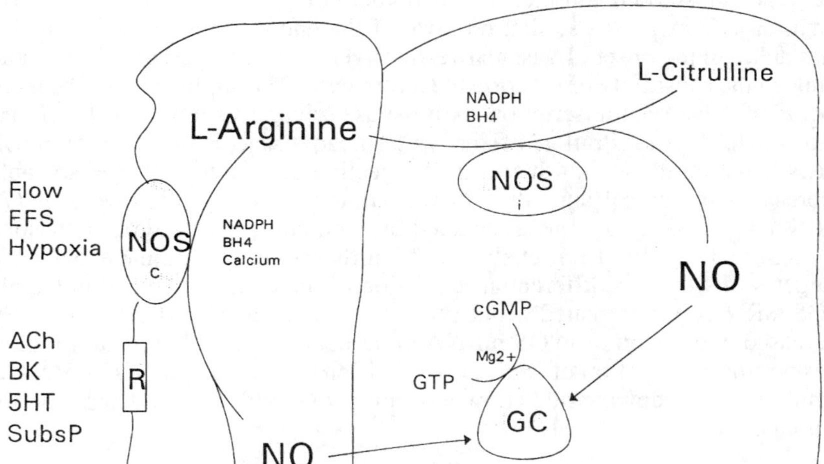

Figure 5. Illustration of the mechanics of production of NO in the vascular smooth muscle cell in endotoxaemia. For simplicity the endothelial cell is shown as only possessing the constitutive form of the enzyme NOS, but in fact it is also capable of producing NO via the inducible form of the enzyme. Abbreviations: ACh, acetylcholine; BK, bradykinin; 5HT, 5-hydroxytryptamine; SubsP, substance P; EFS, electrical field stimulation; BH4, tetrahydrobiopterin; GC, guanylate cyclase; R, receptor.

endothelium and the vascular smooth muscle,[82,83] as well as in the myocardium where the increase in NO production has been shown to reduce contractility.[84] Other cytokines (TNF, IL-1 and -2) also stimulate iNOS activity in vessel walls.

The time course of the increase in NO release in sepsis is the subject of considerable speculation. In isolated endotoxin-treated rat main pulmonary arteries, NOS inhibitors reverse the vascular hyporesponsiveness to phenylephrine,[85] and there is no doubt that in established sepsis NO is largely responsible for this reduced reactivity. The NO-mediated hyporeactivity to noradrenaline starts within 60 min in a rat model of sepsis *in vivo*,[86] and may therefore be too rapid to be explained by the induction of iNOS. It therefore seems likely that this early increase in NO release is explained by an elevation in NO production by endothelial cNOS, but this remains controversial, and in fact in one study, although the administration of L-NAME after 1 h in endotoxin-treated pithed rats did elevate blood pressure and increase vascular responsiveness to catecholamines, this was to no greater degree than in saline-treated animals.[87] This suggests that the early hyporesponsiveness is caused not by NO, but by some other factor(s). What is clear, however, is that from about 3 h after the endotoxic insult, there is massive NO production as a result of iNOS activity in the endothelium, and to an even greater extent in the vascular smooth muscle. The endothelium appears to be required for maximal NO response, so that removal of the endothelium caused a significant delay in the onset of vascular responsiveness (6 compared with 4 h) and reduced the sensitivity of rat aorta to LPS *in vitro*. The application of the technique of reverse transcription polymerase chain reaction (rt-PCR) has allowed the demonstration of the widespread tissue expression of iNOS mRNA in a rat model at 4 h after LPS injection compared with undetectable expression in control animals.[88] In rat pulmonary artery this rise in iNOS mRNA expression could be attenuated by pretreatment with dexamethasone 30 min before the LPS challenge.[89] Furthermore, preliminary evidence suggests that there is differential regulation of the constitutive and inducible NOS mRNAs in rats treated with LPS *in vivo*, such that, whilst there is greatly increased expression of iNOS mRNA in rat heart, lung and aorta at 4 h after intraperitoneal injection of LPS, the expression of endothelial NOS mRNA is simultaneously downregulated when compared with levels from control animals.[90]

NOS inhibitors as therapeutic agents in sepsis

As has already been mentioned, the intravenous administration of L-NMMA was shown to (temporarily) correct systemic hypotension in two patients with septic shock. Another L-arginine analogue that non-specifically blocks NOS, N-nitro-L-arginine (L-NNA) has also been given to critically ill patients with sepsis.[91] This agent did, however, cause a significant increase in both systemic and pulmonary vascular resistance as well as in mean arterial pressure, but with an accompanying reduction in cardiac index. Further research is underway. The main theoretical objection to these non-specific inhibitors of NOS is that NO is known to contribute to basal vascular tone, and in some organ beds (notably renal, mesenteric and pulmonary) there is frequently an overall reduction in regional blood flow in sepsis which could be amplified by NOS inhibition.

A gradual improvement in the understanding of the role of iNOS in sepsis has fuelled investigation into the possibility of the selective blockade of this enzyme in sepsis.[92] The theoretical attractions of this as a therapeutic tool are obvious. In comparative studies between L-NMMA and aminoguanidine, the latter was found to be at least seven times more potent at inhibiting iNOS. L-NMMA was 15 times more potent at inhibiting the constitutive enzyme than aminoguanidine, however. Aminoguanidine produced a dose-dependent increase in phenylephrine-induced tension in intact and endothelium-denuded pulmonary artery rings from endotoxin-treated rats, but it had no effect on sham-treated controls.[93] The aminoguanidine-precipitated contraction in the endothelium-denuded vessels was abolished by L-arginine or L-NMMA pretreatment, thus suggesting that its mechanism of action involves the L-arginine/NO axis. Clinical trials on the use of aminoguanidine in septic patients are already underway.

NO in HPV

A reduction in NO production or a decrease in its target receptor sensitivity could theoretically result in vasoconstriction during hypoxia. Certainly, endothelium-dependent relaxation is impaired by hypoxia in rabbit and rat pulmonary artery rings.[94,95] However, there is no consistency between such *in vitro* results and those obtained in human tissue or in isolated lung experiments. In fact, the contraction induced by hypoxia in isolated human lobar arteries is potentiated by endothelial removal.[96] In isolated perfused lung preparations, inhibition of NO release under hypoxic conditions with eicosatetraynoic acid, nordihydroguaiaretic acid, hydroquinone,[97] methylene blue[98] or L-NMMA[99,100] all potentiate the pressor response, suggesting that NO release may actually increase during HPV. It is therefore tempting to speculate that alterations in this shift of NO production in the most hypoxic areas of lung could disrupt appropriate blood diversion.

In sepsis, the induction of iNOS would be expected to reduce the degree of local HPV. However, recent evidence on pulmonary artery and aortic rings *in vitro* from LPS-treated rats suggests that not only does hypoxia inhibit cNOS, thus producing rapid vasoconstriction, but it also inhibits LPS-induced iNOS.[101]

Endothelins

Background

In 1988 an endothelially derived vasoconstrictor was cloned and sequenced following its isolation from the culture medium of porcine aortic endothelial cells.[102] This substance, termed endothelin (ET), was found to elicit a slow sustained contraction of isolated arteries from many different species. Three similar but distinct ET-related genomic loci have been identified that encode for three similar but distinct 21-amino acid ET peptides (ET-1, ET-2, ET-3).[103] These peptides are produced following cleavage of a prepropeptide via a propeptide. This conversion is mediated by the activity of an endothelin-converting enzyme (ECE). Several types of enzyme with this property have already been demonstrated; two are neutral proteases, one of which is membrane-bound and phosphoramidon-sensitive, and one of which is soluble and insensitive to phosphoramidon.

ET-1 immunoreactivity cannot be demonstrated in homogenates of capillary endothelial cells, and release of ET from cultured endothelial cells can be prevented by the protein synthesis inhibitor cycloheximide, suggesting that ETs are not stored but synthesized *de novo*. Factors that have been found to be capable of stimulating ET release are diverse and include vessel wall shear stress, hypoxia, endotoxin, TNF, interferon, adrenaline, angiotensin, thrombin, activated platelets and some prostanoids. Local ET release would therefore be expected in response to any form of inflammatory response. ET-induced smooth muscle contraction occurs as the result of the action of several second messenger pathways whose final common pathway is to increase free intracellular calcium. Phospholipase C activation with increases in inositol triphosphate and diaglycerol synthesis is thought to be the principal effector system, although since staurosporine, a protein kinase C inhibitor, can attenuate ET-1-induced contraction *in vitro*, this system is presumably also involved[104] (Figure 6).

Two ET receptor subtypes have so far been cloned and expressed. ET_A has a higher affinity for ET-1 than ET-2 or -3, and has widespread expression including on vascular smooth muscle, but has not been found on endothelial cells. ET_B is non-selective and binds all three ETs equally avidly so that they are equipotent in their displacement of [^{125}I]-ET-1. ET_B is found on vascular endothelium and also on smooth muscle in some vascular beds. At first it was thought that ET_A receptor stimulation was responsible for the direct constrictor effects of ET and that ET_B receptor stimulation resulted in properties such as the release of other vasoactive factors from those cells. ET-1 is certainly a potent vasoconstrictor in humans and animals by direct stimulation of ET_A receptors, and the endothelium can modulate this vascular response to ET via ET_B receptor stimulation, but recently it has become apparent that the situation is complicated by the demonstration of ET_B receptors on some vascular smooth muscle that mediate contraction, and ET_A receptors capable of stimulating prostanoid release.[105–107] The importance of endothelial ET_B receptors has been demonstrated in several models. There is now also clear evidence from both *in vitro* and *in vivo* studies that ETs release NO from the endothelium by ET_B receptor stimulation. This gives rise to the characteristic haemodynamic responses of rats (and other species) to intravenous ET-1, when there is an initial transient fall in systemic blood pressure followed by a sustained pressor response.[102] Only the former can be attenuated by L-NMMA pretreatment,[108] and only the latter can be attenuated by ET_A receptor antagonists such as BQ-123.[109] There is also evidence that at least in some species, and in some vascular beds, ET-1 also stimulates the release of prostacyclin and thromboxane from endothelial cells via ET_B receptors (Figure 6).

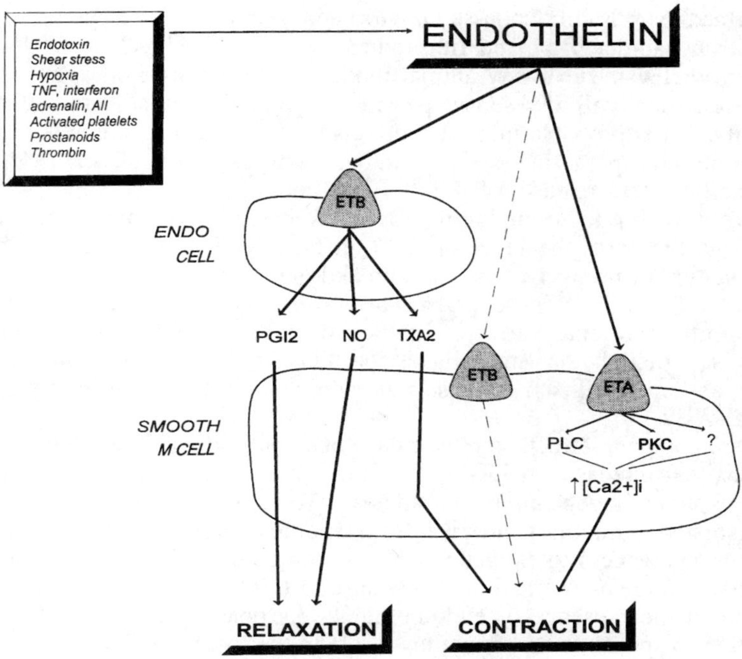

Figure 6. Many of the factors stimulating the release of ET-1 from the vascular endothelium are present as integral components of the early inflammatory response to sepsis, including endotoxin, TNF, adrenaline, prostanoids, and activated platelets and thrombin. It is not surprising therefore to find elevated mRNA expression for ET-1 in vascular tissue and organs such as the heart and lung, nor to be able to measure large rises in the plasma concentration of ET-1 in animals and patients with endotoxaemia or related clinical conditions. ET-1 can act on at least two receptor subtypes (*vide supra*), but the distribution of receptors on the vascular smooth muscle cell membrane, in particular, appears to be highly tissue- and species-specific, and probably also changes according to local inflammatory conditions. Several second-messenger systems have been identified, including phospholipase C (PLC) and protein kinase C (PKC), with alterations in intracellular free calcium ([Ca2+]i) being the final common pathway. Abbreviations: endo cell, endothelial cell; smooth M cell, smooth muscle cell, AII, angiotensin II.

ET-1 is largely removed by the pulmonary vasculature, whilst some is eliminated by the kidneys. The plasma half-life of a bolus of [^{125}I]ET-1 in anaesthetized rats was 40 s in one study, with 82% uptake in the lungs and 10% in the kidneys.[110]

Endothelins in sepsis

Taking into account the factors known to stimulate ET release (*vide supra*), it is inevitable this release is going to increase during the inflammatory response associated with sepsis. ET release in response to endotoxin has been confirmed by radioimmunoassay *in vitro* and *in vivo*, and in response to TNF, interferon gamma, IL-1 and free radical species. The level of ET-1 in the plasma is elevated in many animal models of sepsis, as well as in patients who are critically ill with sepsis, possibly in parallel with indicators of illness severity.[111] It is probable that ET-1 effects on vascular tone are as a result of autocrine and paracrine activity rather than as a circulating hormone, especially since release of ET-1 from endothelial cells appears to be polarized, with release predominantly in the basal (non-luminal) direction.[112] If this is the case, the level of ET-1 in the blood would only reflect the combination of production rate and breakdown/elimination rate. The expression of ET-1 mRNA in several tissues from endotoxin-treated rats (heart, lung, aorta, pulmonary artery) significantly increases when compared with controls, although the time course for this increase varies from tissue to tissue, and no significant increase was seen in skeletal muscle from the same animals.[113,114]

Despite potent effects on vascular tone, both direct and indirect, and unequivocal increases in ET-1 production and release in sepsis, the role of these peptides in sepsis remains unclear. We have previously demonstrated that isolated pulmonary arteries from endotoxaemic rats do demonstrate hyporesponsiveness to exogenous ET-1 when compared with sham animals, and that complete contraction in response to ET-1 in these vessels is dependent upon the presence of endothelium.[115] As potent vasoconstrictors, it is tempting to speculate that they play a role in the local reductions in regional blood flow seen in certain organ beds such as the gut, kidney and lung. This is an area of intense investigation, particularly now that the necessary experimental (and potentially therapeutic) tools are becoming available in the form of selective ET_A/ET_B or combined ET receptor antagonists.

Endothelins in HPV

Normobaric hypoxia stimulates ET-1 gene expression in the rat.[116,117] ET release has also been confirmed in response to hypoxia in cultured bovine endothelial cells[118] and in rat resistance vessels perfused *in vitro*.[119] In addition, the vasoconstrictor response to ET-1 was twice as great in perfused mesentery of pithed rats *in situ* when oxygen levels were reduced by lowering ventilation.[120] ET-1 and ET-3 have both vasoconstrictor and vasodilator properties in the rat lung,[121,122] and can reverse the HPV response in isolated lungs, an effect unchanged by indomethacin or glibenclamide but attenuated by L-NMMA. On the other hand, the hypoxia-induced contraction of isolated canine systemic and pulmonary artery rings *in vitro* was not affected by pretreatment with the ET_A receptor antagonist, BQ-123, even though this agent at the same dose significantly antagonizes exogenous ET-1-induced contractions.[123] This implies that ET-1 is not involved in the HPV response.

As yet there is no clear evidence that ETs are responsible for mediating HPV, especially as the response time course is different for anoxia- and ET-induced contractions.[124] However, hypoxia not only stimulates ET production and release, but also alters the functional response to the peptides so that *in vitro* dose–response curves to ETs-1 and -3 are altered, with an increased maximum pressor response.[125] Importantly, there is also evidence that hypoxia/ischaemia increases the maximum binding capacity for [^{125}I]ET-1 in rat cardiac membranes, probably through externalization of binding sites.[126–128] This evidence implies that the functional role of ETs may be altered in hypoxia, which may be important in the light of their ability to modulate the release and activity of other endothelium-derived vasoactive agents. Thus, ETs are able to stimulate the release of NO from endothelial cells,[129–132] an effect probably mediated via the ET_B receptor.[133–136] ETs also stimulate release of eicosanoids, both vasoconstrictors[137] and vasodilators.[138,139] Interestingly, all these endothelium-derived mediators can also modulate ET production[140,141] and contraction.[142,143]

The precise role of ETs during HPV, and more importantly, in the disrupted responses seen during lung injury, has not yet been elucidated. However, evidence strongly suggests that they have considerable potential to alter the endothelium-mediated pulmonary vascular response to hypoxia in septic conditions. ET-1 expression is elevated, as demonstrated by both immunocytochemical analysis and *in situ* hybridization, in the lungs of patients with pulmonary hypertension,[144] and their other mitogenic and chemotactic properties also put the ETs under suspicion as mediators contributing to the longer-term structural responses to chronic insults in the lung.

Arachidonic acid metabolites

Background

The endothelium produces prostanoids and thromboxane after the conversion of arachidonic acid by the enzyme COX. This enzyme exists in two isoforms; COX-1 is constitutive and is responsible for physiological production, and COX-2 is cytokine-inducible in inflammatory conditions. Endothelial production of the vasodilator and platelet inhibitor, prostacyclin (PGI_2), is important both as an antithrombotic agent and for regulation of basal vascular tone. Activation of membrane phospholipase A_2 results in the generation via the COX pathway of prostaglandins and thromboxane A_2 (TXA_2), and leukotrienes via the lipoxygenase pathway.[145] Clinical studies of patients with ARDS have demonstrated increased serum levels of TXA_2,[146] and leukotrienes in bronchoalveolar lavage fluid.[147] The pulmonary production of COX products is suggested by the finding in endotoxaemic sheep that lung lymph concentrations exceed plasma levels.[148]

Prostacyclin (PGI_2) is a potent vasodilator and inhibitor of platelet aggregation,[149,150] and infusion of this agent in critically ill patients has been shown to improve *V/Q* matching and hence oxygen delivery, although convincing reductions in mortality have yet to be achieved. TXA_2 is a vasoconstrictor, and its inhibition, using specific blockade of its synthesis, has been shown to diminish early pulmonary hypertension significantly, but not the increased vascular permeability, in an experimental model of endotoxin-induced sepsis.[151] Leukotrienes can induce pulmonary vasoconstriction, as well as bronchoconstriction and increased vascular permeability.[152]

COX products in sepsis

Cytokines stimulate prostanoid release both *in vivo* and *in vitro*. During the inflammatory response, this generation of prostanoids and thromboxane (TXA_2) occurs in inflammatory cells such as macrophages as well as in the endothelium. The balance between the local production of vasodilator (PGI_2) and vasoconstrictor (TXA_2 and endoperoxides) agents in this way undoubtedly contributes to the vascular tone in that area.[153] In particular, in the lung, animal studies suggest that TXA_2 production is one of the main factors producing the early elevation in PVR (and probably also increased vascular permeability) following endotoxin challenge. Interestingly, evidence from isolated pulmonary artery rings from endotoxaemic rats suggests that a portion of the ET-1-elicited contraction is dependent on the release of an endothelium-derived COX product.[115] As a result of these findings, several studies have successfully attenuated these changes in pulmonary haemodynamics using COX inhibitors or thromboxane receptor antagonists with a corresponding improvement in survival.[154,155] TXA_2-mediated increases in PVR are also thought to occur in man during sepsis, and trials of COX inhibitors in these patients are currently underway in the USA.

Eicosanoids in HPV

Inhibitors of prostaglandin (PG) synthesis such as indomethacin and meclofenamate can augment HPV,[156,157] implying that the response is modulated by vasodilator PGs. However, one study in human pulmonary artery rings demonstrated inhibition of the hypoxia-induced contraction when another COX inhibitor, flurbiprofen, was used.[158] The relative importance of vasodilator prostaglandins in the vasomotor response to hypoxia appears to vary, not only between species, but also between the type of pulmonary artery studied. Thus, in pig pulmonary artery rings *in vitro*, the reaction of distal and proximal vessels to hypoxia was different as was the response of each to indomethacin.[159] Arachidonic acid infusion into canine pulmonary arteries leads to a decrease in hypoxia-induced elevations in pulmonary vascular resistance,[160] which is accompanied by an increase in the prostacyclin metabolite 6-keto-$PGF_{1\alpha}$.

Thromboxane[161] and leukotriene (LT) B_4 [162] are both potent vasoconstrictors. LTC_4 is released in the rat lung during hypoxia,[163] and induces pulmonary hypertension in the same species.[164] In healthy volunteers after exposure to altitude, TXB_2 and LTB_4 levels were maximally elevated at the same time as the clinical features of acute mountain sickness.[165] Both inhibitors of LT synthesis and an LT receptor antagonist can reduce HPV in the rat.[166] Despite evidence that eicosanoids have a role in HPV, it is unclear whether alterations in eicosanoid production in acute lung injury can disrupt it.

SUMMARY AND CONCLUSIONS

Acute lung injury occurs in association with a variety of pulmonary and extrapulmonary pathologies. Damage to the pulmonary vascular endothelium is a fundamental step in the initiation of the inflammatory process that produces tissue injury. Endothelial activation and injury leads to release of a group of potent vasoactive agents, including NO, ETs and eicosanoids, and the balance of these determine both the local pulmonary vascular tone and the extent of the inflammatory reaction. Research is currently concerned with identifying therapeutic ways of altering the balance of these mediators in a favourable way, to damp the inflammatory response and restore the usually beneficial effects of HPV, which is disrupted in lung injury.

ACKNOWLEDGEMENTS

N.P.C. is an MRC Training Fellow.

REFERENCES

1. Asbaugh DG, Bigelow DB, Petty TL & Levine BE (1967) Acute respiratory distress in adults. *Lancet* **ii:**319–323.
2. Petty TL & Ashbaugh AG (1971) The adult respiratory distress syndrome: clinical features, factors influencing prognosis and principles of management. *Chest* **60:**233–239.
3. Weinberg PF, Matthay MA & Webster RO (1984) Biologically active products of complement and acute lung injury in patients with the sepsis syndrome. *American Review of Respiratory Distress* **130:**791–796.
4. Mizer L, Weisbrode S & Dorinsky PM (1989) Neutrophil accumulation and structural changes in non-pulmonary organs following phorbol myristate acetate-induced acute lung injury. *American Review of Respiratory Disease* **139:**1017–1026.
5. Bone RC, Balk R & Slotman G (1992) Adult respiratory distress syndrome sequence and importance of multiple organ failure. *Chest* **101:**320–326.
6. Griffiths MJD & Evans TW (1996) Adult respiratory distress syndrome. In Brewis RAL, Gibson GJ & Geddes DM (eds) *Respiratory Medicine* (2nd edn), pp 605–629. London: Balliere Tindall.
7. Montgomery AB, Stager MA, Carrico CJ & Hudson LD (1985) Causes of mortality in patients with the adult respiratory distress syndrome. *American Review of Respiratory Disease* **132:**485–489.
8. Fowler AA, Hamman RF, Zerbe GO et al (1985) Adult respiratory distress syndrome: prognosis after onset. *American Review of Respiratory Disease* **132:**472–478.
9. Seidenfeld JJ, Pohl DF, Bell RC et al (1986) Incidence, site and outcome of infection in patients with the adult respiratory distress syndrome. *American Review of Respiratory Disease* **134:**12–16.
10. Vincent J-l & Bihari D (1992) Sepsis, severe sepsis or sepsis syndrome: need for clarification. *Intensive Care Medicine* **18:**255–257
11. Bone RC, Fisher CJ & Clemmer TP (1989) Sepsis syndrome: a valid clinical entity. *Critical Care Medicine* **171:**389–393.
12. Bone RC (1991) The pathogenesis of sepsis. *Annals of Internal Medicine* **115:**457–469.
13. Bringham KL, Bowers R & Haynes J (1979) Increased sheep lung vascular permeability caused by *E. coli* endotoxin. *Circulation Research* **45:**292–297.
14. Snell JS & Ramsay LJ (1969) Pulmonary oedema as a result of endotoxaemia. *American Journal of Physiology* **217:**170–175.

15. Ferrari-Baliviera E, Mealy K, Smith RJ & Wilmore DW (1989) Tumour necrosis factor induces ARDS in rats. *Archives of Surgery* **124:**1400–1405.
16. Vijaykumar E, Raziuddin S & Wardle EN (1991) Plasma endotoxin levels in patients with trauma, sepsis and severe haemorrhage. *Clinical Intensive Care* **2:**4–9.
17. Jacobs RF, Tabor DR, Burks AW, Campbell GD (1989) Elevated IL-l release by human alveolar macrophages during ARDS. *American Review of Respiratory Disease* **140:**1686–1692.
18. Hyers TM, Tricomi SM, Dettenmeier PA & Fowler AA (1991) TNF levels in serum and bronchoalveolar lavage fluid of patients with the adult respiratory distress syndrome. *American Review of Respiratory Disease* **144:**268–271.
19. Smedley JA, Tonnesen MG, Sandhaus RA et al (1986) Neutrophil-mediated injury to endothelial cells. Enhancement by endotoxin and essential role of neutrophil elastase. *Journal of Clinical Investigation* **77:**1233–1243.
20. Weiland JE, Davis WB, Holter JF et al (1986) Lung neutrophils in ARDS. *American Review of Respiratory Disease* **133:**218–225.
21. Lee CT, Fein AM & Lippman M (1981) Elastolytic activity in pulmonary lavage fluid from patients with adult respiratory distress syndrome. *New England Journal of Medicine* **304:**192–194.
22. Christner P, Fein A, Goldberg S et al (1985) Collagenase in the lower respiratory tract of patients with adult respiratory distress syndrome. *American Review of Respiratory Disease* **131:**690–695.
23. Braude SR, Apperley J, Krautz T & Goldman JM (1985) Adult respiratory distress syndrome after allogenic bone marrow transplantation, evidence for a neutrophil-independent mechanism. *Lancet* **i:**1239–1242.
24. Tracey KJ, Lowry SF & Cerami A (1988) Cachectin/TNF in septic shock and septic adult respiratory distress syndrome. *American Review of Respiratory Disease* **138:**1377–1379.
25. Stephens KE, Ishizaka A, Larrick JW & Raffin TA (1988) Tumour necrosis factor causes increased pulmonary permeability and edema. Comparison to septic acute lung injury. *American Review of Respiratory Disease* **137:**1364–1370.
26. Golblum SE, Jay M, Yoneka K et al (1987) Monokine-induced acute lung injury in rabbits. *Journal of Applied Physiology* **63:**2093–2100.
27. Phillips P & Tsan M-F (1992) Cytoarchitectural aspects of endothelial barrier function in response to oxidants and inflammatory mediators. In Johnson A & Ferro TJ (eds) *Lung Vascular Injury*, Chapter 4. New York: Marcel Dekker.
28. Lum H & Malik AB (1994) Regulation of vascular endothelial barrier function. *American Journal of Physiology* **267:**L223–L241.
29. McEver RP (1991) GMP-140: a receptor for neutrophils and monocytes on activated platelets and endothelium. *Journal of Cellular Biochemistry* **45:**156–161.
30. Albelda SM, Smith CW & Ward PA (1994) Adhesion molecules and inflammatory injury. *FASEB Journal* **8:**504–512.
31. Bevilacqua M, Buthcher E, Furie B et al (1991) Selectins: a family of adhesion receptors. *Cell* **67:**223.
32. Rouslahti E (1991) Integrins. *Journal of Clinical Investigation* **87:**1–5.
33. Laurent T, Markert M, Fliedner VV et al (1994) CD11b/CD18 expression, adherence, and chemotaxis of granulocytes in adult respiratory distress syndrome. *American Journal of Respiratory and Critical Care Medicine* **149:**1534–1538.
34. Muller WA, Weigl SA, Deng X & Phillips DM (1993) PECAM-1 is required for transendothelial migration of leukocytes. *Journal of Experimental Medicine* **178:**449–460.
35. MacNaughton PD & Evans TW (1992) Management of adult respiratory distress syndrome. *Lancet* **339:**469–472.
36. Murray VF, Mathay MA, Luce JM et al (1988) Pulmonary perspectives: an expanded

definition of the adult respiratory distress syndrome. *American Review of Respiratory Disease* **138:**720–723.

37. Sloane PJ, Gee MH, Gottlieb JE et al (1992) A multi-center registry of patients with acute respiratory distress syndrome. *American Review of Respiratory Disease* **146:**419–426.
38. Zapol WM & Snider MT (1977) Pulmonary hypertension in severe acute respiratory failure. *New England Journal of Medicine* **296:**476–480.
39. Zapol WM, Snider MT, Rie MA et al (1985) Pulmonary circulation during adult respiratory distress syndrome. In Zapol WM & Falke KJ (eds) *Acute Respiratory Failure*, vol. 24, pp 241–273. New York: Dekker.
40. Leeman M (1991) The pulmonary circulation in acute lung injury: a review of some recent advances. *Intensive Care Medicine* **17:**254–260.
41. Sibbald WJ & Driedger AA (1983) Right ventricular function in disease states: pathophysiologic considerations. *Critical Care Medicine* **11:**339–345.
42. Bernard GR, Rinaldo J, Harris T et al (1985) Early predictors of ARDS reversal in patients with established ARDS. *American Review of Respiratory Disease* **131:**143.
43. Mohsenifar Z, Goldbach P, Tashkin DP & Campisis DJ (1983) Relationship between O_2 delivery and O_2 consumption in the adult respiratory distress syndrome. *Chest* **84:**267–271.
44. Dantzker DR, Foresman B & Gutierrez G (1991) Pulmonary perspective: oxygen supply and utilisation relationships, a reevaluation. *American Review of Respiratory Disease* **143:**675–679.
45. Gutierrez G & Pohil RJ (1986) Oxygen consumption is linearly related to oxygen supply in critically ill patients. *Journal of Critical Care* **1:**45–53.
46. Schoemaker WC, Appel PL, Kram HB et al (1988) Prospective trial of supranormal values of survivors as therapeutic goals in high risk surgical patients. *Chest* **94:**1176–1186.
47. Schoemaker WC, Appel PL & Kram HB (1991) Oxygen transport measurements to evaluate tissue perfusion and titrate therapy: dobutamine and dopamine effects. *Critical Care Medicine* **19:**672–688.
48. Pallares LCM & Evans TW (1992) Oxygen transport in the critically ill. *Respiratory Medicine* **86:**289–295.
49. von Euler UA & Liljestrand G (1946) Observations on the pulmonary artery blood pressure in the cat. *Acta Physiologica Scandinavica* **12:**301–319.
50. Motley HL, Cournand A, Werko L et al (1947) The influence of short periods of induced acute anoxia upon pulmonary artery pressures in man. *American Journal of Physiology* **150:**315–320.
51. Morgan BC, Church SC & Gunteroth WG (1968) Hypoxic constriction of small pulmonary artery and vein in intact dogs. *Journal of Applied Physiology* **25:**356–361.
52. Dawson CA, Forrester TE & Hamilton LH (1975) Effects of hypoxia and histamine infusion on lung blood volume. *Journal of Applied Physiology* **38:**811–818.
53. Kato M & Staub NC (1966) Response of small pulmonary arteries to unilobar hypoxia and hypercapnia. *Circulation Research* **19:**426–440.
54. Glazier JB & Murray JF (1971) Site of pulmonary vasomotor reactivity in the dog during alveolar hypoxia and serotonin, and histamine infusion. *Journal of Clinical Investigation* **50:**2550–2558.
55. Shirai M, Sada K & Ninomiya I (1986) Effects of regional hypoxia and hypercapnia on small pulmonary vessels in cats. *Journal of Applied Physiology* **61:**440–448.
56. Nagasaka Y, Bhattacharya J, Nanjio S et al (1984) Micropuncture measurement of lung microvascular pressure profile during hypoxia in cats. *Circulation Research* **54:**90–95.
57. Hauge A (1968) Role of histamine in hypoxic pulmonary hypertension in the rat. I. Blockade or potentiation of endogenous amine, kinins and ATP. *Circulation Research* **22:**371–383.

58. Hauge A & Melmon KL (1968) Role of histamine in hypoxic pulmonary hypertension in the rat. II. Depletion of histamine, serotonin, and catecholamines. *Circulation Research* **22:**385–392.
59. Robin ED, Theodore J, Burke CM et al (1987) Hypoxic pulmonary vasoconstriction persists in the human transplanted lung. *Clinical Science* **72:**283–287.
60. Malik AB & Kidd BSL (1973) Adrenergic blockade and the pulmonary vascular response to hypoxia. *Respiration Physiology* **19:**96–106.
61. Goldring RM, Turino GM, Cohen G et al (1962) The catecholamines in the pulmonary arterial pressor response to hypoxia. *Journal of Clinical Investigation* **41:**1211–1222.
62. Fishman AP (1961) Respiratory gases in the regulation of the pulmonary circulation. *Physiological Reviews* **41:**214–280.
63. Murray TR, Chen L, Marshall BE & Macarak EJ (1990) Hypoxic contraction of cultured pulmonary vascular smooth muscle cells. *American Journal of Respiratory Cell and Molecular Biology* **3:**457–465.
64. Weir EK, Milczoch J, Reeves JT & Grover RF (1976) Endotoxin and prevention of hypoxic pulmonary vasoconstriction. *Journal of Laboratory and Clinical Medicine* **68:**975–983.
65. Dantzker DR, Brook CJ, Dehart P et al (1979) Ventilation-perfusion distributions in the adult respiratory distress syndrome. *American Review of Respiratory Disease* **120:**1039–1052.
66. Holden WE & McCall E (1984) Hypoxia-induced contractions of porcine pulmonary artery strips depend on intact endothelium. *Experimental Lung Research* **7:**101–112.
67. De Mey JG & Vanhoutte PM (1982) Heterogeneous behaviour of canine arterial and venous wall; importance of the endothelium. *Circulation* **51:**439–447.
68. Rodman DM, Yamaguchi T, Hasanuma K et al (1990) Effects of hypoxia on endothelium-dependent relaxation of rat pulmonary artery. *American Journal of Physiology* **258:**L207–L214.
69. Liu SF, Dewer A, Crawley DE et al (1992) Effect of tumour necrosis factor on hypoxic pulmonary vasoconstriction. *Journal of Applied Physiology* **72:**1044–1049.
70. Hill NS & Rounds S (1983) Vascular reactivity is increased in rat lungs injured with alpha-naphthiourea. *Journal of Applied Physiology* **54:**1693–1701.
71. Magee F, Wright JL, Wiggs BR et al (1988) Pulmonary vascular structure and function in chronic obstructive pulmonary disease. *Thorax* **43:**183–189.
72. Alabaster VA & Bakhle YS (1970) Removal of 5-hydroxytryptamine in the pulmonary circulation of rat lungs. *British Journal Pharmacology* **40:**468–482.
73. Johnson AR & Erdos EG (1977) Metabolism of vasoactive peptides by human endothelial cells in culture. *Journal of Clinical Investigation* **59:**684–695.
74. Moncada S & Higgs A (1993) The L-arginine – nitric oxide pathway. [Review]. *New England Journal of Medicine* **329:**2002–2012.
75. Knowles RG & Moncada S (1994) Nitric oxide synthases in mammals. *Biochemical Journal* **298:**249–258.
76. Fineman JR, Crowley MR, Heymann MA & Soifer SJ (1991) *In vivo* inhibition of endothelium-dependent pulmonary vasodilation by methylene blue in the lamb. *Journal of Applied Physiology* **71:**735–741.
77. Fineman JR, Chang R & Soifer SJ (1991) L-arginine, a precursor of EDRF *in vitro*, produces pulmonary vasodilatation in lambs. *American Journal of Physiology* **261:**H1563–H1569.
78. Vallance P, Collier J & Moncada S (1989) Effects of endothelium-derived nitric oxide on peripheral arteriolar tone in man. *Lancet* **2:**997–1000.
79. Ochoa JB, Udekwu AO, Billiar TR et al (1991) Nitrogen oxide levels in patients after trauma and during sepsis. *Annals of Surgery* **214:**621–626.

80. Petros A, Bennett D & Vallance P (1991) Effect of nitric oxide synthase inhibitors on hypotension in patients with septic shock. *Lancet* **338:**1557–1558.
81. Klabunde RE & Ritger RC (1991) N^G-monomethyl-L-arginine restores arterial blood pressure but reduces cardiac output in a canine model of endotoxic shock. *Biochemical and Biophysical Research Communications* **178:**1135–1140.
82. Busse R, Mulsch A, Fleming I & Hecker M (1993) Mechanisms of nitric oxide release from the vascular endothelium. *Circulation* **87:**V18–V25.
83. Fleming I, Gray GA, Schott C & Stoclet JC (1991) Inducible but not constitutive production of nitric oxide by vascular smooth muscle cells. *European Journal of Pharmacology* **200:**375–376.
84. Brady AJ, Poole-Wilson PA, Harding SE & Warren JB (1992) Nitric oxide production within cardiac myocytes reduces their contractility in endotoxemia. *American Journal of Physiology* **263:**H1963–H1966.
85. Griffiths MJD, Messent M & Evans TW (1993) The role of nitric oxide in the pulmonary vascular response to sepsis. *Thorax* **48:**467(Abstract).
86. Szabo C, Mitchell JA, Thiemermann C & Vane JR (1993) Nitric oxide-mediated hyporeactivity to noradrenaline precedes the induction of nitric oxide synthase in endotoxin shock. *British Journal of Pharmacology* **108:**786–792.
87. Guc MO, Furman BL & Parratt JR (1992) Modification of alpha-adrenoceptor-mediated pressor responses by N^G-nitro-L-arginine methyl ester and vasopressin in endotoxin-treated pithed rats. *European Journal of Pharmacology* **224:**63–69.
88. Liu S, Adcock IM, Old RW, Barnes PJ & Evans TW (1993) Lipopolysaccharide treatment *in vivo* induces widespread tissue expression of inducible nitric oxide synthase mRNA. *Biochemical and Biophysical Research Communications* **196:**1208–1213.
89. Griffiths MJD, Liu SF, Curzen N & Evans TW (1995) *In vivo* treatment with endotoxin induces nitric oxide synthase in rat main pulmonary artery. *American Journal of Physiology* **268:**L509–L518.
90. Liu SF, Adcock IM, Barnes PJ & Evans TW (1995) Differential regulation of the constitutive and inducible NO synthase mRNA by endotoxin *in vivo* in the rat. *American Journal of Respiratory and Critical Care Medicine* **151:**A15.
91. Gold ME, Wood KS, Byrns RE, Buga GM & Ignarro LJ (1990) L-arginine-dependent vascular smooth muscle relaxation and cGMP formation. *American Journal of Physiology* **259:**H1813–H1821.
92. Griffiths MJD, Curzen NP, Sair M & Evans TW (1994) Nitric oxide synthase inhibitors in septic shock: theoretical considerations. *Clinical Intensive Care* **5:**29–36.
93. Griffiths MJD, Messent M, MacAllister RJ & Evans TW (1993) Aminoguanidine selectively inhibits inducible nitric oxide synthase. *British Journal of Pharmacology* **110:**963–968.
94. Johns RA, Linden JM & Peach MJ (1989) Endothelium-dependent relaxation and cyclic GMP accumulation in rabbit pulmonary artery are selectively impaired by moderate hypoxia. *Circulation Research* **65:**1508–1515.
95. Rodman DM, Yamaguchi T, Hasanuma K et al (1990) Effects of hypoxia on endothelium-dependent relaxation of rat pulmonary artery. *American Journal of Physiology* **258:**L207–L214.
96. Ohe M, Ogata M, Shirato K & Takishima T (1987) The role of endothelium in the hypoxic contraction of isolated human pulmonary artery. *Circulation* **76 (Suppl.) II:**467.
97. Brashers VL, Peach MJ & Rose CE (1988) Augmentation of hypoxic pulmonary vasoconstriction in the isolated perfused rat lung by *in vitro* antagonists of endothelium-dependent relaxation. *Journal of Clinical Investigation* **82:**1495–1502.
98. Mazmanian G-M, Baudet B, Brink C et al (1989) Methylene blue potentiates vascular reactivity in isolated rat lungs. *Journal of Applied Physiology* **66:**1040–1045.

99. Archer SL, Tolins JP, Raij L & Weir EK (1989) Hypoxic pulmonary vasoconstriction is enhanced by inhibition of the synthesis of an endothelium derived relaxing factor. *Biochemical and Biophysical Research Communications* **164:**1198–1205.
100. Hasanuma K, Yamaguchi T, Rodman DM et al (1991) Effects of inhibitors of EDRF and EDHF on vasoreactivity of perfused rat lungs. *American Journal of Physiology* **260:**L97–L104.
101. Zelenkov P, McLoughlin T & Johns RA (1993) Endotoxin enhances hypoxic constriction of rat aorta and pulmonary artery through induction of EDRF/NO synthase. *American Journal of Physiology* **265:**L346–L354.
102. Yanagisawa M, Kurihara H, Limura S et al (1988) A novel potent vasoconstrictor peptide produced by vascular endothelial cells. *Nature* **332:**411–415.
103. Haynes WG & Webb DJ (1993) The endothelin family of peptides: local hormones with diverse roles in health and disease. *Clinical Science* **84:**485–500.
104. Kiff RJ, Gardiner SM, Compton AM & Bennett T (1991) The effects of endothelin-1 and NG-nitro-L-arginine methyl ester on regional haemodynamics in conscious rats with streptozotocin-induced diabetes mellitus. *British Journal of Pharmacology* **103:**1321–1326.
105. Bax WA & Saxena PR (1994) The current endothelin receptor classification: time for reconsideration? *Trends in Pharmacological Sciences* **15:**379–386.
106. Filep JG, Clozel M, Fournier A & Foldes-Filep E (1994) Characterization of receptors mediating responses to endothelin-1 in the conscious rat. *British Journal of Pharmacology* **113:**845–852.
107. McMurdo L, Corder R, Thiemermann C & Vane JR (1993) Incomplete inhibition of the pressor effects of endothelin-1 and related peptides in the anaesthetised rat with BQ-123 provides evidence for more than one vasoconstrictor recptor. *British Journal of Pharmacology* **108:**557–561.
108. Gardiner SM, Compton AM, Kemp PA & Bennett T (1990) Regional and cardiac haemodynamic effects of NG-nitro-L-arginine methyl ester in conscious, Long Evans rats. *British Journal Pharmacology* **101:**625–631.
109. Rubanyi GM & Polokoff MA (1994) Endothelins: molecular biology, biochemistry, pharmacology, physiology, and pathophysiology. *Pharmacological Reviews* **46:**325–415.
110. Sirvio ML, Metsarinne K & Fyhrquist F (1990) Tissue distribution and half-life of ^{125}I-endothelin in the rat: importance of pulmonary clearance. *Biochemical and Biophysical Research Communications* **167:**1191–1195.
111. Pittet JF, Morel DR, Hemsen A et al (1991) Elevated plasma endothelin-1 concentrations are associated with the severity of illness in patients with sepsis. *Annals of Surgery* **213:**261–264.
112. Wagner OF, Christ g, Wojta J et al (1992) Polar secretion of endothelin-1 by cultured endothelial cells. *Journal of Biological Chemistry* **267:**16066–16068.
113. Kaddoura S, Curzen N, Firth J, Sugden PH, Poole-Wilson PA & Evans TW (1994) Tissue expression of endothelin-1 expression in endotoxaemia. *Clinical Science* **88:**12P.
114. Curzen N, Kaddoura S, Firth J, Sugden P, Poole-Wilson P & Evans TW (1995) Vascular expression of ET-1 mRNA increases in sepsis. *British Heart Journal* **73:**P46.
115. Curzen NP, Griffiths MJD & Evans TW (1995) Contraction to endothelin-1 in pulmonary arteries from endotoxin-treated rats is modulated by the endothelium. *American Journal of Physiology* **268:**H2260–H2266.
116. Kourembanas S, Marsden PA, McQuillan LP & Faller DV (1991) Hypoxia induces endothelin gene expression and secretion in cultured human endothelium. *Journal of Clinical Investigation* **88:**1054–1057.
117. Elton TS, Oparil S & Taylor GR (1992) Normobaric hypoxia stimulates endothelin-1 gene expression in the rat. *American Journal of Physiology* **263:**R1260–R1264.

118. Hieda HS & Gomez-Sanchez CE (1990) Hypoxia increases endothelin release in bovine endothelial cells in culture, but epinephrine, norepinephrine, serotonin, histamine and angiotensin II do not. *Life Sciences* **47:**247–251.
119. Rakugi H, Tabuchi Y, Nakamaru M et al (1990) Evidence for endothelin-1 release from resistance vessels of rats in response to hypoxia. *Biochemical and Biophysical Research Communications* **169:**973–977.
120. Maclean MR, Randall MD & Hiley CR (1989) Effects of moderate hypoxia, hypercapnia, and acidosis on haemodynamic changes induced by endothelin-1 in the pithed rat. *British Journal Pharmacology* **98:**1055–1065.
121. Crawley DE, Liu SF, Barnes PJ & Evans TW (1992) Endothelin-3 is a potent vasodilator in the rat. *Journal of Applied Physiology* **72:**1425–1431.
122. Hasunuma K, Rodman DM, O'Brien RF & McMurty IF (1990) Endothelin 1 causes pulmonary vasodilatation in rats. *American Journal of Physiology* **259:**H48–H54.
123. Douglas SA, Vickery-Clark LM & Ohlstein EH (1993) Endothelin-1 does not mediate hypoxic vasoconstriction in canine isolated blood vessels. *British Journal Pharmacology* **108:**418–421.
124. Vanhoutte PM, Auch-Schwelk W & Boulanger C et al (1989) Does endothelin-1 mediate endothelium-dependent contractions during anoxia? *Journal of Cardiovascular Pharmacology* **13 (Suppl 5):** S124–128.
125. Douglas SA, James S & Hiley CR (1991) Endothelial modulation and changes in endothelin pressor activity during hypoxia in the rat isolated perfused superior mesenteric arterial bed. *British Journal Pharmacology* **103:**1441–1448.
126. Liu J, Gu XH, Casley DJ & Nayler WG (1990) Reoxygenation, but neither hypoxia nor intermittent ischaemia, increases [^{125}I]endothelin-1 binding to rat cardiac membrances. *Journal of Cardiovascular Pharmacology* **15:**436–443.
127. Liu J, Chen R, Casley DJ & Nayler WG (1990) Ischaemia and reperfusion increase ^{125}I-labelled endothelin-1 binding in rat cardiac membranes. *American Journal of Physiology* **258:**H829–H835.
128. Liu J, Casley DJ & Nayler WG (1989) Ischaemia causes externalisation of endothelin-1 binding sites in rat cardiac membranes. *Biochemical and Biophysical Research Communications* **164:**1220–1225.
129. Warner TD, Mitchell JA, De Nucci G & Vane JR (1989) Endothelin-1 and endothelin-3 release EDRF from isolated perfused arterial vessels of the rat and rabbit. *Journal of Cardiovascular Pharmacology* **13:**S85–S88.
130. Warner TD, De Nucci G & Vane JR (1989) Rat endothelin is a vasodilator in the isolated perfused mesentery of the rat. *European Journal of Pharmacology* **159:**325–326.
131. Fukuda N, Soma M, Izumi Y et al (1991) Low doses of endothelin-3 elicit endothelium-dependent vasodilatation which is accompanied by elevation of cyclic GMP. *Japanese Circulation* **55:**617–622.
132. Fukuda N, Izumi Y, Soma M et al (1990) L-N^G-monomethyl-arginine inhibits the vasodilating effects of low dose of endothelin-3 on rat mesenteric arteries. *Biochemical and Biophysical Research Communications* **167:**739–745.
133. Fukuroda T, Nishikibe M, Ohta Y et al (1992) Analysis of responses to endothelins in isolated porcine blood vessels by using a novel endothelin antagonist, BQ-153. *Life Sciences* **50:**107–112.
134. Hirata Y, Emori T, Eguchi S et al (1993) Endothelin receptor subtype B mediates synthesis of nitric oxide by cultures of bovine endothelial cells. *Journal of Clinical Investigation* **91:**1367–1373.
135. Karaki H, Sudjarwo SA & Hori M (1993) ETB receptor antagonist, IRL 1038, selectively inhibits the endothelin-induced endothelium-dependent vascular relaxation. *European Journal of Pharmacology* **231:**371–374.

136. Masaki T (1991) Tissue specificity of the endothelin-induced responses. *Journal of Cardiovascular Pharmacology* **17 (Suppl.7):**S1–S4.
137. Michael JR, Yang J, Farrukh IS & Gurtner GH (1993) Protein kinase C-mediated pulmonary vasoconstriction in rabbit: role of Ca^{2+}, AA metabolites, and vasodilators. *Journal of Applied Physiology* **74:**1310–1319.
138. Dohi Y & Luscher TF (1991) Endothelin in hypertensive resistance arteries: intraluminal and extraluminal dysfunction. *Hypertension* **18:**543–549.
139. Rae GA, Trybulec M, de Nucci G & Vane JR (1989) Endothelin-1 releases eicosanoids from rabbit isolated kidney and spleen. *Journal of Cardiovascular Pharmacology* **13 (Suppl.5):**89–92.
140. Boulanger C & Luscher TF (1990) Endothelin is released from porcine aorta: inhibition by endothelium-derived nitric oxide. *Journal of Clinical Investigation* **85:**587–590.
141. Yokokawa K, Kohno M, Yasunari K et al (1991) Endothelin-3 regulates endothelin-1 production in cultured human endothelial cells. *Hypertension* **18:**304–315.
142. De Nucci G, Thomas R, D'Orleans-Juste P et al (1988) Pressor effects of circulating endothelin are limited by its removal in the pulmonary circulation and by the release of prostacyclin and endothelium-derived relaxing factor. *Proceedings of the National Academy of Sciences US.* **85:**9797–9800.
143. Rapoport RM & Murad F (1983) Agonist induced endothelium-dependent relaxation in rat thoracic aorta may be mediated through cGMP. *Circulation Research* **52:**352–357.
144. Giaid A, Yanagisawa M, Langleben D et al (1993) Expression of endothelin-1 in the lungs of patients with pulmonary hypertension. *New England Journal of Medicine* **328:**1732–1739.
145. Gerrard JM (1985) The structures and functional properties of prostaglandins and related chemicals. In *Prostaglandins and Leukotrienes. Blood and vascular cell function*, Chapter 2. New York: Marcel Dekker.
146. Leeman M, Boeynaems JM, Degaute JP et al (1985) Administration of dazoxiben, a selective thromboxane synthesis inhibitor, in the adult respiratory distress syndrome. *Chest* **87:**726–730.
147. Matthay MA, Eschenbacher WL & Goetzel EJ (1984) Elevated concentrations of leukotriene D_4 in pulmonary oedema fluid of patients with the adult respiratory distress syndrome. *Journal of Clinical Immunology* **4:**479–483.
148. Ogletree M, Begley C, King G & Brigham K (1986) Influence of steroidal and non-steroidal anti-inflammatory agents on accumulation of arachidonic acid metabolites in plasma and lung lymph after endotoxaemia in awake sheep: measurements of prostacyclin and thromboxane metabolites and 12-HETE. *American Review of Respiratory Disease* **133:**55–61.
149. Moncada S & Vane JR (1979) Pharmacology and endogenous roles of prostaglandins, endoperoxides, thromboxane A_2 and prostacyclin. *Pharmacological Review* **30:**293–331.
150. Radomski MW, Palmer RMS & Moncada S (1987) Comparative pharmacology of endothelium-derived relaxing factor, nitric oxide and prostacyclin in platelets. *British Journal of Pharmacology* **92:**181–187.
151. Winn R, Harlan J, Nadir B et al (1983) Thromboxane A_2 mediates vasoconstriction but not permeability after endotoxin. *Journal of Clinical Investigation* **72:**911–918.
152. Samuelsson B, Dahlen SE, Lindgren JA et al (1987) Leukotrienes and lipoxins: structures, biosynthesis, and biological effects. *Science* **237:**1171–1176.
153. Petrak RA, Balk RA & Bone RC (1989) Prostaglandins, cyclo-oxygenase inhibitors, and thromboxane synthetase inhibitors in the pathogenesis of multiple systems organ failure. *Critical Care Clinics* **5:**303–314.
154. Ahmed T, Wasserman MA, Muccitelli R, Tucker S, Gazeroglu H & Marchette B

(1986) Endotoxin-induced changes in pulmonary hemodynamics and respiratory mechanics: role of lipoxygenase and cyclooxygenase products. *American Review of Respiratory Diseases* **134:**1149–1157.

155. Harlan RWJ, Harker BNL & Hilderbrandt J (1983) Thromboxane A_2 mediates lung vasoconstriction but not permeability after endotoxin. *Journal of Clinical Investigation* **72:**911–918.
156. Hales CA, Rouse ET & Slate JL (1978) Influence of aspirin and indomethacin on variability of alveolar hypoxic vasoconstriction. *Journal of Applied Physiology* **45:**33–39.
157. Weir EK, McMurtry IF, Tucker A et al (1976) Prostaglandin synthetase inhibitors do not decrease hypoxic pulmonary vasoconstriction. *Journal of Applied Physiology* **41:**714–718.
158. Demiryurek AT, Wadsworth RM, Kane KA & Peacock AJ (1993) The role of the endothelium in hypoxic constriction of human pulmonary artery rings. *American Review of Respiratory Disease* **147:**283–290.
159. Kovitz KL, Aleskowitch TD, Sylvester JT & Flanahan NA (1993) Endothelium-derived contracting and relaxing factors contribute to hypoxic responses of pulmonary arteries. *American Journal of Physiology* **265:**H1139–H1148.
160. Gerber JG, Voelkel N, Nies AS et al (1980) Moderation of hypoxic vasoconstriction by infused arachidonic acid: role of PGI_2. *Journal of Applied Physiology* **49:**107–112.
161. Auch-Schwelk W, Katusic ZS & Vanhoutte PM (1990) Thromboxane A_2 receptor antagonists inhibit endothelium-dependent contractions. *Hypertension* **15:**699–703.
162. Voelkel NF (1985) Species variations in the pulmonary responses to arachidonic acid metabolites. *Prostaglandins* **29 :** 867–889.
163. Morganroth ML, Stenmark KR, Zirrolli JA et al (1984) Leukotriene C_4 production during hypoxic pulmonary vasoconstriction in isolated rat lungs. *Prostaglandins* **28:**867–875.
164. Voelkel NF, Stenmark KR, Reeves JT et al (1984) Action of lipoxygenase metabolites in isolated rat lungs. *Journal of Applied Physiology* **57:**860–867.
165. Richalet J-P, Hornych A, Rathat C et al (1991) Plasma prostaglandins, leukotrienes and thromboxane in acute high altitude hypoxia. *Respiration Physiology* **85:**205–215.
166. Morganroth ML, Reeves JH, Murphy RC & Voelkel NF (1984) Leukotriene synthesis and receptor blockers block hypoxic pulmonary vasoconstriction. *Journal of Applied Physiology* **56:**1340–1346.

6

Pathophysiology of the Perinatal Pulmonary Circulation

Jean-Christophe Mercier
John P. Kinsella
A. Tuan Dinh-Xuan
Steven H. Abman

FETAL AND PERINATAL CIRCULATION

Fetal pulmonary circulation is characterized by high resistance and low flow, accepting less than 10% of the combined ventricular output.[1] This unique physiologic state ensures enough pulmonary blood flow to provide for lung growth and development,[2] yet allows blood to shunt right-to-left at the levels of the ductus arteriosus and foramen ovale to perfuse the placenta, the fetal organ of gas exchange. *Mechanisms* that contribute to the maintenance of high resting tone in the fetal lung are not completely understood but include mechanical factors such as the lack of rhythmic distension, the absence of an air–liquid interface, the presence of a low resting alveolar and arteriolar oxygen tension, and a different 'balance', when compared with the postnatal lung, between vasodilating and vasoconstricting mediators.[3–6]

A second feature of fetal pulmonary circulation, in addition to high resting tone, is its capacity for autoregulation. Upon exposure to several dilating stimuli including shear stress, oxygen, and several pharmacologic agents that act on endothelium, the fetal pulmonary vasculature exhibits a time-limited response.[7–10] Initial vasodilation is followed by a return of vascular resistance to its resting state despite continued exposure to the vasodilating stimulus. This time-limited vasodilatory response limits excessive pulmonary blood flow, which is detrimental to the developing fetus, and allows preservation of placental perfusion. In contrast, agents that act directly on the vascular smooth muscle cell, such as atrial natriuretic peptide and 8-bromo-cGMP, cause sustained vasodilation in the fetal lung.[11] This suggests that factors responsible for the autoregulatory response include the inability of the endothelial cell to sustain the release of locally acting vasodilatory mediators, an 'uncoupling' of these mediators from the adjacent smooth muscle cell, or alternatively, enhanced release of vasoconstricting mediators by the endothelial cell to counterbalance vasodilation.

At birth, as the lungs assume the function of gas exchange, pulmonary blood flow increases 8–10-fold, and pulmonary vascular resistance (PVR) rapidly drops.[3–12] The fall in PVR reflects both structural adaptation of the pulmonary bed to lung inflation and the effects of locally acting vasoactive mediators released at birth. Central to this transition from the high-resistance bed *in utero* to the low-resistance circuit *ex utero* is the endothelial cell which acts as a paracrine modulator of vascular resistance by releasing various vasoactive products.[13] Therefore, the intimate relationship between the endothelial cell and smooth muscle cell and the mechanisms that elicit vasodilation are essential in understanding the transitional circulation.

The role of the endothelial cell in regulating vascular tone

The endothetial cell produces and releases several mediators which act on the subjacent smooth muscle cell to modulate local vascular tone. Several stimuli influence the release of these mediators, and complex mechanisms determine the overall balance between endothelial-derived vasoconstricting and vasodilating factors. For example, the onset of ventilation at birth directly lowers PVR, presumably by recruitment and a change in the geometry of small pulmonary vessels.[14] Ventilation and oxygenation also stimulate the release of the endothelial-derived vasodilators, prostacyclin and nitric oxide (NO).[15,16] This chapter will focus on the major endothelium-derived mediators, i.e. eicosanoids, NO, and endothelin (Figure 1).

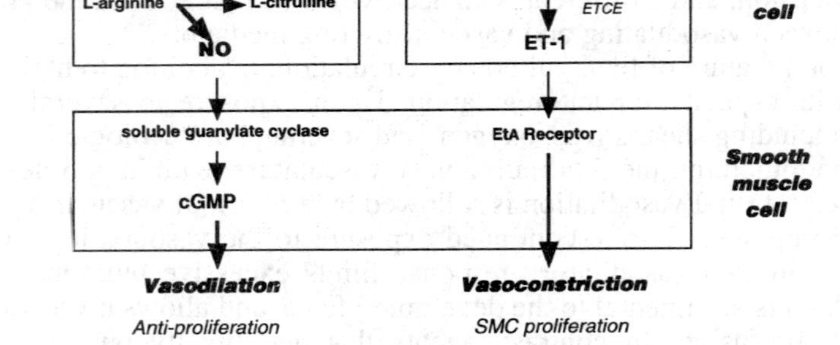

Figure 1. Schematic diagram showing the balance between the NO–cGMP pathway leading to vasodilation and anti-proliferation of the smooth vascular muscle cells (SMC), and the endothelin-1 (ET-1) leading to vasoconstriction and SMC proliferation.

Eicosanoids

Eicosanoids are locally produced vasoactive lipid metabolites of arachidonic acid. Within the endothelial cell, arachidonic acid can be metabolized through the lipoxygenase pathway to form leukotrienes or through the cyclo-oxygenase pathway to form various prostaglandins. In the fetal and transitional circulations, the cyclooxygenase pathway predominates with release of PGI_2 (prostacyclin), the most potent prostanoid mediator formed.[17]

Leukotrienes

Early work suggested that the leukotrienes, powerful vasoconstrictors when infused into the fetal pulmonary circulation, played an important role in maintaining high tone within the fetal pulmonary vascular bed. It was further suggested that leukotriene production decreased at birth contributing to the drop in PVR during postnatal transition. These hypotheses were based on two findings: (1) the administration of nonspecific leukotriene antagonists caused fetal pulmonary vasodilation and blocked the pressor response to exogenous administration of leukotrienes;[18] (2) leukotrienes were detected in tracheal aspirates from human newborns with persistent pulmonary hypertension of the newborn (PPHN), but not in intubated newborns without pulmonary hypertension.[19] However, the nonspecificity of the leukotriene blockers used made speculations regarding leukotriene importance in the fetal circulation questionable.[20] Furthermore, leukotriene levels in lung fluid in newborns with PPHN remain detectable even after resolution of pulmonary hypertension.[21] Cassin et al[22] measured leukotriene content in fetal lamb tracheal fluid and demonstrated very low leukotriene activity. To further clarify the role of leukotrienes in fetal and transitional pulmonary vascular regulation, Abman & Stenmark[23] measured leukotriene concentrations in fetal and postnatal lambs in both lung liquid and lung tissues. Leukotriene content in fetal lung liquid was found to be extremely low, in comparison with adult ewes. Fetal lung tissue levels of leukotrienes were also very low. In addition, no significant change in lung leukotriene levels was observed during the transition in normal or hypertensive ovine fetuses. Thus, direct measurement of leukotriene levels in the fetal lung fails to support leukotriene activity as a major determinant of fetal or transitional pulmonary vascular tone.

Prostaglandins

The prostaglandins comprise a family of chemically related compounds formed via the cyclooxygenase pathway of arachidonic acid metabolism. Although several of these compounds display a vasoactive effect when infused into the fetal pulmonary circulation, prostacyclin appears to be the major prostanoid metabolite within the fetal lung.

Prostacyclin is produced by fetal pulmonary blood vessels *in vitro,*[17,24] and when infused into the fetal lung *in vivo* causes very potent vasodilation.[25] Several studies have demonstrated an increase in prostacyclin production during the normal transition, suggesting that prostacyclin synthesis is stimulated by birth-related events.[26,27] In accordance with this hypothesis, acute cyclooxygenase inhibition with indomethacin or meclofenamate attenuates the drop in PVR at birth in term animals.[28] However, this attenuation is modest, and postnatal adaptation is not significantly changed suggesting that, although increased production of prostacyclin contributes to the pulmonary vascular changes during the transition, prostacyclin is not essential for postnatal adaptation. Increased prostacyclin synthesis at birth was suggested to be primarily stimulated by the onset of breathing. To determine further which type of event at birth accounted for increased prostacyclin production, Velvis et al[29] performed a series of experiments independently evaluating the effects of static distention, rhythmic distention, and oxygenation on prostacyclin production in near-term animals. These investigators demonstated that cyclooxygenase inhibition abolished the drop in PVR associated with rhythmic distention of the lungs after birth but had no effect on PVR during static distention or during rhythmic distention *with* oxygenation. Thus, under normal circumstances, i.e. ventilation with oxygenation, prostacyclin is not essential for normal postnatal transition.

Prostaglandins of the D and E series manifest vasodilatory activity when infused into the fetal lung.[30,31] Prostaglandin E_1 is also important in maintaining patency of the ductus arteriosus. A switch in the production of local prostaglandins stimulated by a change in the oxygen environment at birth is likely to close the ductus arteriosus postnatally. Prostaglandins of the F series induce vasoconstriction in the fetal pulmonary vasculature,[32] but these prostaglandins are probably not important.

Finally, thromboxane is a prostaglandin mediator with potent vasoconstricting and platelet-aggregation properties. This prostanoid is increased in experimental models of PPHN associated with group B streptococcal sepsis, and cyclooxygenase inhibition attenuates the marked pulmonary hypertension that accompanies experimental neonatal group B streptococcal sepsis.[33,34] It is thus feasible that thromboxane, or other prostaglandins with vasopressor activity, may contribute to failed postnatal adaptation.

Nitric oxide (NO)

In the early 1980s, the obligatory role of endothelial cells in the relaxation of arterial smooth muscle by several dilating stimuli including acetylcholine was recognized, and the production and release of an endothelial-derived relaxing factor (EDRF) was hypothesized.[35] This labile compound was identified as NO in 1987.[36,37] Since then, much has been learned about the mechanisms of NO release and activity, and its importance in several vascular beds, including the perinatal circulation, has been established.

Catalyzed by a constitutive enzyme endothelial NO synthase (cNOS), NO and L-citrulline are produced from L-arginine and molecular oxygen.[38,39] Owing to its high lipophilicity, NO rapidly diffuses to the subjacent smooth muscle cell where it activates soluble guanylate cyclase resulting in an increased smooth muscle cell concentration of cyclic guanosinemonophosphate (cGMP).[40] cGMP then initiates a cascade of intracellular events resulting in smooth muscle relaxation.[41] cGMP is rapidly hydrolyzed and inactivated within the smooth muscle cell by phosphodiesterase (PDE) enzymes.[42,43] Thus, continuous release of NO and production of cGMP are important in maintaining low basal tone. This basal production of NO increases in response to endothelial-dependent vasodilators.

Using molecular and immunostaining techniques, Halbower et al[44] have found endothelial NOS protein in the ovine fetal pulmonary vasculature as early as 0.29 term. In addition, intrapulmonary infusion of L-nitroarginine (LNA), an inhibitor of NOS and thus NO production, results in an increase in pulmonary vascular tone as early as 0.77 term.[45] Thus, endogenous NO release is physiologically important in modulating basal fetal pulmonary vascular tone, early in gestation.

In contrast, a diminished ability of the pulmonary vascular endothelial cell to increase production of NO has been found *in vitro* in isolated rings[46] and *in vivo* in whole animals[47] in response to endothelial-dependent dilators, early in gestation. For instance, the endothelial-dependent agonists acetylcholine and oxygen exhibit progressive vasodilator potency between 115 and 140 days gestation (term is 150 days).[8,48] Unlike endothelial-dependent dilators, the early fetus normally responds to endothelial-independent agonists such as inhaled NO or the direct NO donor, sodium nitroprusside.[9] These findings suggest that the ability of developing smooth muscle cells to respond to NO precedes the ability of the immature endothelium to increase and sustain the stimulated production and release of NO.

At birth, ventilation with rhythmic distention of the lungs and increased oxygenation and shear stress contribute to the normal postnatal decline in PVR. The vasodilatory response to these birth-related stimuli is markedly attenuated by pretreatment with LNA suggesting that increased release of endogenous NO is necessary for a smooth transition of the pulmonary circulation at birth.[49–51] To confirm these findings, the effects of exogenous NO have been studied in the ovine transitional circulation.[52] Without changing fetal PaO_2, inhaled NO causes potent and selective pulmonary vasodilation equivalent to that achieved with the combination of ventilation plus 100% oxygen. It is thus tempting to speculate that endothelial cell dysfunction and inability to sustain the release of NO in response to birth-related stimuli might contribute to failure of postnatal adaptation and result in the clinical state, PPHN. This hypothesis was supported by findings in a hypertensive fetal model.[53] Late-gestation ovine fetuses made hypertensive by partial ductal compression or ligation develop histologic changes of pulmonary hypertension including right ventricular hypertrophy and pulmonary vascular remodeling.[54] Upon delivery, the hypertensive animals demonstrate a much smaller increase in pulmonary blood flow and a failure to decrease PVR compared with the controls, i.e. non-hypertensives,[55] as well as hypoxic episodes contemporary of suprasystemic pulmonary arterial pressure very similar to the ones observed in newborns with severe PPHN.[56] Furthermore, they exhibit preferential impairment of endothelial-dependent vasodilation, while responsiveness to exogenous NO remains relatively intact.[52]

Although exogenous NO causes vasodilation in the hypertensive ovine fetus, the degree of vasodilation achieved is less than in controls. This difference in maximal vasodilation between hypertensive and control animals might be explained on the basis of structural changes within the pulmonary vascular bed. However, the NO response can be pharmacologically increased by the use of cGMP PDE inhibitors, such as zaprinast and dipyridamole.[57,58]

Much remains to be learned about the NO–cGMP system. Recent work has suggested that NO may have a direct effect on the smooth muscle cell,[59,60] independent of guanylate cyclase activation, and further elucidation of the interaction of NO with the smooth muscle cell is an active area of research. Other areas include the mechanisms of NO expression and regulation, the intracellular interactions between NO, cGMP, cAMP, and the PDE enzymes, as well as the mechanisms of cGMP-induced vasodilation.

Endothelin

Recognition of the important role of the endothelial cell in regulating vascular tone, and the identification of EDRF, prompted the search for counter-balancing endothelial-derived vasoconstrictor substances. In 1988, a novel potent vasoconstrictor peptide produced by vascular endothelial cells was isolated and named endothelin.[61] Further work established that this agent was one of a family of three structurally similar peptides, endothelin-1, -2, and -3 (ET-1, ET-2, and ET-3), each produced by a separate gene.[62] Investigations of the perinatal circulation have focused primarily on ET-1.

Within the endothelial cell, ET-1 is formed during a two-step reaction. Preproendothelin-1, a 212-amino acid precursor, is cleaved by an endo-peptidase to form proendothelin-1 or big ET-1, a 38-amino acid peptide. Big ET-1 is then cleaved by a putative endothelin-converting enzyme (ECE) to the biologically active ET-1, a 21-amino acid peptide. ET-1 is primarily formed and released at the abluminal surface of the endothelial cell. ET-1 then binds to specific receptors to elicit its physiologic effect.

Two different receptors (ET_A and ET_B) for endothelin have been characterized[63,64] (Figure 2). The ET_A receptor displays much greater binding affinity for ET-1 and ET-2, and is generally present on the smooth muscle cell in fetal lung. Binding of ET-1 to this receptor results in vasoconstriction through a complex series of intracellular events involving activation of phospholipase C, production of inositol trisphosphate, and release of intracellular stores of calcium.[65] In the fetal and newborn lung, the ET_B receptor is located on the endothelial cell. ET_B receptor binding results in vasodilation which may be mediated by endogenous NO,[66,67] or prostacyclin release,[68] or via ATP-gated potassium channels.[69]

The hemodynamic response to ET-1 in the fetus depends on the dose and route of administration, the vascular bed examined, and resting vascular tone. Pulmonary infusion of ET-1 in the fetus and newborn results in a biphasic response with initial potent vasodilation followed by vasoconstriction.[70] Prolonged or repeated infusions of ET-1 cause progressively increased vaso-constriction. Systemic administration of ET-1 in the fetus and newborn results in a sustained vasoconstriction without preceding vasodilation.[70,71] The mech-anisms responsible for this difference between the fetal pulmonary and systemic response to exogenous ET-1 are unknown but probably involve

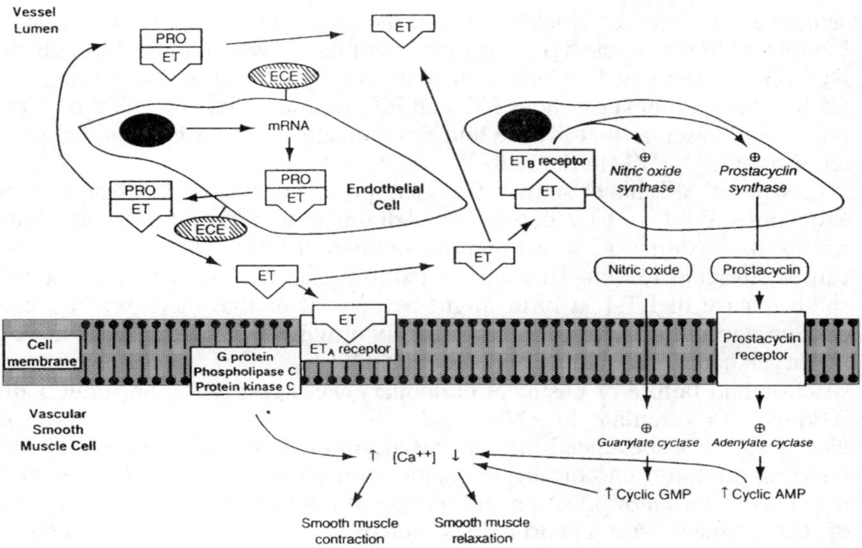

Figure 2. Generation and actions of ET-1 in the blood vessel wall. ET-1 is generated via cleavage of its precursor proendothelin-1 (PRO ET) by membrane-bound endothelin-converting enzyme (ECE). The mature peptide can then act locally either at vascular smooth muscle cell ET_A receptors to directly cause vasoconstriction, or at endothelial cell ET_B receptors to stimulate production of endothelium-derived vasodilators, NO and prostacyclin. ET_A receptors may also be present on smooth vascular cells, where they cause vasoconstriction. (From Haynes WG & Webb DJ (1993) The endothelin family of peptides. Local hormones with diverse roles in health and disease? *Clinical Science* **84:**491; with permission).

differential expression of receptor subtypes within these vascular beds. The hemodynamic response to big ET-1 in the fetal lung differs from the response to ET-1.[72,73] Big ET-1 causes vasoconstriction without vasodilation. Since big ET-1 requires processing by the endothelial cell before release as ET-1, the response to the exogenous administration of big ET-1 may be more representative of the physiologic response to endogenous ET-1. It also suggests that ET-1 is preferentially released abluminally by the endothelial cell where it is more likely to bind to smooth muscle cell ET_A receptors and cause vasoconstriction.

To clarify further the physiologic role of ET_A and ET_B receptor activity within the fetal lung, the hemodynamic effects of BQ-123, a selective ET_A receptor antagonist, and Sarafotoxin S6c, a selective ET_B receptor agonist were studied.[74] Blockade of the ET_A receptor with BQ-123 caused a dose-dependent increase in pulmonary blood flow and decrease in PVR; stimulation of the ET_B receptor with Sarafotoxin S6c also resulted in vasodilation. Both of these vasodilatory responses were blocked by LNA, suggesting that selective ET_A receptor blockade within the fetal lung allows for preferential binding of ET-1 to the ET_B receptor resulting in vasodilation through the NO–cGMP pathway.[74,75] Consistent with this hypothesis is the finding that CGS 27830, a blocker of both ET_A and ET_B receptors, has no effect on basal pulmonary vascular tone. These findings indicate a role for ET-1 in the maintenance of high PVR in the fetus.[74,76]

Cassin et al[77] have shown that the pulmonary vascular response to exogenous ET-1 is tone-dependent. Administration of ET-1 to the fetus results in vasodilation whereas after ventilation with 100% oxygen, ET-1 causes vasoconstriction. This finding led to the interesting speculation that a spike release of ET-1 at birth might be one factor that increases NO production during the transition. However, abnormally sustained release of ET-1 might 'exhaust' NO stores and stimulate ET_A receptors causing vasoconstriction and failure of postnatal pulmonary vascular adaptation. Endothelin is known to stimulate fibroblast and smooth muscle cell proliferation *in vitro*,[78] and it is speculated that increased production and release of ET-1 *in utero* might cause chronic hypertension with pulmonary vascular remodeling. This abnormal production and release of ET-1 might account for several of the characteristic abnormalities noted in PPHN. This hypothesis is supported by the fact that elevated immunoreactive ET-1 levels are present in newborns with PPHN.[79]

In summary, ET-1 is physiologically active in the fetal and transitional pulmonary circulations. ET-1 may play an important role in modulating fetal and transitional vascular tone. Abnormal production and/or release of ET-1 or a change in the normal balance between the two receptors, i.e. ET_A eliciting vasoconstriction and ET_B inducing vasodilation, may contribute to abnormal postnatal adaptation of the pulmonary vascular bed. However, much remains to be learned about the mechanisms controlling ET-1 expression by the endothelial cells.

PERSISTENT PULMONARY HYPERTENSION OF THE NEWBORN

Some newborns fail to achieve or sustain this normal decrease in PVR at birth, leading to severe hypoxemia due to continued right-to-left shunting of desaturated blood across the ductus arteriosus or foramen ovale.[80] This entity is now designated persistent pulmonary hypertension of the newborn (PPHN).[81,82] Biomolecular mechanisms underlying these findings are still unclear, but may include downregulation of endothelial NO synthase (eNOS), loss of smooth muscle responsiveness due to decreased soluble guanylate cyclase or increased cGMP PDE activities, upregulation of ET_A receptors or inability to release NO and prostacyclin in response to ET_B stimulation. Preliminary results from Western blot analysis have found that type III eNOS protein was reduced by nearly 50% in the nitrophen-induced model of congenital diaphragmatic hernia,[83] as well as in constricted ductus hypertensive lungs in comparison with controls. Loss of smooth muscle responsiveness in this hypertensive model can also be due to increased cGMP PDE activity and decreased activity of phosphatase, the enzyme responsible for smooth muscle relaxation.[84] Nevertheless, increased PVR in this model may be partly due to vasoconstriction through enhanced or unopposed stimulation of the ET_A receptors,[74] as suggested by the high levels of ET-1 found in the blood of neonates with PPHN requiring extracorporeal membrane oxygenation (ECMO).[79]

NO inhalation

Recent studies have suggested that inhaled NO causes marked improvement in oxygenation in many newborn infants with PPHN. Roberts et al[85] reported that brief (30 min) inhalation of NO at 80 ppm improved oxygenation in patients with PPHN, but this response was sustained in only one patient after NO was discontinued. Kinsella et al[86] demonstrated rapid improvement in oxygenation in six neonates with severe PPHN with inhaled NO, using doses of 20 ppm for 4 h, then decreasing the dose to 6 ppm, with sustained improvement in oxygenation for the duration of the treatment. In a subsequent study, this low-dose NO strategy was used in an additional nine infants with severe PPHN, including two with congenital diaphragmatic hernia.[87] The management incorporated the use of high-frequency oscillatory ventilation (HFOV) to optimize lung inflation during NO therapy. All neonates showed resolution of the underlying PPHN, but two infants with overwhelming sepsis subsequently required treatment with ECMO for hemodynamic support. Thus, in this pilot study, 13 of 15 infants with severe PPHN recovered without the need for ECMO.[88] Finer et al[89] randomly evaluated the improvement in oxygenation with doses of NO ranging from 5 to 80 ppm, and found that the acute improvement in oxygenation in PPHN was similar at all doses of NO studied. They also found that oxygenation increased in patients who did not have extrapulmonary shunting by echocardiography, suggesting that NO could improve oxygenation in some cases of neonatal hypoxemic respiratory failure without severe PPHN.

A large open trial including 29 preterm and 121 term (≥34 weeks) newborns with severely hypoxemic respiratory failure was conducted by the French pediatric study group on inhaled NO.[90] Improvement in oxygenation in response to inhaled NO was found to be disease-specific. The reduction in the oxygenation index (OI) was marked and sustained in most of the newborns with hyaline membrane disease, acute or adult respiratory distress syndrome (ARDS), idiopathic 'persistent fetal circulation' (PPHN) or sepsis provided that there was no evolving shock. The decrease in OI was slower and not always sustained in neonates with meconium aspiration syndrome (MAS). In contrast, the response to inhaled NO was very inconsistent, often marginal and transient in infants with congenital diaphragmatic hernia (CDH) and was more or less associated with lung hypoplasia. Survival due to NO depended mainly upon the gestational age, the associated diagnosis, i.e. all associated diagnosis versus CDH, and the magnitude of the improvement in oxygenation. More striking was the fact that inhaled NO, in combination with exogenous surfactant, and possibly better general care, has, as in other centers, dramatically decreased the numbers of newborns requiring ECMO in France over the last 2 years.

Management strategies in PPHN

A few infants do not respond well to inhaled NO, and the reasons for this failure remain speculative. In cases complicated by severe lung disease, inhaled NO alone is unlikely to be effective without optimal pulmonary management and adequate alveolar recruitment. There is some evidence that surfactant deficiency contributes to decreased lung compliance and atelectasis in some patients with PPHN.[92,93] Recent studies have suggested that exogenous surfactant therapy can cause sustained clinical improvement in term infants with pneumonia and MAS,[94] and in infants with CDH,[95] and can reduce the duration of ECMO.[96] Another mode of recruiting non-ventilated lung areas while minimizing baro/volu-trauma is to decrease air–liquid surface tension area using perfluorocarbon derivatives, e.g. total or partial liquid ventilation. This has been successfully tested in animals, and used in a few infants with refractory hypoxemic respiratory failure.[97]

For many years, alkalosis-induced mechanical hyperventilation with the hope of decreasing pulmonary arterial pressure and improving oxygenation has been the cornerstone of management of infants with PPHN.[98–100] However, concerns have been raised over the potential complications associated with baro/volu-trauma. Thus, alternative approaches to mechanical ventilation of the newborn infant with PPHN have attracted considerable interest. HFOV allows effective alveolar ventilation and recruitment, while reducing the potential parenchymal and airway injury associated with large phasic pressure and lung volume changes.[101] High end-inspiratory lung volume, as it occurs during conventional ventilation, has been implicated in the development of pulmonary edema and lung injury.[102] However, the strategy employed during HFOV is critically important to optimize lung inflation and minimize the risk of adverse cardiopulmonary interactions.[103] Without a strategy to adequately recruit and sustain lung volume, HFOV was found to be somewhat ineffective.[104] In contrast, with a strategy designed to recruit atelectatic lung and sustain lung volume, HFOV was more efficacious than conventional mechanical ventilation in severe neonatal hypoxemic respiratory failure.[105]

Perspectives in the modulation of vasodilation

In some infants, the effects of inhaled NO may be time-dependent, with gradual improvement in oxygenation over several hours. The rate of response to inhaled NO is likely to depend upon many factors, including the nature of the underlying lung disease, the presence of circulating vasoconstrictor agents, cardiac performance, and structural changes in the pulmonary vasculature. The potential mechanisms for suboptimal NO responses and loss of NO responsiveness require further study. Excess concentrations of vasoconstrictor mediators could potentially abate the vasodilatory effects of inhaled NO. Moreover, both functional changes in the pulmonary vascular smooth muscle cell, i.e. decreased soluble guanylate cyclase activity and structural alterations in the pulmonary vascular tree, may alter responsiveness to exogenous NO. It is thus possible that the combination of other agents, such as the PDE inhibitors zaprinast and dipyridamole, with inhaled NO could reinforce the pulmonary vasodilation[57,58] or lower the doses of NO required,[106] thereby reducing its potential toxicity.[107]

SUMMARY

Our understanding of fetal and transitional pulmonary circulation has greatly improved over recent years. Of the many neurohumoral mechanisms in place, regulation of the pulmonary vascular tone is insured by two finely balanced endothelial-derived systems, including prostaglandins and leukotrienes, and more importantly NO and endothelin. At birth, rhythmic distension of the lung, drainage of fetal lung liquid, establishment of a gas–liquid interface, increased oxygenation, and shear stress all contribute to the normal decline in PVR. Altered production of vasoactive products appears to mediate or modulate the effects of these birth-related stimuli. These include increased production of vasodilators, such as NO, PGI_2, other dilator prostaglandins and adenosine, and perhaps stimulation of K^+ channels. Decreased production of endogenous vasoconstrictors may also participate in the fall in PVR at birth. Although the pathophysiologic events that culminate in PPHN remain poorly understood, PPHN likely results from endothelial cell dysfunction and the inability to release endogenous dilators, including endothelium-derived NO and prostaglandins, contributing to failure of postnatal adaptation. Inhaled NO should normally overcome this failure, reverse PPHN, and markedly improve oxygenation, provided that optimal lung inflation has been achieved and adequate cardiovascular function maintained. Nevertheless, only ongoing randomized controlled studies will definitely demonstrate the potential value, and limitations, of this very promising therapy.

REFERENCES

1. Teitel DF, Iwamoto HS & Rudolph AM (1987) Effects of birth-related events on central blood flow patterns. *Pediatric Research* **22:**557–566.
2. Wallen LD, Perry SF, Alston JT & Maloney JE (1990) Morphometric study of the role of pulmonary arterial flow in fetal lung growth in sheep. *Pediatric Research* **27:**122–127.
3. Dawes GS, Mott JC, Widdicombe JG, Wyatt DG & Wyatt DG (1953) Changes in the lungs of the newborn lamb. *Journal of Physiology (London)* **121:**141–162.
4. Cassin S, Dawes GS & Ross BB (1964) Pulmonary blood flow and vascular resistance in immature foetal lambs. *Journal of Physiology (London)* **171:**80–89.
5. Enhorning G, Adams FH & Norman A (1966) Effects of lung expansion on the fetal lamb circulation. *Acta Paediatrica Scandinavica* **55:**441–451.
6. Walker AM, Ritchie BC, Adamson TM & Maloney JE (1988) Effect of changing lung volume on the pulmonary circulation of fetal lambs. *Journal of Applied Physiology* **64:**61–67.
7. Abman SH, Accurso FJ, Ward RM & Wilkening RB (1986) Adaptation of fetal pulmonary blood flow to local infusions of tolazoline. *Pediatric Research* **20:**1131–1135.

8. Accurso FJ, Alpert B, Wilkening RB, Petersen RG & Meschia G (1986) Time-dependent response of fetal pulmonary blood flow to an increase in fetal oxygen tension. *Respiration Physiology* **63:**43–52.
9. Accurso FJ & Wilkening RB (1988) Temporal response of the fetal pulmonary circulation to pharmacologic vasodilators. *Proceedings of the Society of Experimental Biology and Medicine* **187:**89–98.
10. Abman SH & Accurso FJ (1989) Acute effects of partial compression of the ductus arteriosus in the fetal pulmonary circulation. *American Journal of Physiology* **257:**H626–H634.
11. Abman SH, & Accurso FJ (1991) Sustained fetal pulmonary vasodilation during prolonged infusion of atrial natriuretic factor and 8-bromo-GMP. *American Journal of Physiology* **266:**H183–H192.
12. Cassin S, Dawes GS, Mott JC & Strang LB (1964) The vascular resistance of the foetal and newly ventilated lung of the lamb. *Journal of Physiology (London)* **171:**61–79.
13. Vane Änggard EE & Botting RM (1990) Regulatory functions of the vascular endothelium. *New England Journal of Medicine* **323:**27–36.
14. Haworth SG (1988) Pulmonary vascular remodeling in neonatal pulmonary hypertension: state of the art. *Chest* **93:**133S–138S.
15. Velvis H, Moore R & Heymann MA (1991) Prostaglandin inhibition prevents the fall in pulmonary vascular resistance as a result of rhythmic distention of the lungs in fetal lambs. *Pediatric Research* **30:**62–68.
16. Fineman JR, Heymann MA & Soifer SJ (1991) N^{ω}-nitro-L-arginine attenuates endothelium-dependent pulmonary vasodilation in lambs. *American Journal of Physiology* **260:**H1299–H1306.
17. Terragno NA & Terragno A (1979) Prostaglandin metabolism in fetal and maternal vasculature. *Federation Proceedings* **38:**75–77.
18. Soifer SJ, Loitz RD, Roman C & Heymann MA (1985) Leukotriene end organ antagonists increase pulmonary blood flow in fetal lambs. *American Journal of Physiology* **249:**H570–H570.
19. Stenmark KR, James SL, Voelkel NF, Toews WH, Reeves JT & Murphy RC (1983) Leukotriene C4 and D4 in neonates with hypoxemia and pulmonary hypertension. *New England Journal of Medicine* **309:**77–80.
20. Gause GE, Baker R & Cassin S (1988) Specificity of RPL 57231 for leukotriene D4 receptors in fetal pulmonary circulation. *American Journal of Physiology* **254:**H120–H125.
21. Kulik TJ & Lock JE (1987) Leukotrienes and the immature circulation. *American Review of Respiratory Disease* **136:**220–222.
22. Cassin S, Stenmark KR, Gause G, Zapp LM, Kuck H & Westcott JY (1990) Leukotrienes and prostaglandins in fetal lung liquid. *Journal of Applied Physiology* **68:**2214–2222.
23. Abman SH & Stenmark KR (1992) Changes in lung eicosanoid content during normal and abnormal transition in perinatal lambs. *American Journal of Physiology* **262:**L214–L222.
24. Remuzzi G, Misiani R, Muratore D et al (1979) Prostacyclin and human fetal circulation. *Prostaglandins* **18:**341–348.
25. Cassin S, Winikor I, Tod ML et al (1981)The effects of prostacyclin on the fetal pulmonary circulation. *Pediatric Pharmacology* **1:**197–203 .
26. Leffler CW, Hessler JR & Terragno NA (1980) Ventilation-induced release of prostaglandin-like material from fetal lungs. *American Journal of Physiology* **238:**H282–H286.
27. Leffler CW, Hessler JR & Green RS (1984) The onset of breathing at birth stimulates pulmonary vascular prostacyclin synthesis. *Pediatric Research* **18:**938–942.

28. Davidson D (1988) Pulmonary hemodynamics at birth: effects of acute cyclo-oxygenase inhibition in lambs. *Journal of Applied Physiology* **64:**1676–1682.
29. Velvis H, Moore P & Heymann MA (1991) Prostaglandin inhibition prevents the fall in pulmonary vascular resistance as a result of rhythmic distention of the lungs in fetal lambs. *Pediatric Research* **30:**62–68.
30. Cassin S, Tyler T, Leffler C & Wallis R (1979) Pulmonary and systemic vascular responses of perinatal goats to prostaglandin E_1 and E_2. *American Journal of Physiology* **236:**H828–H832.
31. Cassin S, Tod ML, Phillips J, Frisinger J, Jordan J & Gibbs C (1981) Effects of prostaglandin D_2 on the perinatal circulation. *American Journal of Physiology* **240:**H755–H760.
32. Kadowitz PJ, Joiner PD & Hyman AL (1974) Influence of prostaglandins E_1 and F_2alpha on pulmonary vascular resistance in the sheep. *Proceedings of the Society of Experimental Biology and Medicine* **145:**1257–1262.
33. Rojas J, Larson LE, Ogletree ML, Brigham KL & Stahlman MT (1983) Effects of cyclooxygenase inhibition on the response to Group B streptococcal toxin in sheep. *Pediatric Research* **17:**107–110.
34. Runkle B, Goldberg RN, Streiffeld MM et al (1984) Cardiovascular changes in Group B streptococcal sepsis in the piglet: response to indomethacin and relationship to prostacyclin and thromboxane A_2. *Pediatric Research* **18:**874–8.
35. Furchgott RF & Zawadski JV (1980) The obligatory role of endothelial cells in the relaxation of arterial smooth muscle by acetylcholine. *Nature* **288:**373–376.
36. Palmer RMJ, Ferrige AG & Moncada S (1987) Nitric oxide release accounts for the biological activity of endothelium-derived relaxing factor. *Nature* **327:**524–526.
37. Ignarro LJ, Buga GM, Wood KS, Byrns RE & Chaudhuri G (1987) Endothelium-derived relaxing factor produced and released from artery and vein is nitric oxide. *Proceedings of the National Academy of Sciences USA* **84:**9265–9269.
38. Forstermann U, Schmidt HHHW, Pollock JS et al (1991) Isoforms of nitric oxide synthase: characterization and purification from different cell types. *Biochemical Pharmacology* **42:**1849–57.
39. Busse R, Mulsch A, Fleming I & Hecker M (1993) Mechanisms of nitric oxide release from the vascular endothelium. *Circulation* **87 (Suppl. V):**18–25.
40. Moncada S, Palmer RMJ & Higgs EA (1991) Nitric oxide: physiology, pathophysiology, and pharmacology. *Pharmacological Reviews* **43:**109–142.
41. Somlyo AP & Somlyo AV (1994) Signal transduction and regulation in smooth muscle. *Nature* **372:**231–236.
42. Lugnier C, Schoeffter P, LeBec A, Strouthou E & Stoclet JC (1986) Selective inhibition of cyclic nucleotide phosphodiesterases of human, bovine, and rat aorta. *Biochemical Pharmacology* **35:**1743–1751.
43. Thomas MK, Francis SH & Corbin JD (1990) Characterization of a purified bovine lung cGMP-binding cGMP phosphodiesterase. *Journal of Biological Chemistry* **265:**14964–14970.
44. Halbower AC, Tuder RM, Franklin WA, Pollock JS, Föstermann U & Abman SH (1994) Maturation-related changes in endothelial nitric oxide synthase immunolocalization in developing ovine lung. *American Journal of Physiology* **267:**L585–L591.
45. Kinsella JP, Ivy DD & Abman SH (1994) Ontogeny of NO activity and response to inhaled NO in the developing ovine pulmonary circulation. *American Journal of Physiology* **267:**H1955–H1961.
46. Abman SH, Chatfield BA, Rodman DM, Hall SL & McMurtry IF (1991) Maturational changes in endothelial-derived relaxing factor activity in ovine pulmonary arteries *in vitro*. *American Journal of Physiology* **260:**L280–L285.

47. Morin FC III, Egan EA, Ferguson W & Lundgren CEG (1988) Development of pulmonary vascular response to oxygen. *American Journal of Physiology* **254:**H542–H546.
48. Abman SH, Chatfield BA, Hall SL & McMurtry IF (1990) Role of endothelium-derived relaxing factor during transition of pulmonary circulation at birth. *American Journal of Physiology* **259:**H1921–H1927.
49. Cornfield DN, Chatfield BA, McQueston JA, McMurtry IF & Abman SH (1992) Effects of birth-related stimuli on L-arginine-dependent pulmonary vasodilation in ovine fetus. *American Journal of Physiology* **262:**H1474–H1481.
50. Moore P, Velvis H, Fineman JR, Soifer SJ & Heymann MA (1992) EDRF inhibition attenuates the increase in pulmonary blood flow due to oxygen ventilation in fetal lambs. *Journal of Applied Physiology* **73:**2151–2157.
51. Fineman JR, Wong J, Morin FC III, Wild LM & Soifer SJ (1994) Chronic nitric oxide *in utero* produces persistent pulmonary hypertension in newborn lambs. *Journal of Clinical Investigation* **93:**2675–2683.
52. Kinsella JP, McQueston JA, Rosenberg M & Abman SH (1992) Hemodynamic effects of exogenous nitric oxide in ovine transitional pulmonary circulation. *American Journal of Physiology* **263:**H875–H880.
53. McQueston JA, Kinsella JP, lvy DD, McMurtry IF & Abman SH (1995) Chronic pulmonary hypertension *in utero* impairs endothelium-dependent vasodilation. *American Journal of Physiology* **268:**H288–H294.
54. Morin FC III (1989) Ligating the ductus arteriosus before birth remodels the pulmonary vasculature of the lamb. *Pediatric Research* **25:**251–257.
55. Abman SH, Shanley PF & Accurso FJ (1989) Failure of postnatal adaptation of the pulmonary circulation after chronic intrauterine pulmonary hypertension in fetal lambs. *Journal of Clinical Investigation* **83:**1849–1858.
56. Morin FC III (1989) Ligating the ductus arteriosus before birth causes persistent pulmonary hypertension in the newborn lamb. *Pediatric Research* **25:**245–250.
57. Steinhorn RH, Thusu KG, Russell JA, Gugino SF, Paradisis M & Morin FC (1994) The cGMP specific phosphodiesterase inhibitor M&B 22948 enhances the effect of nitric oxide in newborn lambs with persistent pulmonary hypertension. *Pediatric Research* **35:**89A.
58. Ziegler JW, lvy DD, Kinsella JP, Fox JJ, Kinsella JP, Clarke WR & Abman SH (1995) Dipyridamole, a cGMP phospodiesterase inhibitor, causes pulmonary vasodilation in the ovine fetus. *American Journal of Physiology* **269:**H473–9.
59. Archer SL, Huang JMC, Hampl V, Nelson DP, Shultz PJ & Weir EK (1994) Nitric oxide and cGMP cause vasorelaxation by activation of a charybdotoxin-sensitive K channel by cGMPdependent protein kinase. *Proceedings of the National Academy of Sciences USA* **91:**7583–7587.
60. Bolotina VM, Najibi S, Palacino JJ, Pagano PJ & Cohen RA (1994) Nitric oxide directly activates calcium-dependent potassium channels in vascular smooth muscle. *Nature* **368:**850–853.
61. Yanagisawa M, Kurihara H, Kimura S et al (1988) A novel potent vasoconstrictor peptide produced by vascular endothelial cells. *Nature* **332:**411–415.
62. Inoue A, Yanagisawa M, Kimura S et al (1989) The human endothelin family: structurally and pharmacologically distinct isopeptides predicted by three separated genes. *Proceedings of the National Academy of Sciences USA* **86:**2863–2867.
63. Arai H, Hari S, Aramori I, Ohkubo H & Nakanishi S (1990) Cloning and expression of a cDNA encoding endothelin receptor. *Nature* **348:**730–732.
64. Sakurai T, Yanagisawa M, Takuwa Y et al (1990) Cloning of a cDNA encoding a non-isopeptide-selective subtype of the endothelin receptor. *Nature* **348:**732–735.

65. Masaki T, Kimura S, Yanagisawa M & Goto K (1991) Molecular and cellular mechanism of endothelin regulation. Implications for vascular function. *Circulation* **84:**1457–1468.
66. Hirata Y, Emori T, Eguchi S et al (1993) Endothelin receptor subtype B mediates synthesis of nitric oxide by cultured bovine endothelial cells. *Journal of Clinical Investigation* **91:**1367–1373 .
67. Wong J, Vanderford PA, Fineman JR & Soifer SJ (1993) Endothelin-1 produces pulmonary vasodilation in the intact newborn lamb. *American Journal of Physiology* **265:**H1318–H1325.
68. D'Orleans P, Telemaque S, Claing A et al (1992) Human big-endothelin-1 and endothelin-1 release prostacyclin via the activation of ET-1 receptors in the rat perfused lung. *British Journal of Pharmacology* **103:**773–776.
69. Wong J, Fineman JR & Heymann MA (1994) The role of endothelin and endothelin receptor subtypes in regulation of fetal pulmonary vascular tone. *Pediatric Research* **35:**664–670.
70. Chatfield BA, McMurtry IF, Hall SL & Abman SH (1991) Hemodynamic effects of endothelin-1 on ovine fetal pulmonary circulation. *American Journal of Physiology* **261:**R182–R187.
71. Bradley LM, Czaja JF & Goldstein RE (1990) Circulatory effects of endothelin in newborn piglets. *American Journal of Physiology* **259:**H1613–H1617.
72. Liben S, Stewart DS, De Marte J & Perreault T (1993) Ontogeny of Big-Endothelin-1 effects in the newborn piglet pulmonary vasculature. *American Journal of Physiology* **265:**H139–H145.
73. Jones OW III & Abman SH (1994) Systemic and pulmonary hemodynamic effects of Big endothelin-1 and phosphoramidon in the ovine fetus. *American Journal of Physiology* **266:**R929–R935.
74. Ivy DD, Kinsella JP & Abman SH (1994) Physiologic characterization of endothelin A and B receptor activity in the ovine fetal pulmonary circulation. *Journal of Clinical Investigation* **93:**2141–2148.
75. Tod ML & Cassin S (1992) Endothelin-1-induced pulmonary arterial dilation is reduced by *N*-nitro-L-arginine in fetal lambs. *Journal of Applied Physiology* **72:**1730–1734.
76. Wang Y & Coceani F (1992) Isolated pulmonary resistance vessels from fetal lambs. Contractile behavior and responses to indomethacin and endothelin-1. *Circulation Research* **71:**320–327.
77. Cassin S, Kristova V, Davis T, Kadowitz P & Gause G (1991) Tone-dependent responses to endothelin in the isolated perfused fetal sheep pulmonary circulation *in situ*. *Journal of Applied Physiology* **70:**1228–1234.
78. Janakidevi K, Fisher MA, Del Vecchio PJ, Tiruppathi C, Figge J & Malik AB (1992) Endothelin-1 stimulates DNA synthesis and proliferation of pulmonary artery smooth muscle cells. *American Journal of Physiology* **263:**C1295–C1301.
79. Rosenberg M, Kennaugh J, Koppenhafer SL, Loomis M, Chatfield BA & Abman SH (1993) Elevated immunoreactive endothelin-1 levels in infants with persistent pulmonary hypertension of the newbom. *Journal of Pediatrics* **123:**109–114.
80. Gersony WM, Duc GV & Sinclair JC (1969) 'PPHN' syndrome (persistence of the fetal circulation). *Circulation* **40 (Suppl 3):**87a.
81. Levin D, Heymann M, Kitterman J, Gregory G, Phibbs R & Rudolph A (1976) Persistent pulmonary hypertension of the newborn infant. *Journal of Pediatrics* **88:** 626–630.
82. Gersony WM (1984) Neonatal pulmonary hypertension: pathophysiology, classification, and etiology. *Clinical Perinatology* **11:**517–524.
83. Shaul P (1995) Decreased eNOS in nitrophen-induced CDH model. *FASEB Journal* **9:**A599. .

84. Belik J (1995) Phosphatase, the enzyme responsible for smooth muscle relaxation is decreased in the ovine hypertensive model. *Pediatric Research* **36:**326A.
85. Roberts JD, Polaner DM, Lang P & Zapol WM (1992) Inhaled nitric oxide in persistent pulmonary hypertension of the newborn. *Lancet* **340:**818–819.
86. Kinsella JP, Neish SR, Shaffer E & Abman SH (1992) Low-dose inhalational nitric oxide in persistent pulmonary hypertension of the newborn. *Lancet* **340:**819–820.
87. Kinsella JP, Neish SR, Ivy DD, Shaffer E & Abman SH (1993) Clinical responses to prolonged treatment of persistent pulmonary hypertension of the newborn with low doses of inhaled nitric oxide. *Journal of Pediatrics* **123:**103–108.
88. Kinsella JP & Abman SH (1993) Inhalational nitric oxide therapy for persistent pulmonary hypertension of the newborn. *Pediatrics* **91:**997–998.
89. Finer NN, Etches PC, Kamstra B, Tierney AJ, Peliowski A & Ryan CA (1994) Inhaled nitric oxide in infants referred for extracorporeal membrane oxygenation: dose response. *Journal of Pediatrics* **124:**302–308.
90. Dehan M & the Groupe français pédiatrique d'étude du NO inhalé (1940 Inhalational nitric oxide in persistent pulmonary hypertension of the newborn (PPHN). Results of the French multicenter open study. *American Journal of Respiratory and Critical Care Medicine* **149:**A545.
92. Hallmann M & Kankaanpaa K (1980) Evidence of surfactant deficiency in persistence of the fetal circulation. *European Journal of Pediatrics* **134:**129–134.
93. Lotze A, Whitsett JA, Kammerman LA, Ritter M, Taylor GA & Short BL (1990) Surfactant protein A concentrations in tracheal aspirate fluid from infants requiring extracorporeal membrane oxygenation. *Journal of Pediatrics* **116:**435–440.
94. Auten RL, Notter RH, Kendig JW, Davis JM & Shapiro DL (1991) Surfactant treatment of full-term newborns with respiratory failure. *Pediatrics* **87:**101–107.
95. Glick PL, Leach CL, Besner GE et al (1992) Pathophysiology of congenital diaphragmatic hernia III: exogenous surfactant therapy for the high-risk neonate with CDH. *Journal of Pediatrics Surgery* **27:**866–869.
96. Lotze A, Knight FR, Martin GR et al (1993) Improved pulmonary outcome after exogenous surfactant therapy for respiratory failure in term infants requiring extracorporeal membrane oxygenation. *Journal of Pediatrics* **122:**261–268.
97. Leach CL, Fuhrman BP, Morin FC & Rath MG (1993) Perfluorocarbon associated gas exchange (partial liquid ventilation) in respiratory distress syndrome. *Critical Care Medicine* **21:**1270–1278.
98. Peckham GJ & Fox WW (1978) Physiologic factors affecting pulmonary artery pressure in infants with persistent pulmonary hypertension. *Journal of Pediatrics* **93:**1005–1010.
99. Drummond WH, Gregory GA, Heymann MA & Phibbs RA (1981) The independent effects of hyperventilation, tolazoline, and dopamine on infants with persistent pulmonary hypertension. *Journal of Pediatrics* **98:**603–611.
100. Schreiber MD, Heymann MA & Soifer SJ (1986) Increased arterial pH, not decreased PaCO2, attenuates hypoxia induced pulmonary vasoconstriction in newborn lambs. *Pediatric Research* **20:**113–117.
101. Clark RH (1994) High-frequency ventilation. *Journal of Pediatrics* **124:**661–670.
102. Dreyfuss D & Saumon G (1993) Role of tidal volume, FRC, and end-inspiratory volume in the development of pulmonary edema following mechanical ventilation. *American Review of Respiratory Disease* **148:**1194–1203.
103. Meredith KS, deLemos RA, Coalson JJ et al (1989) Role of lung injury in the pathogenesis of hyaline membrane disease in premature baboons. *Journal of Applied Physiology* **66:**2150–2158.
104. Froese AB, McCulloch PR, Sugiura M, Vaclavik S, Possmayer F & Moller F (1989) A comparison of ventilation strategies for the use of high-frequency oscillatory ventilation in the treatment of hyaline membrane disease. *Acta Anaesthesiologica Scandinavica* **33:**102–107.

105. Clark RH, Yoder BA & Sell MS (1994) Prospective, randomized comparison of high frequency oscillation and conventional ventilation in candidates for extracorporeal membrane oxygenation. *Journal of Pediatrics* **124:**447–454.
106. Braner DA, Fineman JR, Change R & Soifer SJ (1993) M&B 22948, a cGMP phosphodiesterase inhibitor, is a pulmonary vasodilator in lambs. *American Journal of Physiology* **264:**H252–H258.
107. Freeman B (1994) Free radical chemistry of nitric oxide. *Chest* **150:**79S–84S.

7

Role of Nitric Oxide in Hypoxic Pulmonary Vasoconstriction

A. Tuan Dinh-Xuan
Jean-Christophe Mercier

INTRODUCTION

The vascular endothelium is not just a simple layer of cells that interposes a physical barrier between the underlying vascular smooth muscle and the circulating blood. It plays a major role in the regulation of vascular tone and platelet function through release of its products of synthesis, namely the nonprostanoid endothelium-derived vasoactive factors.[1] These products are distinct from the arachidonic acid metabolites, prostacyclin and thromboxane A_2, since endothelium-dependent relaxation and contraction occur in tissues pretreated with indomethacin, a potent cyclooxygenase inhibitor. Two major nonprostanoid endothelium-derived vasoactive factors were identified in the early- and mid-1980s, and were initially termed endothelium-derived relaxing factor (EDRF)[2] and endothelium-derived contracting factor (EDCF)[3] respectively. The chemical nature of both factors has now been elucidated, EDRF being identified as the radical gas, nitric oxide (NO),[4,5] and the peptides, endothelins, representing the major EDCF.[6] In the paragraphs that follow, we shall only review the biology and physiology of EDRF (NO). In the last few years, there has been an explosion of information about NO, which is not only involved in the modulation of vascular tone, as initially thought, but also appears to have major roles in neurotransmission, host defense mechanisms, nonspecific immunity, and inflammation.[7–10] As this chapter is about hypoxic pulmonary vasoconstriction, only the effects of NO on the pulmonary vasculature will be reviewed here. After a brief description of endothelium-dependent relaxation mediated by EDRF (NO) in the pulmonary circulation, we shall review evidence showing that NO might play a role in the modulation of pulmonary vascular tone, with a special emphasis on acute hypoxia. Finally, issues that remain either unanswered or controversial will also be briefly discussed at the end. Neither the molecular mechanisms by which NO induces vascular relaxation, nor the physiology of the free radical gas NO, which is used in a new therapy for acute pulmonary hypertension, are going to be discussed here, as these topics are covered in other chapters of this book.

EFFECTS OF HYPOXIA ON THE PULMONARY CIRCULATION

Acute hypoxic pulmonary vasoconstriction (HPV)

The pulmonary vasculature exhibits an enormous capacity for adaptation to general and local changes in blood flow. During exercise, pulmonary blood flow may increase fourfold without raising mean pulmonary artery pressure.[11] Local alveolar hypoxia can cause regional pulmonary vasoconstriction resulting in a reduction in pulmonary perfusion.[12] This regulation of pulmonary vascular tone is probably localized and does not necessarily require neural and/or humoral influences,[13] but the exact mechanisms causing HPV have not as yet been uncovered.[14] In healthy subjects, one can rightly consider that the effects of HPV are usually more beneficial than detrimental. Indeed, by diverting pulmonary blood flow away from poorly ventilated areas of the lungs, HPV reduces ventilation/perfusion mismatching thereby improving gas exchange and arterial oxygenation. In diseased lungs, however, repeated episodes of HPV may pave the way for subsequent development of chronic pulmonary hypertension, a hallmark of chronic obstructive pulmonary disease (COPD). Indeed the latter is the most common group of lung diseases that lead to the development of pulmonary hypertension.[15]

Chronic hypoxic pulmonary hypertension

There is evidence from epidemiological studies to suggest that pulmonary hypertension is an important source of morbidity and a cause of mortality in man.[16] Furthermore, the occurrence and severity of pulmonary hypertension, in turn, determine the prognosis of COPD.[17] Indeed, the higher the pulmonary artery pressure, the poorer the prognosis.[18] It is thought that prolonged alveolar hypoxia, the main characteristic of COPD, is the major determinant of the increased pulmonary vascular tone.[12,13,15] However, the mechanism by which prolonged alveolar hypoxia causes pulmonary hypertension remains unknown.[19] What is known is that structural changes in the pulmonary vessels gradually develop in hypoxic conditions.[20,21] Structural changes involve all three coats of the pulmonary arteries, i.e. the adventitia, the media, and the intima. However, intimal thickening occurs early in the course of the disease, prior to structural alterations in the media and the adventitia. This holds true for both human disease and experimental conditions. Indeed, it is known from detailed histopathological studies that ultrastructural changes in the endothelial cells of pulmonary vessels always occur and can be detected as early as 3 days after exposure to hypoxia.[22] These changes consist of intimal thickening of pulmonary arteries from both the hilum and the lung periphery of rats.[22] The characteristic ultrastructural changes in endothelial cells include a flocculent cytoplasm, small elongated mitochondria, a rough endoplasmic reticulum, and numerous pinocytic vesicles.

That structural changes in the intima may contribute to the rise in pulmonary vascular tone in chronic hypoxia is hardly a surprise, as this can be suspected from what is known about endothelial function. Indeed, a wide variety of vasoactive substances are synthesized or inactivated by the endothelium. For example, the potent vasodilators prostacyclin[23] and platelet-activating factor,[24] and the vasoconstrictor peptides endothelins[6] are synthesized and released by endothelial cells which can also take up, metabolize and inactivate vasoconstrictor substances like serotonin,[25] norepinephrine[26] and prostaglandin $F_{2\alpha}$.[27] The endothelium also produces and expresses on its plasma membrane surface the enzyme that converts angiotensin I into the potent vasoconstrictor angiotensin II.[28] However, the physiological role of these various vasoactive factors is as yet uncertain. It is also unclear as to how these metabolic functions of the endothelium could be affected in disease. Still, disturbance of endothelial-cell metabolism in chronic hypoxia is very likely. For example, pulmonary uptake of propranolol is reduced in patients with emphysema,[29] and in endothelial cells cultured under conditions of chronic hypoxia, the production of thrombomodulin is suppressed and a novel activator of factor X is formed.[30]

PHYSIOLOGICAL ROLES OF NO IN THE PULMONARY CIRCULATION

Endothelium-dependent relaxation of isolated pulmonary artery

As with other vascular beds, endothelium-dependent relaxation mediated by NO also occurs in the pulmonary circulation (Table 1). This was first reported by Furchgott and Zawadzki[2] who described, in their seminal paper, endothelium-dependent relaxation of the isolated cat pulmonary artery in response to acetylcholine. A year later, Chand and Altura[31] were among the first to suggest that impaired pulmonary-artery endothelium-dependent relaxation could lead to increased pulmonary vascular resistance which is seen in various forms of pulmonary hypertension. Since these first two reports, different authors[32–48] have consistently demonstrated endothelium-dependent relaxation of isolated pulmonary arterial rings or strips in various animal species using a large variety of pharmacological agonists (Table 1).

In man, there have been only three reports of endothelium-dependent relaxation in isolated pulmonary arteries obtained from patients undergoing thoracic surgery for lung carcinoma.[49–51] None of these patients were

Table 1. Pulmonary-artery endothelium-dependent relaxation *in vitro* with various agonists in different animal species.

Agonist	Species	Authors	Reference
Acetylcholine & other cholinergic agonists	Cat	Furchgott & Zawadzki	2
	Dog	Chand & Altura	31
		Cherry et al	32
		De Mey & Vanhoutte	33
	Cattle	Ignarro et al	34, 35
	Guinea-pig	Bolton & Clapp	36
	Rat	McMurtry & Morris	37
		Chen & Suzuki	38
	Pig	Pepke-Zaba et al	39
Arachidonic acid	Dog	Chand & Altura	40
		De Mey et al	41
	Cattle	Ignarro et al	35
Bradykinin	Dog	Altura & Chand	42
		Chand & Altura	31, 40
		Cherry et al	32
	Cattle	Ignarro et al	35
Substance P	Rabbit	Tanaka & Grunstein	43
	Guinea-pig	Bolton & Clapp	36
Histamine	Guinea-pig	Satoh & Inui	44
		Abacioglu et al	45
	Rat	Chen & Suzuki	38
ADP/ATP	Dog	De Mey & Vanhoutte	33
Thrombin	Dog	De Mey & Vanhoutte	33
		Christie et al	46
Platelet-activating factor	Rat	McMurtry & Morris	37
Leukotrienes	Guinea-pig	Sakuma et al	47
Norepinephrine	Dog	Miller & Vanhoutte	48
Clonidine	Pig	Pepke-Zaba et al	39

considered to have pulmonary hypertension, thus rendering difficult the evaluation of the role of NO in pulmonary vascular disease in man.[52] However, *in vivo* vasodilatory effects of acetylcholine on the human pulmonary circulation have been known for decades,[53] and since the late 1950s, several reports have convincingly demonstrated impairment of pulmonary vasodilatation in response to infused acetylcholine in patients with various forms of pulmonary hypertension.[54–56] In recent years, a large body of evidence has accumulated to suggest that NO might play a crucial role in the modulation of pulmonary vascular tone in health and disease. Indeed, there are, to date, two main lines of evidence suggesting that NO is produced by various pulmonary cell types and its presence can be detected in the lung. First, both the constitutive and inducible isoforms of the NO synthases have been localized in human lung using immunocytochemical and histochemical methods.[57] Secondly, endothelial cells, epithelial cells, airway and vascular smooth muscle cells, mast cells, macrophages, fibroblasts, and nonadrenergic noncholinergic nerves in the lung are all capable of synthesizing NO in certain conditions.[58] Finally, several authors have recently found the presence of NO in the exhaled air from healthy volunteers and asthmatic patients.[59–62]

NO and basal pulmonary vascular tone

The demonstration of basal release of NO in the pulmonary circulation is important because it might provide the physiological support for the normally low normoxic pulmonary vascular tone at rest. Since NO is extremely labile, direct assessment of its activity in the human pulmonary circulation *in vivo* is difficult. An attractive means of circumventing this difficulty is to study the effects of NO synthase inhibitors, which might provide indirect evidence to better define the role of NO in the modulation of pulmonary vascular tone. However, bearing in mind the potential toxicity of these inhibitors, such studies were initially thought to be only feasible *ex vivo* in isolated perfused lungs. Infusion of both methylene blue and the arginine analog, N^{ω}-nitro-L-arginine methyl ester (L-NAME), into the main pulmonary artery significantly increases basal normoxic pulmonary vascular resistance of isolated perfused lungs from humans, whereas indomethacin has no effect.[63] Recently, two groups of investigators have infused *N*-monomethyl-L-arginine (L-NMMA) directly into the pulmonary circulation of living adults[64] and infants.[65] Both groups found that inhibition of NO release by the L-arginine analog significantly increased pulmonary vascular resistance and decreased pulmonary blood flow velocity in healthy adults[64] as well as in infants with congenital heart disease but normal pulmonary arterial pressure at rest.[65] These results are consistent with those obtained by Cremona et al[63] and suggest that basal release of NO but not of prostanoid products might account at least in part for the low pulmonary vascular tone in humans. The architecture of the pulmonary vascular tree is probably also important, however, and further investigations are needed to assess the respective importance of NO and the particular anatomic disposition of the pulmonary circulation. Also, whether NO is the only paracrine nonprostanoid substance involved is still uncertain. Neither is it known to what extent the role of NO is more (or less) important in the pulmonary circulation than in various systemic vascular beds. Although NO certainly contributes in an important manner to the active vasodilator tone of the systemic vascular bed,[64, 66] the probability remains, however, that NO modulates pulmonary vasoreactivity in normoxia. Indeed, recent evidence suggests that prevention of NO production, either mechanically by rubbing the intimal surface or biochemically by use of NO synthase inhibitors, significantly increases the tension developed in isolated pulmonary vascular rings from humans in response to the α_1-adrenergic vasoconstrictor agonist, phenylephrine.[67–69] Electrical field stimulation causes contraction of vascular tissues through release of norepinephrine from perivascular adrenergic nerve endings. Electrical-field-stimulation-induced contractile response of guinea-pig pulmonary arteries is significantly potentiated by L-NMMA, suggesting that endogenous NO (released from either nerve endings or endothelium) also modulates adrenergic neural pulmonary vasoconstriction.[70]

NO AND THE HYPOXIC PULMONARY VASCULAR BED

Acute alveolar hypoxia

The modulation of pulmonary vascular tone by NO is even more marked during acute alveolar hypoxia. Indeed, in isolated perfused rat lungs, treatment with various NO synthase inhibitors also markedly enhances the pulmonary pressor response to acute hypoxic challenges.[71–76] These results rule out the hypothesis that a blunted NO production causes acute hypoxic pulmonary vasoconstriction. Instead, they suggest that NO activity is increased during acute alveolar hypoxia. They also point out that production of NO by pulmonary endothelium possibly acts as a brake to limit excessive vasoconstriction induced by various chemical and physical stimuli.[77,78] This protective mechanism of NO, modulating pulmonary vasoreactivity and preventing disproportionate pulmonary vasoconstriction, might be of significance in health and pulmonary vascular disease.

Chronic hypoxia

The effect of acute hypoxia has to be clearly differentiated from that of chronic hypoxic conditions. Acute hypoxia likely causes pulmonary vasoconstriction through a direct effect on vascular smooth muscle[79] (Figure 1A). This in turn increases endothelial release of NO, which acts as a protecting mechanism against excessive hypoxic pulmonary vasoconstriction (Figure 1A). But the metabolic effect of hypoxia might, by itself, result in impairment of NO synthesis.[80,81] With prolonged hypoxia, impairment of NO release ensues as a result of reduced synthesis (Figure 1B), depriving the pulmonary circulation of a physiologic protecting mechanism (Figure 1B). Thus, it is reasonable to hypothesize that impairment of NO production, by predisposing the pulmonary vascular bed to excessive and prolonged vasoconstriction, could pave the way for subsequent development of pulmonary hypertension (Figure 1B).[82,83]

In both human[63] and rat[84–87] lungs, basal release of NO seems to be preserved in chronic hypoxia. This conclusion stems from the observation of a raised basal pulmonary vascular tone after inhibition of either NO activity by methylene blue[63] or NO synthesis by various L-arginine analogs.[84–87] Isaacson et al[85] have even found a greater effect of L-NAME in raising basal pulmonary vascular tone in rats with chronic pulmonary hypertension than in normoxic controls. These results suggest that background NO activity is increased in the pulmonary circulation of the chronically hypoxic rats, and that NO participates in a critical manner in the modulation of pulmonary vascular tone in hypoxic pulmonary hypertension. Until we have new methods allowing accurate measurement of NO from pulmonary artery endothelial cells, it will always be difficult to tell whether endothelial NO synthesis is indeed reduced or, on the contrary, enhanced by chronic hypoxia. Instead of speculating on the differences between species, i.e. rats versus humans, it seems reasonable to speculate that during chronic hypoxia, background release of NO is enhanced whereas agonist-stimulated release of NO

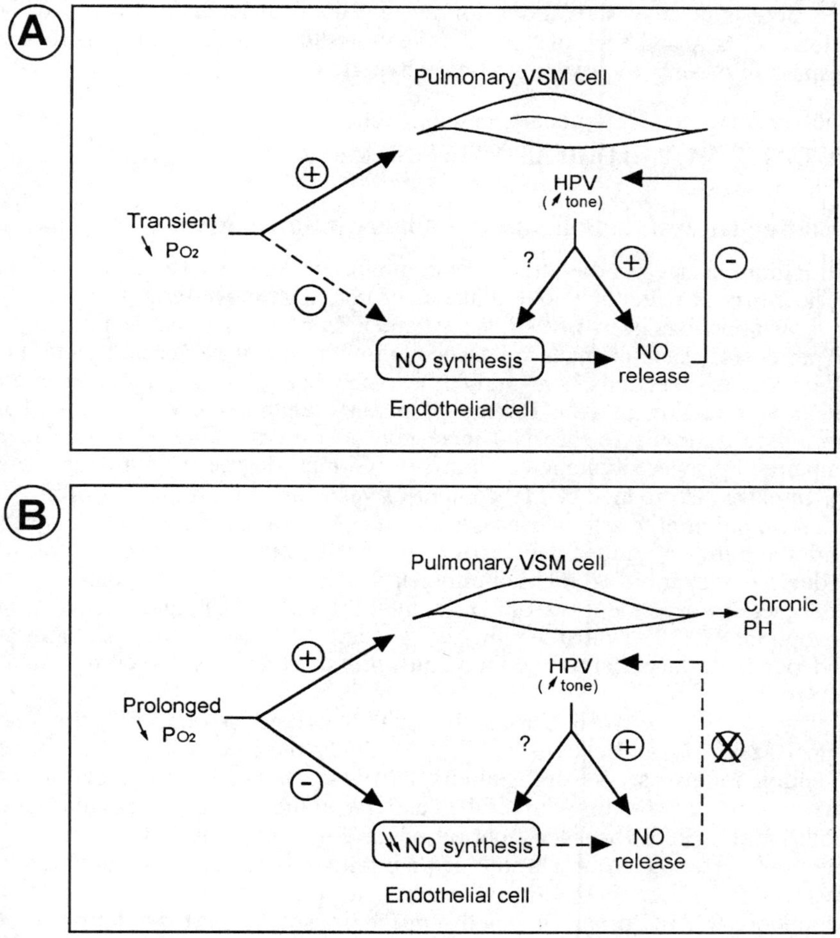

Figure 1. Acute and chronic effects of hypoxia on pulmonary vascular tone and NO release. (A) A transient decrease in partial pressure of oxygen (Po_2) stimulates constriction of pulmonary vascular smooth muscle (VSM) cells, a phenomenon known as hypoxic pulmonary vasoconstriction (HPV). The increase in tone that ensues stimulates NO release which, in turn, modulates pulmonary vascular tone. However, the metabolic effect of hypoxia might already alter NO synthesis. (B) If prolonged, hypoxia eventually causes impairment of NO release as a result of reduced NO synthesis, depriving the pulmonary circulation of a physiologic protecting mechanism, therefore permitting the setting-up of chronic pulmonary hypertension (PH). (From reference 83).

is impaired. It is likely that background release of NO is related to the increased shear stress and pulmonary blood flow which, in turn, stimulate a calcium-activated potassium channel on the endothelial cell membrane that ultimately leads to the release of NO.[88] Thus, it is likely that agonist-activated and flow-induced vasodilations follow two quite different pathways to the release of NO, and each of these pathways could be affected in a distinctive manner in chronic hypoxic pulmonary hypertension.

PUTATIVE PATHOLOGICAL MECHANISMS

Endothelial dysfunction and pulmonary vasoreactivity

Structural changes in the intima are common in pulmonary arteries obtained at necropsy of patients with end-stage chronic obstructive lung disease.[89,90] A logical approach is to investigate whether, in chronic hypoxic pulmonary hypertension, such changes are associated with altered paracrine function of the pulmonary endothelium and, more specifically, with a reduced endothelial production of NO. Bovine pulmonary endothelial cells cultured in normoxia normally release NO in response to bradykinin.[81] This release is impaired by severe hypoxia (15 mmHg).[80] Similar degrees of hypoxia (3 and 17 mmHg) also reduce cGMP content of vascular smooth muscle from isolated rat pulmonary arterial rings as a result of impaired NO release from the endothelium.[91] A milder degree of hypoxia (42 mmHg) is also capable of reducing relaxation of rabbit pulmonary arterial rings in response to the endothelium-dependent vasodilators methacholine, ATP and the calcium ionophore A23187, whilst leaving the relaxant responses to the endothelium-independent vasodilators sodium nitroprusside and isoproterenol unaffected.[80]

The relation between chronic hypoxia and development of pulmonary hypertension is well established.[12,13,15] To study the role of endothelial dysfunction in disease, several authors have assessed the effects of chronic hypoxia on endothelium-derived NO activity in the pulmonary circulation of both animals kept for a long period of time in a hypoxic environment and humans suffering from chronic hypoxic lung disease. Pulmonary endothelium-dependent relaxation in response to acetylcholine and the calcium ionophore A23187 progressively disappears in isolated perfused lungs of rats kept in hypoxic chambers for 1–3 weeks.[92] Similar impairment of relaxation in response to acetylcholine is also reported with pulmonary arterial rings from rats kept in hypoxia from 10 days[93] to 6 weeks.[94] Remarkably, this blunted response is reversed as early as 48 h after the animals are put back to normoxia,[92] and normal relaxation is completely restored 1 week after recovery.[95] However, restoration of normal agonist-induced NO release takes place before regression of pulmonary hypertension on return to normoxia, since on day 2 of recovery normal endothelium-dependent relaxation is seen in rats still having high levels of pulmonary artery pressure.[92] On day 7 of recovery, both NO activity and pulmonary hemodynamics are back to normal.[95] This suggests that normal release of NO from pulmonary endothelial cells is important to maintain a low pulmonary vascular tone. The physiologic importance of NO could probably be further investigated by looking at its basal release both under chronic hypoxia and after normoxic recovery.

Role of hypoxia

Several lines of evidence suggest that appropriate O_2 tension is critical for NO production in the lung. First, acute severe reduction of O_2 tension *in vitro* blunts, or markedly reduces, NO release and/or activity in cultured bovine pulmonary endothelial cells,[81] as well as adult rabbit,[80] rat,[91] and fetal ovine[96] isolated pulmonary arteries. The latter observation is consistent with reports of reduced NO activity in fetal pulmonary circulation[97] where high vascular resistance is thought to be related to low arterial O_2 tension. Secondly, the more hypoxemic the patients with chronic hypoxic pulmonary hypertension, the less the endothelium-dependent relaxation of pulmonary arterial rings.[67,68] Thirdly, in rats kept in hypoxic chambers, normal pulmonary endothelium-dependent relaxation is restored when the animals are put back to normoxia.[92] These results suggest that lack of O_2 probably accounts for reduced NO release in chronic hypoxic pulmonary hypertension, and are consistent with the fact that O_2 is involved in NO synthesis. Altered NO synthase activity could be another explanation for the reduced NO synthesis by pulmonary artery endothelial cells exposed to chronic hypoxia.[98] The mechanisms of this alteration could be at the transcriptional level between the gene encoding the constitutive endothelial NO synthase, which has been recently assigned to the 7q35–7q36 region of chromosome 7,[99,100] and its messenger RNA.

REFERENCES

1. Vane JR, Änggård EE & Botting RM (1990) Regulatory functions of the vascular endolhelium. *New England Journal of Medicine* **323:**27–36.
2. Furchgott RF & Zawadzki JV (1980) The obligatory role of endothelial cells in the relaxation of arterial smooth muscle by acetylcholine. *Nature* **288:** 373–376.
3. Hickey KA, Rubanyi GM, Paul RJ & Highsmith RF (1985) Characterization of a coronary vasoconstrictor produced by cultured endothelial cells. *American Journal of Physiology* **248:**C550–C556.
4. Ignarro LJ, Buga GM, Wood KS, Byrns RE & Chaudhuri G (1987) Endothelium-derived relaxing factor produced and released from artery and vein is nitric oxide. *Proceedings of the National Academy of Sciences USA* **84:**9265–9269.
5. Palmer RMJ, Ferrige AG & Moncada S (1987) Nitric oxide release accounts for the biological activity of endothelium-derived relaxing factor. *Nature* **327:**524–526.
6. Yanagisawa M, Kurihara H, Kimura S, Tomobe Y, Kobayashi M, Mitsui Y, Yazaki Y, Goto K & Masaki T (1988) A novel vasoconstrictor peptide produced by vascular endothelial cells. *Nature* **332:**411–415.
7. Änggård E (1994) Nitric oxide: mediator, murderer, and medicine. *Lancet* **343:**1199–1206.
8. Henry Y, Lepoivre M, Drapier J-C, Ducrocq C, Boucher J-L & Guissani A (1993) EPR characterization of molecular targets for NO in mammalian cells and organelles. *FASEB Journal* **7:**1124–1134.
9. Moncada S & Higgs EA (1993) The L-arginine–nitric oxide pathway. *New England Journal of Medicine* **329:**2002–2012.
10. Nathan CF (1992) Nitric oxide as a secretory product of mammalian cells. *FASEB Journal* **6:**3051–3064.
11. Ehrasam RE, Perruchoud A, Oberholzer M, Burkhart F & Herzog H (1983) Influence of age on pulmonary haemodynamics at rest and during supine exercise. *Clinical Science* **65:**653–660.

12. Fishman AP (1961) Respiratory gases in the regulation of the pulmonary circulation. *Physiological Reviews* **41:**214–280.
13. Fishman AP (1976) Hypoxia on the pulmonary circulation: how and where it acts. *Circulation Research* **38:**221–231.
14. Voelkel NF (1986) Mechanisms of hypoxic pulmonary vasoconstriction. *American Review of Respiratory Disease* **133:**1186–1195.
15. Fishman AP (1976) Chronic cor purmonale. *American Review of Respiratory Disease* **114:** 775–794.
16. Bishop JM (1975) Hypoxia and pulmonary hypertension in chronic bronchitis. *Progress in Respiratory Research* **9:**10–16.
17. Burrows B, Kettel LJ, Niden AH, Rabinowitz M & Diener CF (1972) Patterns of cardiovascular dysfunction in chronic obstructive lung disease. *New England Journal of Medicine* **286:**912–918.
18. Weitzenblum E, Hirth C, Ducolone A, Mirhom R, Rasaholinjanahary J & Ehrhart M (1981) Prognostic value of pulmonary artery pressure in chronic obstructive pulmonary disease. *Thorax* **36:**752–758.
19. Reeves JT & Voelkel NF (1989) Mechanisms of chronic pulmonary hypertension: basic considerations. In Wagenvoort CA & Denolin H (eds) *Pulmonary Circulation: Advances and Controversies*, pp 27–39. Amsterdam: Elsevier.
20. Reid LM (1979) The pulmonary circulation: remodeling in growth and disease. *American Review of Respiratory Disease* **119:**531–546.
21. Reid LM (1986) Structure and function in pulmonary hypertension: new perceptions. *Chest* **89:**279–288.
22. Meyrick B & Reid LM (1978) The effect of continued hypoxia on rat pulmonary arterial circulation: an ultrastructural study. *Laboratory Investigation* **38:**188–200.
23. Moncada S, Gryglewski R, Bunting S & Vane JR (1976) An enzyme isolated from arteries transforms prostaglandin endoperoxides to an unstable substance that inhibits platelet aggregation. *Nature* **263:**663–665.
24. Whatley RE, Lewis MS, Zimmerman GA, McIntyre TM, Parker CJ & Stevens DL (1988) The regulation of synthesis of platelet-activating factor by endothelial cells. *Chest* **93:**110S–111S.
25. Strum JM & Junod AF (1972) Radioautographic demonstration of 5-hydroxytryptamine-^{3}H uptake by pulmonary endothelial cells. *Journal of Cell Biology* **54:**456–467.
26. Hughes J, Gillis CN & Bloom FE (1969) The uptake and disposition of dl-norepinephrine in perfused rat lungs. *Journal of Pharmacology and Experimental Therapeutics* **169:**237–248.
27. Ferreira SH & Vane JR (1967) Prostaglandins: their disappearance from and release into the circulation. *Nature* **216:**868–873.
28. Caldwell PR, Seegal BC, Hsu KC, Das M & Soffer RL (1976) Angiotensin-converting enzyme: vascular endothelial localization. *Science* **191:**1050–1051.
29. Pang JA, Butland RJA, Brooks N, Cattell M & Geddes DM (1982) Impaired lung uptake of propranolol in human pulmonary emphysema. *American Review of Respiratory Disease* **125:**194–198.
30. Ogawa S, Shreeniwas R, Brett J, Clauss M, Furie M & Stern DM (1990) The effect of hypoxia on capillary endothelial cell function: modulation of barrier and coagulant function. *British Journal of Haematology* **75:**517–524.
31. Chand N & Altura BM (1981) Acetylcholine and bradykinin relax intrapulmonary arteries by acting on endothelial cells: role in lung vascular diseases. *Science* **213:**1376–1379.
32. Cherry PD, Furchgott RF, Zawadzki JV & Jothianandan D (1982) Role of endothelial cells in relaxation of isolated arteries by bradykinin. *Proceedings of the National Academy of Sciences USA* **79:**2106–2110.

33. De Mey JG & Vanhoutte PM (1982) Heterogeneous behaviour of the canine arterial and venous wall: importance of the endothelium. *Circulation Research* **51:**439–447.
34. Ignarro LJ, Burke TM, Wood KS, Wolin MS & Kadowitz PJ (1984) Association between cyclic GMP accumulation and acetylcholine elicited relaxation of bovine intrapulmonary artery. *Journal of Pharmacology and Experimental Therapeutics* **228:**682–690.
35. Ignarro LJ, Harbison RG, Wood KS & Kadowitz PJ (1986) Activation of purified soluble guanylate cyclase by endothelium-derived relaxing factor from intrapulmonary artery and vein: stimulation by acetylcholine, bradykinin and arachidonic acid. *Journal of Pharmacology and Experimental Therapeutics* **237:**893–900.
36. Bolton TB & Clapp LH (1986) Endothelial-dependent relaxant actions of carbachol and substance P in arterial smooth muscle. *British Journal of Pharmacology* **87:**713–723.
37. McMurtry IF & Morris KG (1986) Platelet-activating factor causes pulmonary vasodilation in the rat. *American Review of Respiratory Disease* **134:**757–762.
38. Chen GF & Suzuki H (1989) Direct and indirect actions of acetylcholine and histamine on intra pulmonary artery and vein muscles of the rat. *Japanese Journal of Physiology* **39:**51–65.
39. Pepke-Zaba J, Higenbottam TW, Dinh-Xuan AT, Ridden C & Kealey T (1993) α-adrenoceptor stimulation of porcine pulmonary arteries. *European Journal of Pharmacology* **235:**169–175.
40. Chand N & Altura BM (1981) Bradykinin and arachidonic acid, but not β-adrenergic or H_2-histaminergic vasorelaxation is mediated by intact endothelial cells. *Clinical Research* **29:**443–447.
41. De Mey JG, Claeys M & Vanhoutte PM (1982) Endothelium dependent inhibitory effects of acetylcholine, adenosine triphosphate, thrombin and arachidonic acid in the canine femoral artery. *Journal of Pharmacology and Experimental Therapeutics* **222:**166–173.
42. Altura BM & Chand N (1981) Bradykinin-induced relaxation of renal and pulmonary arteries is dependent on intact endothelial cells. *British Journal of Pharmacology* **74:**10–11.
43. Tanaka DT & Grunstein MM (1985) Vasoactive effects of substance P on isolated rabbit pulmonary artery. *Journal of Applied Physiology* **58:**1291–1297.
44. Satoh H & Inui J (1984) Endothelial cell-dependent relaxation and contraction induced by histamine in the isolated guinea-pig pulmonary artery. *European Journal of Pharmacology* **97:**321–324.
45. Abacioglu N, Ercan ZS, Kanzik L, Zengil H, Demiryurek T & Turker RK (1987) Endothelium-dependent relaxing effect of histamine on the isolated guinea pig main pulmonary artery strips. *Agents and Action* **22:**30–35.
46. Christie MI, Griffith TM & Lewis MJ (1989) A comparison of basal and agonist-stimulated release of endothelium-derived relaxing factor from different arteries. *British Journal of Pharmacology* **98:**397–406.
47. Sakuma I, Gross SS & Levi R (1987) Peptidoleukotrienes induce an endothelium-dependent relaxation of guinea pig main pulmonary artery and thoracic aorta. *Prostaglandins* **34:**685–696.
48. Miller VM & Vanhoutte PM (1985) Endothelial α_2-adrenoceptors in canine pulmonary and systemic blood vessels. *European Journal of Pharmacology* **118:**123–129.
49. Greenberg B, Rhoden K & Barnes PJ (1987) Endothelium-dependent relaxation of human pulmonary arteries. *American Journal of Physiology* **252:**H434–H438.
50. Thom S, Hughes A, Martin G & Sever PS (1987) Endothelium-dependent relaxation in isolated human arteries and veins. *Clinical Science* **73:**547–552.
51. Dinh-Xuan AT, Higenbottam TW, Clelland CA, Pepke-Zaba J, Wells FC & Wallwork J (1990) Acetylcholine and adenosine diphosphate cause endothelium-dependent

relaxation of isolated human pulmonary arteries. *European Respiratory Journal* **3:**633–638.
52. McCormack D (1990) Endothelium-derived relaxing factors and the human pulmonary circulation. *Lung* **168 (Suppl):**35–42.
53. Fritts HW Jr, Harris P, Clauss RH, Odell JE & Cournand A (1958) The effect of acetylcholine on the human pulmonary circulation under normal and hypoxic conditions. *Journal of Clinical Investigation* **37:**99–108.
54. Harris P (1957) Influence of acetylcholine on the pulmonary arterial pressure. *British Heart Journal* **19:**272–278.
55. Marshall RJ, Helmholz HF & Shepherd JT (1959) Effect of acetylcholine on pulmonary vascular resistance in a patient with idiopathic pulmonary hypertension. *Circulation* **20:**391–395.
56. Wood P (1958) Pulmonary hypertension with special reference to the vasoconstrictive factor. *British Heart Journal* **20:**557–570.
57. Kobzik L, Bredt DS, Lowenstein CJ, Drazen JM, Gaston B, Sugarbaker D & Stamler JS (1993) Nitric oxide synthase in human and rat lung: immunocytochemical and histochemical localization. *American Journal of Respiratory Cell and Molecular Biology* **9:**371–377.
58. Barnes PJ & Belvisi MG (1993) Nitric oxide and lung disease. *Thorax* **48:**1034–1043.
59. Alving K, Weitzberg E & Lundberg JM (1993) Increased amount of nitric oxide in exhaled air of asthmatics. *European Respiratory Journal* **6:**1368–1370.
60. Borland CDR, Cox Y & Higenbottam TW (1993) Measurement of exhaled nitric oxide in man. *Thorax* **48:**1160–1162.
61. Gustafsson LE, Leone AM, Persson MG, Wiklund NP & Moncada S (1991) Endogenous nitric oxide is present in exhaled air of rabbits, guinea pigs and humans. *Biochemical and Biophysical Research Communications* **181:**852–857.
62. Persson MG, Wiklund NP & Gustafsson LE (1993) Endogenous nitric oxide in single exhalations and the change during exercise. *American Review of Respiratory Disease* **148:**1210–1214.
63. Cremona G, Higenbottam TW, Dinh-Xuan AT, Wells FC, Large SR, Stewart S & Wallwork J (1991) Inhibitors of endothelium-derived relaxing factor increase pulmonary vascular resistance in isolated perfused human lungs (abstract). *European Respiratory Journal* **4 (Suppl 14):**336s.
64. Stamler JS, Loh E, Roddy M-A, Currie KE & Creager MA (1994) Nitric oxide regulates basal systemic and pulmonary vascular resistance in healthy humans. *Circulation* **89:**2035–2040.
65. Celermajer DS, Dollery C, Burch M & Deanfield JE (1994) Role of endothelium in the maintenance of low pulmonary vascular tone in normal children. *Circulation* **89:**2041–2044.
66. Vallance P, Leone A, Calver A, Collier J & Moncada S (1992) Accumulation of an endogenous inhibitor of nitric oxide synthesis in chronic renal failure. *Lancet* **339:**572–575.
67. Dinh-Xuan AT, Higenbottam TW, Clelland CA, Pepke-Zaba J, Cremona G, Butt AY, Large SR, Wells FC & Wallwork J (1991) Impairment of endothelium-dependent pulmonary-artery relaxation in chronic obstructive lung disease. *New England Journal of Medicine* **314:**1539–1547.
68. Dinh-Xuan AT, Higenbottam TW & Wallwork J (1992) Relationship between chronic hypoxia and *in vitro* pulmonary relaxation mediated by endothelium-derived relaxing factors in human chronic obstructive lung disease. *Angiology* **43:**350–356.
69. Dinh-Xuan AT, Pepke-Zaba J, Butt AY, Cremona G & Higenbottam TW (1993) Impairment of pulmonary-artery endothelium-dependent relaxation in chronic obstructive lung disease is not due to dysfunction of endothelial cell membrane

receptors nor to L-arginine deficiency. *British Journal of Pharmacology* **109:**587–591.

70. Liu SF, Crawley DE, Evans TW & Barnes PJ (1991) Endogenous nitric oxide modulates adrenergic neural vasoconstriction in guinea-pig pulmonary artery. *British Journal of Pharmacology* **104:**565–569.
71. Archer SL, Tolins JP, Raij L & Weir EK (1989) Hypoxic pulmonary vasoconstriction is enhanced by inhibition of the synthesis of an endothelium-derived relaxing factor. *Biochemical and Biophysical Research Communications* **164:**1198–1205.
72. Brashers VL, Peach MJ & Rose CE Jr (1988) Augmentation of hypoxic pulmonary vasoconstriction in the isolated perfused rat lung by *in vitro* antagonists of endothelium-dependent relaxation. *Journal of Clinical Investigation* **82:** 1495–1502.
73. Liu SF, Crawley DE, Barnes PJ & Evans TW (1991) Endothelium-derived relaxing factor inhibits hypoxic pulmonary vasoconstriction in rats. *American Review of Respiratory Disease* **143:**32–37.
74. Mazmanian GM, Baudet B, Brink C, Cerrina J, Kirkiacharian S & Weiss M (1989) Methylene blue potentiates vascular reactivity in isolated rat lungs. *Journal of Applied Physiology* **66:**1040–1045.
75. Persson MG, Gustafsson LE, Wiklund NP, Moncada S & Hedqvist P (1990) Endogenous nitric oxide as a probable modulator of pulmonary circulation and hypoxic pressor response *in vivo*. *Acta Physiologica Scandinavica* **140:**449–457.
76. Robertson BE, Warren JB & Nye PCG (1990) Inhibition of nitric oxide synthesis potentiates hypoxic vasoconstriction in isolated rat lungs. *Experimental Physiology* **75:**255–257.
77. Crawley DE, Liu SF, Evans TW & Barnes PJ (1990) Inhibitory role of endothelium-derived relaxing factor in rat and human pulmonary arteries. *British Journal of Pharmacology* **101:**166–170.
78. Yamaguchi T, Rodman DM, O'Brien RF & McMurtry IF (1989) Modulation of pulmonary artery contraction by endothelium-derived relaxing factor. *European Journal of Pharmacology* **161:**259–262.
79. Murray TR, Chen L, Marshall BE & Macarak EJ (1990) Hypoxic contraction of cultured pulmonary vascular smooth muscle cells. *American Journal of Respiratory Cell and Molecular Biology* **3:**457–465.
80. Johns RA, Linden JM & Peach MJ (1989) Endothelium-dependent relaxation and cyclic GMP accumulation in rabbit pulmonary artery are selectively impaired by moderate hypoxia. *Circulation Research* **65:**1508–1515.
81. Warren JB, Maltby NH, McCormack D & Barnes PJ (1989) Pulmonary endothelium-derived relaxing factor is impaired in hypoxia. *Clinical Science* **77:** 671–676.
82. Dinh-Xuan AT (1992) Endothelial modulation of pulmonary vascular tone. *European Respiratory Journal* **5:**757–762.
83. Dinh-Xuan AT (1993) Disorders of endothelium-dependent relaxation in pulmonary disease. *Circulation* **87(Suppl V):**V81–V87.
84. Hampl V, Archer SL, Nelson DP & Weir EK (1993) Chronic EDRF inhibition and hypoxia: effects on pulmonary circulation and systemic blood pressure. *Journal of Applied Physiology* **75:**1748–1757.
85. Isaacson TC, Hampl V, Weir EK, Nelson DP & Archer SL (1994) Increased endothelium-derived NO in hypertensive pulmonary circulation of chronically hypoxic rats. *Journal of Applied Physiology* **76:**933–940.
86. Russell P, Wright C, Kapeller G, Barer G & Howard P (1993) Attenuation of chronic hypoxic pulmonary hypertension in rats by cyclooxygenase products and by nitric oxide. *European Respiratory Journal* **6:**1501–1506.
87. Zhao L, Crawley DE, Hughes JMB, Evans TW & Winter RJD (1993) Endothelium-derived relaxing factor activity in rat lung during hypoxic pulmonary vascular remodeling. *Journal of Applied Physiology* **74:**1061–1065.

88. Cooke JP, Rossitch E Jr, Andon NA, Loscalzo J & Dzau VJ (1991) Flow activates an endothelial potassium channel to release an endogenous nitrovasodilator. *Journal of Clinical Investigation* **88:**1663–1671.
89. Magee F, Wright JL, Wiggs BR, Paré PD & Hogg JC (1988) Pulmonary vascular structure and function in chronic obstructive pulmonary disease. *Thorax* **43:**183–189.
90. Wilkinson M, Langhorne CA, Health D, Barer GR & Howard P (1988) A pathophysiological study of 10 cases of hypoxic cor pulmonale. *Quarterly Journal of Medicine* **66:**65–85.
91. Rodman DM, Yamaguchi T, Hasunuma K, O'Brien RF & McMurtry IF (1990) Effects of hypoxia on endothelium-dependent relaxation of rat pulmonary artery. *American Journal of Physiology* **258:**L207–L214.
92. Adnot S, Raffestin B, Eddahibi S, Braquet P & Chabrier P-E (1991) Loss of endothelium-dependent relaxant activity in the pulmonary circulation of rats exposed to chronic hypoxia. *Journal of Clinical Investigation* **87:**155–162.
93. Maruyama J & Maruyama K (1994) Impaired nitric oxide-dependent responses and their recovery in hypertensive pulmonary arteries of rats. *American Journal of Physiology* **266:**H2476–H2478.
94. Leach RM, Twort CHC, Ward JPT & Cameron IR (1990) Endothelial dysfunction in isolated pulmonary arteries from chronically hypoxic rats (abstract). *Thorax* **45:**808.
95. Tozzi CA & Riley DJ (1990) Impaired endothelium-dependent relaxation of pulmonary artery rings is restored after recovery from hypoxic pulmonary hypertension (abstract). *American Review of Respiratory Disease* **141(Suppl):**A350.
96. Shaul PW, Farrar MA & Zellers TM (1992) Oxygen modulates endothelium-derived relaxing factor production in fetal pulmonary arteries. *American Journal of Physiology* **31:**H355–H364.
97. Abman SH, Chatfield BA, Rodman DM, Hall SL & McMurtry IF (1991) Maturational changes in endothelium-derived relaxing factor activity of ovine pulmonary arteries *in vitro*. *American Journal of Physiology* **260:**L280–L285.
98. Giaid A & Saleh D (1995) Reduced expression of endothelial nitric oxide synthase in the lungs of patients with pulmonary hypertension. *New England Journal of Medicine* **333:**214–221.
99. Marsden PA, Heng HHQ, Scherer SW, Stewart RJ, Hall AV, Shi X-M, Tsui L-C & Schappert KT (1993) Structure and chromosomal localization of the human constitutive endothelial nitric oxide synthase gene. *Journal of Biological Chemistry* **268:**17478–17488.
100. Robinson LJ, Weremowicz S, Morton CC & Michel T (1994) Isolation and chromosomal localization of the human endothelial nitric oxide synthase (NOS3) gene. *Genomics* **19:**350–357.

8

Role of Nitric Oxide in Chronic Obstructive Pulmonary Disease

Joan Albert Barberà

INTRODUCTION

Nitric oxide (NO) is a ubiquitous molecule involved in numerous physiological functions as well as in the pathogenesis of different diseases. It acts as a signaling molecule in endothelial and nerve cells and as a cytotoxic agent when released by macrophages and neutrophils.[1] When administered by inhalation, NO has a selective pulmonary vasodilator action[2,3] which can also improve pulmonary gas exchange in patients with adult (or acute) respiratory distress syndrome (ARDS)[4] and in persistent pulmonary hypertension of the newborn.[5] NO has also been identified as an endogenous neurotransmitter of nonadrenergic noncholinergic inhibitory nerves of human airways with bronchodilator effect when assessed *in vitro*.[6] Experimental studies in guinea-pigs and rabbits have shown that inhaled NO can modulate the increase in airway tone induced by methacholine.[7,8]

All of the above actions of NO may be particularly relevant in the pathogenesis of and therapeutical approach to patients with chronic obstructive pulmonary disease (COPD), a disorder characterized by nonreversible airflow obstruction, impairment of gas exchange and, eventually, pulmonary hypertension.

REDUCED SYNTHESIS OF NO IN COPD

Reduced synthesis of NO by the endothelial cells of pulmonary vessels may be involved in the development of pulmonary hypertension in patients with COPD. Dinh-Xuan and co-workers[9] studied the endothelium-dependent relaxation of pulmonary artery rings in patients who had undergone heart–lung transplantation for end-stage obstructive lung disorders (cystic fibrosis and α_1-antitrypsin deficiency). They showed a lower relaxation in response to both acetylcholine and ADP in this group of patients than in subjects with normal lung function. Moreover, the arteries of patients with airflow obstruction responded normally to nitroprusside, whereas *N*-monomethyl-L-arginine (L-NMMA) (a competitive inhibitor of NO synthesis) further impaired the vascular relaxation induced by acetylcholine and ADP. These findings are consistent with impairment of the endothelial synthesis of NO in chronic obstructive lung disorders. The underlying mechanism of the endothelial impairment is not completely understood, but it has been suggested that it might be related to the chronic hypoxemia that these patients show, as the pulmonary endothelial production of NO is dependent on the alveolar $P\text{O}_2$.[10]

Moreover, Giaid & Saleh[11] have recently shown a reduced expression of endothelial NO synthase in pulmonary arteries of patients with pulmonary hypertension. Contrasting with the conspicuous expression of NO synthase in the lungs of control subjects, little or no expression was found in the endothelium of pulmonary arteries with severe histologic abnormalities in patients with pulmonary hypertension. Patients with primary pulmonary hypertension and plexogenic arteriopathy had the lowest expression of NO synthase. COPD patients with secondary pulmonary hypertension showed greater expression of the enzyme than those with primary pulmonary hypertension, but significantly lower than control cases.[11]

Interestingly, the severity of the morphological abnormalities in pulmonary muscular arteries of COPD patients is inversely related to the expression of NO synthase[11] and the relaxation response to acetylcholine.[9] These observations are in agreement with previous data reported by our group showing that in COPD patients the enlargement of the intima in small arteries may interfere with the vascular regulation of the balance between ventilation and perfusion.[12]

Increased concentrations of NO in exhaled air have been shown in patients with untreated bronchial asthma,[13] bronchiectasis,[14] and during upper respiratory tract infections.[15] In contrast, patients with bronchial asthma treated with corticosteroids exhibit NO concentrations in exhaled air that are similar to healthy subjects.[13] The most likely source of the increase in exhaled NO is the activation of the inducible isoform of NO synthase in epithelial and infiltrating inflammatory cells (macrophages, neutrophils) of the airways of patients with bronchial asthma or bronchiectasis. Nevertheless, it cannot be excluded that NO synthesized by the pulmonary vascular endothelium might also contribute to the NO found in exhaled air.[16]

Unfortunately, at the present time there are no data available on the concentrations of NO in exhaled air of COPD patients. However, it has been shown that smokers exhibit reduced concentrations of NO in exhaled air.[17,18] The reason for such a reduction is not clear, but it has been suggested that it may be related to the toxic damage to the NO-producing epithelial cells of the airways caused by tobacco smoke or by an increase in endogenous inhibitors of NO synthase.[17,18] Accordingly, it could be speculated that patients with COPD might also exhibit a reduced concentration of exhaled NO as a result of both diminished synthesis in endothelial cells of pulmonary arteries and the effects of tobacco smoke on airway epithelium.

EFFECT OF INHALED NO ON RESPIRATORY SYSTEM RESISTANCE

The identification of NO as a mediator of nonadrenergic noncholinergic regulation of airway tone[6] and its bronchodilator effect in experimental animals after methacholine-induced bronchoconstriction[7,8] has provided the rationale for its use as a potential bronchodilator in airway obstructive disorders.

In patients with bronchial asthma, Högman and co-workers[19] have shown that inhaled NO, at a concentration of 80 parts per million (ppm), exerted a moderate bronchodilator effect increasing specific airway conductance (G_{aw}) from 0.4±0.2 to 0.6±0.2 (kPa s^{-1}). However, such a bronchodilatory effect was much lower than that induced by salbutamol, indicating that inhaled NO caused only modest bronchodilation in patients with bronchial asthma, even when used at high concentrations.

In patients with COPD, the same group of investigators[19] showed that the inhalation of 80 ppm of NO over 10 min exerted no effect on the specific airway conductance, measured 10–20 s after termination of the NO inhalation. Since the lack of bronchodilator effect of NO could be due to its instantaneous loss of activity when returning the inspired concentration to baseline values, our group has used the forced oscillation technique to assess the changes in respiratory system resistance simultaneous with NO inhalation.[20] We studied eight patients with COPD (7M/1F; mean age 66±7 years; forced expiratory volume in 1 s (FEV_1) 37±17% of predicted) and eight healthy subjects (7M/1F; mean age 33±4 years; FEV_1 108±14% pred) during the inhalation of NO (40 ppm). Total resistance (Rrs) and reactance (Xrs) of the respiratory system were continuously recorded at baseline, during NO inhalation, and after its termination. At baseline, patients with COPD showed higher Rrs than healthy subjects (4.97±2.19 versus 2.29±0.65 hPa/ls). During NO inhalation, no significant change in Rrs or in Xrs was observed (Figure 1). The mean variation in Rrs while NO was being inhaled was negligible and similar in the two groups (–0.10±0.13 hPa/l s in COPD patients and –0.02±0.13 hPa/l s in healthy subjects). Accordingly, the results of our study[20] and those of Högman et al[19] show that NO exerts no effect on bronchial tone in patients with COPD, at concentrations of both 40 and 80 ppm.

EFFECT OF INHALED NO ON PULMONARY HEMODYNAMICS AND GAS EXCHANGE

Rossaint and co-workers[4] have shown that inhaled NO improved arterial oxygenation in patients with ARDS. This effect was attributed to a selective increase in perfusion of ventilated lung areas accessible to inhaled NO, which ameliorated the ventilation–perfusion ($\dot{V}_A/\dot{Q}$) imbalance. However, this is not an invariable effect, as arterial oxygen desaturation may develop in a

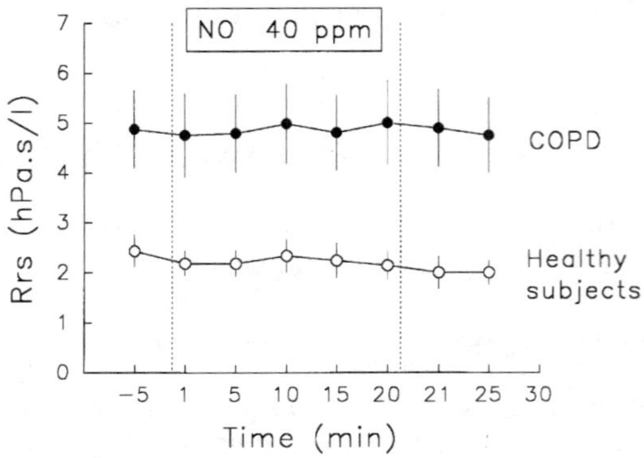

Figure 1. Time course of respiratory system resistance (Rrs) before, during, and after the inhalation of NO (40 ppm) in healthy subjects (○) and in patients with COPD (●). Dotted lines delimit the period of NO inhalation. Patients with COPD showed higher Rrs values than healthy subjects ($P<0.05$). However, no changes in Rrs were observed during NO inhalation in either of the two groups.

proportion of patients inhaling NO.[21] It is well known that vasodilator agents may worsen pulmonary gas exchange by reversing hypoxic vasoconstriction, a mechanism that plays an important role in improving the matching of ventilation and perfusion in COPD.[22] Accordingly, it can be speculated that the detrimental effect of NO on gas exchange observed in some patients could be due to the reversal of hypoxic vasoconstriction in those cases where this mechanism contributes to the maintenance of adequate $\dot{V}_A/\dot{Q}$ balance.

The effect of inhaled NO on COPD was first investigated by Adnot and associates,[23] who performed a dose–response study of the hemodynamic and gas exchange effects of inhaled NO, as compared with intravenous acetylcholine. They showed that inhaled NO produced a significant decrease in pulmonary artery pressure (PAP) at concentrations as low as 5 ppm, and that higher concentrations resulted in a further decrease in PAP in a dose-dependent manner. In contrast, changes in arterial $P\text{O}_2$ were observed only at concentrations of 40 ppm (from 57±3 to 60±3 mmHg), and not at lower concentrations. Moinard and co-workers[24] evaluated the effect of 15 ppm NO, inhaled over 10 min, in 14 COPD patients with severe airflow obstruction. PAP decreased moderately with NO inhalation (from 24.3±10.4 to 19.2±8.6 mmHg), whereas arterial $P\text{O}_2$ did not change (59.4±9.5 and 59.0±10.2, breathing room air and NO respectively). The latter was consistent with the absence of changes in $\dot{V}_A/\dot{Q}$ distributions (logS.D. Q, 1.2±0.3 and 1.1±0.3 means ± S.D.). This lack of effect of NO on gas exchange could be explained by the low dose of NO used. However, it is interesting to note that, whereas the mean value of $P\text{aO}_2$ increased during NO inhalation in the study by Adnot et al,[23] and it did not change in the study by Moinard et al,[24] the individual responses in both studies were quite variable, some patients showing a decrease in $P\text{aO}_2$ during NO inhalation.

To investigate further the effects of inhaled NO on gas exchange in COPD, specifically the effect on hypoxic pulmonary vasoconstriction, we studied 13 patients with advanced COPD (FEV_1, 28±2% pred.) while breathing NO (40 ppm) and 100% oxygen.[25] NO inhalation decreased the mean PAP, from 25.9±2.0 to 21.5±1.7 mmHg (Figure 2), and the $Pa\text{O}_2$, from 56±2 to 53±2 mmHg. The latter resulted from worsening of $\dot{V}_A/\dot{Q}$ distributions, as shown by a greater dispersion of the blood flow distribution (logS.D. Q, from 1.11±0.1 to 1.22±0.1) (Figure 3) and an increased proportion of lung units with low $\dot{V}_A/\dot{Q}$ ratio (from 5.3±1.7% to 8.3±3.0% of blood flow) (Figure 4). Oxygen breathing reduced the mean PAP to 23.4±2.1 mmHg and caused greater $\dot{V}_A/\dot{Q}$ mismatch than NO (logS.D. Q, 1.49±0.12; blood flow to low $\dot{V}_A/\dot{Q}$ units, 17.4±3.8% (Figures 3 and 4). The intrapulmonary shunt on breathing room air was small (2.7±0.9%) and did not change when breathing NO or O_2. These

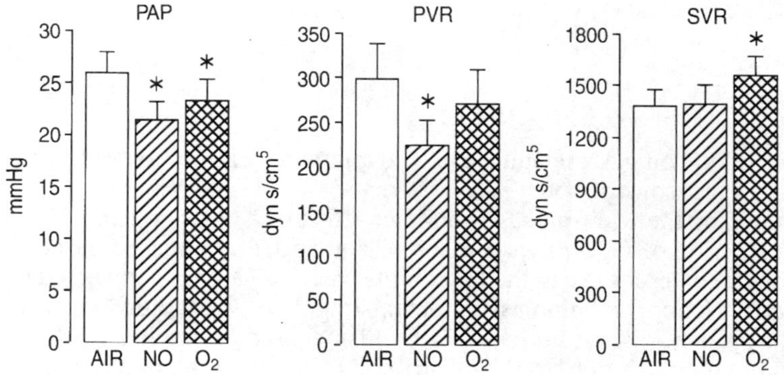

Figure 2. Effects of 40 ppm NO and 100% O_2 breathing on PAP, pulmonary vascular resistance (PVR) and systemic vascular resistance (SVR). * $P<0.05$ compared with room air values.

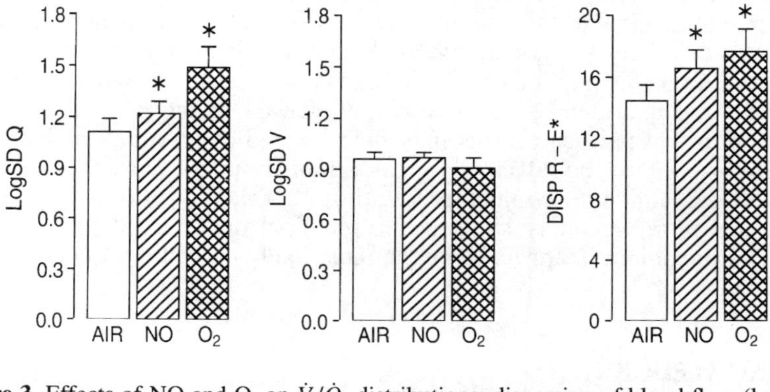

Figure 3. Effects of NO and O_2 on $\dot{V}_A/\dot{Q}$ distributions: dispersion of blood flow (logS.D. Q, normal <0.6) and ventilation (logS.D. V, normal <0.6) distributions, and dispersion of retention minus excretion of inert gases (DISP R-E*, normal <3). * $P<0.05$ compared with room air values.

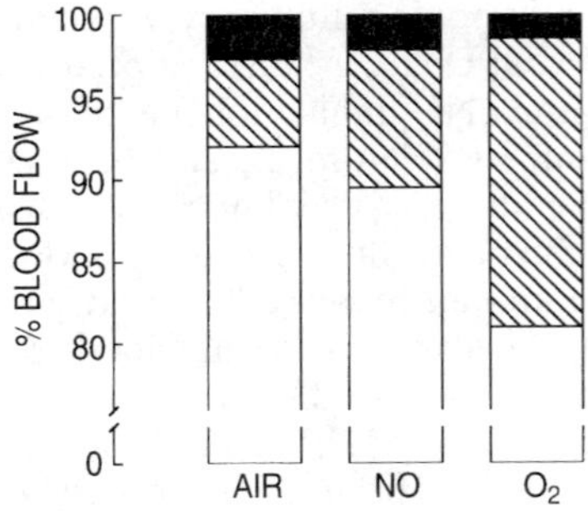

Figure 4. Percentage of blood flow perfusing alveolar units with normal $\dot{V}_A/\dot{Q}$ (ratio 0.1–10; □), low $\dot{V}_A/\dot{Q}$ (ratio 0.005–0.1; ▧), and shunt (ratio <0.005;■), during breathing of room air, NO, and O_2.

effects of NO on gas exchange can be explained by inhibition of hypoxic pulmonary vasoconstriction. The differences between NO and O_2 can be explained by the widespread vasodilator effect of NO, as opposed to the more limited action of O_2 on hypoxic alveolar units with increased vascular tone. The higher alveolar $P\text{O}_2$ in the latter units when breathing O_2 reversed hypoxic vasoconstriction and unmasked preexisting low $\dot{V}_A/\dot{Q}$ ratio areas, thereby exerting a major deterioration of $\dot{V}_A/\dot{Q}$ mismatch. By contrast, the detrimental effect of NO inhalation on $\dot{V}_A/\dot{Q}$ distributions, through dilation of vessels constricted by hypoxia, might well be balanced by concomitant vasodilation in units with normal $\dot{V}_A/\dot{Q}$ ratios, thus minimizing the overall gas exchange impairment. Accordingly, it can be concluded that, in COPD, inhaled NO causes a moderate decrease in PAP, but at the same time it can worsen gas exchange due to the reversal of hypoxic pulmonary vasoconstriction.

A potential clinical implication of these results is that, in patients in whom hypoxemia is caused essentially by $\dot{V}_A/\dot{Q}$ imbalance rather than by shunt (COPD, idiopathic pulmonary fibrosis), inhaled NO can worsen gas exchange due to the impairment of the hypoxic regulation of the matching between ventilation and perfusion. This may help in predicting which patients with respiratory failure should show a greater improvement of gas exchange with inhaled NO. Patients without preexisting chronic lung disease, in whom increased intrapulmonary shunt is the principal determinant of hypoxemia (ARDS, pneumonia), appear to be the most likely candidates to benefit from NO inhalation.

ACKNOWLEDGEMENTS

This work was supported by the Fondo de Investigaciones Sanitarias (FIS 94/1009), the Sociedad Española de Neumología y Cirugía Torácica (SEPAR/1992), and the Fundació Catalana de Pneumologia (FUCAP/1993).

REFERENCES

1. Moncada S & Higgs A (1993) The L-arginine–nitric oxide pathway. *New England Journal of Medicine* **329:**2002–2012.
2. Pepke-Zaba J, Higenbottam TW, Dinh-Xuan AT, Stone D & Wallwork J (1991) Inhaled nitric oxide as a cause of selective pulmonary vasodilation in pulmonary hypertension. *Lancet* **338:**1173–1174.
3. Frostell C, Fratacci MD, Wain JC, Jones R & Zapol WM (1991) Inhaled nitric oxide: a selective pulmonary vasodilator reversing hypoxic pulmonary vasoconstriction. *Circulation* **83:**2038–2047.
4. Rossaint R, Falke KJ, López F, Slama K, Pison U & Zapol WM (1993) Inhaled nitric oxide for the adult respiratory distress syndrome. *New England Journal of Medicine* **328:**399–405.
5. Roberts JD, Polaner DM, Lang P & Zapol WM (1992) Inhaled nitric oxide in persistent pulmonary hypertension of the newborn. *Lancet* **340:**819–820.
6. Belvisi MG, Stretton CD, Yacoub M & Barnes PJ (1992) Nitric oxide is the endogenous neurotransmitter of bronchodilator nerves in humans. *European Journal of Pharmacology* **210:**221–222.
7. Dupuy PM, Shore SA, Drazen JM, Frostell C, Hill A & Zapol WM (1992) Bronchodilator action of inhaled nitric oxide in guinea pigs. *Journal of Clinical Investigation* **90:**421–428.
8. Högman M, Frostell C, Arnberg H & Hedenstierna G (1993) Inhalation of nitric oxide modulates methacholine-induced bronchoconstriction in the rabbit. *European Respiratory Journal* **6:**177–180.
9. Dinh-Xuan AT, Higenbottam TW, Clelland CA, Pepke-Zaba J, Cremona G, Butt AY, Large SR, Wells FC & Wallwork J (1991) Impairment of endothelium-dependent pulmonary-artery relaxation in chronic obstructive pulmonary disease. *New England Journal of Medicine* **324:**1539–1547.
10. McQuillan LP, Leung CK, Marsden PA, Kotsky SK & Kourembanas S (1994) Hypoxia inhibits expression of eNOS via transcriptional and posttranscriptional mechanisms. *American Journal of Physiology* **267:**1921–1927.
11. Giaid A & Saleh D (1995) Reduced expression of endothelial nitric oxide synthase in the lungs of patients with pulmonary hypertension. *New England Journal of Medicine* **333:**214–221.
12. Barberà JA, Riverola A, Roca J, Ramírez J, Wagner PD, Ros D, Wiggs BR & Rodriguez-Roisin R (1994) Pulmonary vascular abnormalities and ventilation-perfusion relationships in mild chronic obstructive pulmonary disease. *American Journal of Respiratory and Critical Care Medicine* **149:**423–429.
13. Kharitonov SA, Yates D, Robbins RA, Logan-Sinclair R, Shinebourne EA & Barnes PJ (1994) Increased nitric oxide in exhaled air of asthmatic patients. *Lancet* **343:**133–135.
14. Kharitonov SA, Wells AU, O'Connor BJ, Cole PJ, Hansell DM, Logan-Sinclair RB & Barnes PJ (1995) Elevated levels of exhaled nitric oxide in bronchiectasis. *American Journal of Respiratory and Critical Care Medicine* **151:**1889–1893.
15. Kharitonov SA, Yates D & Barnes PJ (1995) Increased nitric oxide in exhaled air of normal human subjects with upper respiratory tract infections. *European Respiratory Journal* **8:**295–297.
16. Cremona G, Higenbottam T, Takao M, Hall L & Bower EA (1995) Exhaled nitric oxide in isolated pig lungs. *Journal of Applied Physiology* **78:**59–63.
17. Persson MG, Zetterström O, Agrenius V, Ihre E & Gustafsson LE (1994) Single-breath nitric oxide measurements in asthmatic patients and smokers. *Lancet* **343:**146–147.

18. Schilling J, Holzer P, Guggenbach M, Gyurech D, Marathia K & Geroulanos S (1994) Reduced endogenous nitric oxide in the exhaled air of smokers and hypertensives. *European Respiratory Journal* **7:**467–471.
19. Högman M, Frostell CG, Hedenström H & Hedenstierna G (1993) Inhalation of nitric oxide modulates adult human bronchial tone. *American Review of Respiratory Diseases* **148:**1474–1478.
20. Roger N, Barberà JA, Farré R, Cobos A, Roca J & Rodriguez-Roisin R (1996) Effect of nitric oxide inhalation on respiratory system resistance in chronic obstructive pulmonary disease. *European Respiratory Journal* **9:**190–195.
21. Mira JP, Monchi M, Brunet F, Fierobe L, Dhainaut JF & Dinh-Xuan AT (1994) Lack of efficacy of inhaled nitric oxide in ARDS. *Intensive Care Medicine* **20:**532.
22. Agustí AGN, Barberà JA, Roca J, Wagner PD, Guitart R & Rodriguez-Roisin R (1990) Hypoxic pulmonary vasoconstriction and gas exchange during exercise in chronic obstructive pulmonary disease. *Chest* **97:**268–275.
23. Adnot S, Kouyoumdjian C, Defouilloy C, Andrivet P, Sediame S, Herigault R & Fratacci MD (1993) Hemodynamic and gas exchanges responses to infusion of acetylcholine and inhalation of nitric oxide in patients with chronic obstructive lung disease and pulmonary hypertension. *American Review of Respiratory Diseases* **148:**310–316.
24. Moinard J, Manier G, Pillet O & Castaing Y (1994) Effect of inhaled nitric oxide on hemodynamics and $\dot{V}_A/\dot{Q}$ inequalities in patients with chronic obstructive pulmonary disease. *American Journal of Respiratory Critical Care Medicine* **149:**1482–1487.
25. Barberà JA, Roger N, Roca J, Rovira I, Higenbottam TW & Rodgriguez-Roisin R (1996) Worsening of pulmonary gas exchange with nitric oxide inhalation in chronic obstructive pulmonary disease. *Lancet* **347:**436–440.

9

Effect of Inhaled Nitric Oxide on Right Ventricular Function

R. Rossaint
U. Kaisers
I. Schulze-Neick

INTRODUCTION

Right ventricular dysfunction due to increased afterload may complicate acute (or adult) respiratory distress syndrome (ARDS), cardiac surgery and heart transplantation. Under normal physiological conditions, the functional significance of the right ventricle seems to be minimal, because the right ventricle acts more or less as a passive conduit responsible for accepting venous blood and propelling it through the pulmonary system to the left ventricle.[1] However, development of sudden pulmonary hypertension induces a decreased right ventricular ejection fraction (RVEF) and increased right ventricular volumes. As long as the right ventricular contractile function is not depressed, the right ventricle may be able to pump sufficiently to maintain a normal cardiac output, and a severely reduced RVEF indicates right ventricular dysfunction rather than right ventricular failure. However, if pulmonary hypertension further increases and/or if the right ventricular contractile function is depressed, the right ventricle may not be able to generate sufficient pressure output resulting in right ventricular failure. Moreover, in this situation an increased right ventricular end-diastolic volume may cause a shift of the septum to the left which, in turn, may alter left ventricular performance. Thereby, right ventricular failure may influence systemic circulation and may even limit survival.[2] Besides these secondary alterations in left ventricular performance, the shift of the septum to the left may result in wedge pressure increases, possibly enhancing the development of interstitial pulmonary edema.

Intravenous infusions of vasodilators have been shown to lower pulmonary artery pressure (PAP) as well as effective pulmonary capillary pressure[3–6] and thereby might improve right ventricular function.[7–8] However, the use of conventional vasodilators, like nitroglycerin or prostacyclin (PGI_2) is limited because intravenously infused vasodilators produce diffuse dilation of the whole vasculature. Global vasodilation in the pulmonary vasculature increases blood flow to areas of intrapulmonary shunt, which, especially in ARDS patients, further reduces the already compromised arterial partial pressure of oxygen (Pa_{O_2}).[4,5,9,10] Concomitant dilation of the systemic vasculature leads to a dose-dependent arterial hypotension which possibly causes ventricular ischemia and consequent heart failure.[4,5,11]

In contrast, inhalation of low concentrations of gaseous nitric oxide (NO) causes selective vasodilation of ventilated lung regions. Inhaled NO relaxes smooth muscles in arteries and veins like endogenous NO by activating soluble guanylate cyclase and increasing guanosine cyclic 3′,5′-monophosphate. Since NO is inactivated by hemoglobin as soon as it enters the bloodstream, the dilatory effect of low concentrations of inhaled NO is restricted to the pulmonary vasculature of ventilated lung areas.[12,13] Thereby, the elevated PAP is decreased in various diseases and, in addition, in patients with high intrapulmonary shunt the ratio of the partial pressure of arterial oxygen to the fraction of inspired oxygen ($Pa_{O_2}/F_{I}O_2$) may be increased.[14]

EFFECT OF INHALED NO ON RIGHT VENTRICULAR FUNCTION IN ARDS

In patients with ARDS, pulmonary hypertension may result from the combined effects of hypoxic pulmonary vasoconstriction, release of mediators and microthrombosis in the pulmonary circulation. This pulmonary hypertension represents an increase in the outflow pressure load on the right ventricle, which may cause a decrease in right ventricular ejection fraction and increases in right ventricular volumes. When inhaled NO was given for the first time to a patient with severe ARDS, the selective pulmonary vasodilation was preceded by an increased RVEF.[8] Recently, this observation was confirmed by Fierobe and co-workers.[15] In 13 patients with severe ARDS, they investigated whether inhaled NO improves right ventricular function and whether the changes in pulmonary hemodynamics and right ventricular function were related to changes in arterial oxygenation. Inhaled NO (5 ppm) caused a decrease in PAP from 36 ± 5 to 31 ± 6 mmHg ($P < 0.01$) and in pulmonary vascular resistance (PVR) from 211 ± 43 to 180 ± 59 dyn s/cm^5 ($P < 0.05$) which was associated with an increase in RVEF from 32 ± 5 to $36 \pm 6\%$ ($P < 0.05$) and a trend toward decreased right ventricular volumes. The increase in $Pa_{O_2}/F_{I}O_2$ (103 ± 47 versus 142 ± 63 mmHg) was not related to hemodynamic changes. Similar findings were described in a study by Rossaint et al.[16] These investigators compared the effects of inhaled NO and infused PGI_2 on right ventricular function parameters assessed by the thermodilution technique in patients with ARDS. Ten patients inhaled 18 and 36 ppm NO, randomized preceded or followed by an intravenous infusion of

PGI_2 (4 ng/kg per min). Inhaling 18 ppm NO reduced the PAP from 33 ± 2 to 28 ± 1 mmHg ($P = 0.008$), increased RVEF, as assessed by the thermodilution technique, from 28 ± 2 to 32 ± 2% ($P = 0.005$), decreased right ventricular end-diastolic volume index from 114 ± 6 to 103 ± 8 ml/m^2 ($P = 0.005$) and right ventricular end-systolic volume index from 82 ± 4 to 70 ± 5 ml/m^2 ($P = 0.009$). Mean arterial pressure and cardiac index did not change significantly. The effects of 36 ppm NO were not different from the effects of 18 ppm NO. Infusion of PGI_2 also reduced PAP from 34 ± 2 to 30 ± 2 mmHg ($P = 0.02$) and increased RVEF from 29 ± 2 to 32 ± 2% ($P = 0.02$), but in contrast with inhaled NO, right ventricular end-diastolic and end-systolic volume indices did not change significantly, mean arterial pressure decreased from 80 ± 4 to 70 ± 5 mmHg ($P = 0.03$), and cardiac index increased from 4.0 ± 0.5 to 4.5 ± 0.5 liters/min per m^2 ($P = 0.02$).

Both studies demonstrate that, in a group of hemodynamically stable ARDS patients, inhaled NO slightly improved the RVEF, which was not followed by an increase in cardiac index. Since during NO inhalation the increase in RVEF was accompanied by decreased right ventricular volumes at a constant cardiac index, these changes reflect the fact that the right ventricle is working on another part of its pressure–volume loop, indicating a normal physiological response of the right ventricle in the presence of different loading conditions. However, these data also show that cardiac index could not be influenced by the alterations in right ventricular parameters obtained in this group of hemodynamically stable ARDS patients. The increase in cardiac index observed during the intravenous infusion of vasodilators, such as PGI_2, is probably due to reduction in systemic vascular resistance, since in the study by Rossaint et al[16] the decrease in PAP and the corresponding increase in RVEF were similar during the administration of either vasodilator. The right ventricular end-diastolic volume did not decrease during the infusion of PGI_2, probably because of augmented venous return.[17] However, even if in these studies the increased RVEF during NO inhalation did not result in an augmented cardiac index, one should be well aware that, in another group of patients suffering from severe ARDS, inhaled NO may cause an increased RVEF which will be followed by a rise in cardiac index as demonstrated in four patients by Wysocki et al.[18] Furthermore, it cannot be excluded that higher concentrations of inhaled NO, which have been described to decrease PAP more effectively,[19] would have decreased PAP further in both studies, possibly resulting in a greater increase in RVEF and also an increase in cardiac index.

In general, these studies do not allow us to determine when and for what reasons acute pulmonary artery hypertension limits cardiac index in patients with severe ARDS. However, using a selective gaseous pulmonary vasodilator demonstrates that a reduction in PAP secondary to a pharmacological intervention may increase RVEF but not necessarily cardiac index, whereas infused PGI_2 augments cardiac index, presumably due to a decrease in systemic vascular resistance. These results suggest that either the rises in RVEF were not high enough to cause an increase in cardiac index or that the altered right ventricular function was not a limiting factor to the oxygen delivery to the tissues.

EFFECT OF INHALED NO ON RIGHT VENTRICULAR FUNCTION IN CONGENITAL HEART DISEASE

In patients with congenital heart disease, pulmonary hypertension may result from increased pulmonary blood flow or from pulmonary venous obstruction resulting in pulmonary artery smooth muscle hypertrophy and hyperplasia and pulmonary vasoconstriction. After corrective cardiac surgery, the pulmonary vascular bed may not be able to regress sufficiently to accommodate the post-operative hemodynamic changes which, finally, may lead to right ventricular failure. Therefore, right ventricular failure from pulmonary hypertension is a common cause of death after surgical correction of congenital heart diseases with left to right shunt. In order to determine the vasodilatory capacity of the pulmonary vascular bed and thereby to predict the postoperative risk of life-threatening suprasystemic pulmonary hypertension, NO inhalation has been used during preoperative cardiac catheterization.[20,21] Wessel et al[22] and Schulze-Neick and co-workers[21] demonstrated that inhaled NO exhibits a far greater vasodilatory effect than hyperoxic breathing. Moreover, adding inhaled NO to the commonly used test for pulmonary vascular reactivity during preoperative cardiac catheterization allowed identification of patients with preserved vascular reactivity who did not respond to infused PGI_2 or inhaled pure oxygen but responded to inhaled NO. If inhaled NO given before surgery causes pulmonary vasodilation, this gas might be used to relieve severe pulmonary hypertension after surgical correction of congenital diseases as well. Moreover, transient endothelial dysfunction due to cardiopulmonary bypass followed by a lack of endogenous NO may cause or aggravate pulmonary hypertension.[22]

Therefore, recently, inhaled NO was instituted to treat pulmonary hypertension in patients undergoing open heart surgery. Wessel[23] successfully treated several children with moderate pulmonary hypertension after cardiac surgery with inhaled NO. These results are in accordance with the findings of Beghetti et al[24] who also investigated the effects of inhaled NO on severe postoperative hypertension in children after surgical repair of a congenital heart defect. In six of seven patients, NO inhalation decreased PAP and the arteriovenous difference in oxygen content while mean systemic pressure remained unchanged and the $Pa{O_2}$ increased. An increase in pulmonary blood flow and thereby an improvement in right ventricular pump function could be measured in one child who was monitored with a thermodilution catheter, and was indicated in the other children by the decrease in arteriovenous oxygen content. Berner et al[25] reported that NO inhalation selectively reduced suprasystemic pulmonary hypertension following closure of a large ventricular septal defect in a 16-month-old girl. In this child, administration of NO resulted in an effective increase in pulmonary blood flow demonstrated by a simultaneous increase in CO_2 elimination, improvement in arterial oxygenation, progressive weaning from epinephrine and reversal of oligoanuria. Schranz et al[26] described the successful use of inhaled NO in a newborn in whom suprasystemic pulmonary hypertension persisted following surgical valvulotomy for a critical aortic valve stenosis. Again, inhalation of NO was associated with a simultaneous rise in end-tidal CO_2 and $Pa{O_2}$, indicating an improvement in right ventricular function with consecutive increase in pulmonary blood flow.

In summary, inhaled NO is also a potent selective vasodilator in pediatric patients with congenital heart disease complicated by pulmonary artery hypertension. It may help to determine before surgery the vasodilatory capacity of the pulmonary vascular bed and to treat postoperative right ventricular failure due to increased PAP.

EFFECT OF INHALED NO ON RIGHT VENTRICULAR FUNCTION IN ADULTS UNDERGOING CARDIAC SURGERY

In cardiac surgical patients, Girard et al[27] and Rich et al[28,29] investigated the effects of inhaled NO (20–40 ppm) on patients with pulmonary artery hypertension. They found that inhaled NO decreased PAP and PVR but did not affect central venous pressure, cardiac output, and systemic hemodynamics. These observations are in agreement with the results of Pepke-Zaba et al[30] who demonstrated that 40 ppm inhaled NO did not increase cardiac output despite a decrease in PVR and a constant central venous pressure in human volunteers with chronic pulmonary hypertension. Therefore it is suggested that, in general, inhaled NO does not influence right ventricular function in patients with chronic pulmonary hypertension despite its effect on PVR. However, in a small group of these patients inhaled NO may also have a beneficial effect on right ventricular function. Rich et al[28] reported the effects of inhaled NO in five patients receiving circulatory support with a ventricular assist device. In this group of patients, 20 ppm NO decreased PAP from 68 ± 12 to 55 ± 9 mmHg and PVR from 1085 ± 229 to 752 ± 130 dyn s/cm^5 ($P < 0.05$) as well as increasing $P\text{aO}_2$, mean arterial pressure and mixed venous O_2 saturation. It is believed that these alterations reflect an improved right ventricular function and an increase in cardiac output from the natural heart. Therefore, these authors conclude that inhaled NO may improve systemic hemodynamics when right ventricular failure and an elevated PVR are limiting factors. This is supported by a recently published case report which described the reversal of right ventricular failure in a 54-year-old man after implantation of a left ventricular assist system by inhalation of 50 ppm NO.[31] After implantation of the assist device as bridging for heart transplantation, the PAP increased from 40 to 65 mmHg which was associated with a decrease in RVEF from 17 to 6% and a persistence of low cardiac output below 3 liters/min. A therapeutic breakthrough could only be achieved when NO inhalation was started. Inhaled NO caused a decrease in PAP to 35 mmHg, an increase in RVEF to 17% and cardiac output to 5 liters/min. Using continuous NO inhalation for several days, PAP further decreased to 27 mmHg while RVEF rose to 23% avoiding institution of extracorporeal right ventricular support.

EFFECT OF INHALED NO ON RIGHT VENTRICULAR FUNCTION IN ADULTS UNDERGOING HEART TRANSPLANTATION

Inhaled NO was also evaluated in the pre- and post-operative treatment of patients receiving orthotopic heart transplantation. In this group of patients preoperative pulmonary hypertension is a common feature. However, an increased PVR may induce right ventricular failure after implantation of the donor heart. Therefore, the extent of the elevated PVR as well as the prospect of pharmacological treatment should be evaluated in transplant candidates before surgery. If an increased PVR is reversible, the patients can be accepted for orthotopic heart transplantation, otherwise a heart–lung transplantation may be considered more suitable. Currently used vasodilators are intravenous PGI_2, prostaglandin E_1, and sodium nitroprusside. Recently, Kieler-Jensen et al[32] described the use of inhaled NO during preoperative cardiac catheterization of heart transplant candidates with elevated PVR. In this group of patients, NO did not change systemic or pulmonary arterial pressure, cardiac output, right ventricular function, or systemic vascular resistance but increased pulmonary capillary wedge pressure and decreased PVR. These changes are explained by the induction of pulmonary vasodilation, presumably most pronounced on the pulmonary veins, in patients suffering from chronic left ventricular failure. In contrast, Snell et al[33] described a 40-year-old woman with end-stage pulmonary hypertension who was treated with 40–106 ppm NO as a bridge to heart–lung transplantation in order to manage right ventricular failure with consecutive systemic hypoperfusion resulting in low systemic blood pressure, despite intravenous infusion of PGI_2. With the onset of inhaled NO, a rapid increase in mean systolic blood pressure and arterial oxygen saturation combined with a decrease in central venous pressure occurred, suggesting an improvement in right ventricular function. In this patient, the treatment with inhaled NO was continued until the heart–lung transplant could be performed on day 68 after initiation of NO therapy.

After heart transplantation, vasodilator therapy is often required in order to treat pulmonary hypertension. Currently used vasodilators such as intravenous PGI_2, prostaglandin E_1, and sodium nitroprusside are only of limited value because they also lower systemic arterial pressure. Therefore, inhaled NO with its selective pulmonary vasodilatory effect has also been used in the management of pulmonary hypertension with right-sided ventricular failure in heart transplant recipients.[34,35] These investigators report an improvement in right ventricular performance followed by an increase in cardiac output and mean systemic arterial pressure. In addition, Kieler-Jensen et al[36] assessed the effects of inhaled NO shortly after heart transplantation in nine patients without hemodynamic signs of acute right heart failure, as reflected by normal values of right ventricular end-diastolic volume, central venous pressure, stroke volume, cardiac output, and whole-body oxygen extraction. In this study, inhaled NO induced a dose-dependent decrease in PAP, PVR, and central venous pressure and an increase in cardiac output with no changes in right ventricular function parameters and systemic vascular resistance. Since inhaled NO induced an 11% increase in cardiac output, these authors believe that, despite no change in right ventricular function parameters assessed by the thermodilution technique, inhaled NO must have reduced right ventricular outflow impedance in this group of patients with transplanted right ventricles sensitive to changes in PVR. They conclude that this NO-induced decrease in right ventricular outflow impedance most likely resulted in an improvement in right ventricular function. However, comparing in this group of patients the effects of inhaled NO with the effects of intravenously infused vasodilators such as PGI_2, prostaglandin E_1, and sodium nitroprusside, the same authors found that in most patients PGI_2 is the best choice for intravenous vasodilator therapy after heart transplantation, because it reduces both right and left ventricular outflow impedance which is a desired effect in most of the transplanted patients. Nevertheless, in cases of pulmonary hypertension and right ventricular failure associated with systemic hypotension, the selectively acting vasodilator NO could be the drug of choice.

REFERENCES

1. Weber KT, Janicki JS, Shroff SG, Likoff MJ & Sutton MJ (1983) The right ventricle: physiologic and pathophysiologic considerations. *Critical Care Medicine* **11:**323–328.
2. Zapol WM & Snider MT (1977) Pulmonary hypertension in severe acute respiratory failure. *New England Journal of Medicine* **296:**476–480.
3. Gottlieb SS, Wood LD, Hansen DE & Long GR (1987) The effect of nitroprusside on pulmonary edema, oxygen exchange, and blood flow in hydrochloric acid aspiration. *Anesthesiology* **67:**203–210.
4. Radermacher P, Huet Y, Pluskwa F, Herigault R, Mal H, Teisseire B & Lemaire F (1988) Comparison of ketanserin and sodium nitroprusside in patients with severe ARDS. *Anesthesiology* **68:**152–157.
5. Radermacher P, Santak B, Becker H & Falke KJ (1989) Prostaglandin E_1 and nitroglycerin reduce pulmonary capillary pressure but worsen ventilation–perfusion distributions in patients with adult respiratory distress syndrome. *Anesthesiology* **70:**601–606.
6. Zapol WM, Snider MT, Rie MA, Frikker M & Quinn DA (1985) Pulmonary circulation during adult respiratory distress syndrome. In Zapol WM & Falke KJ (eds) *Acute Respiratory Failure*, pp 241–273. New York: Dekker.
7. Radermacher P, Santak B, Wust HJ, Tarnow J & Falke KJ (1990) Prostacyclin and right ventricular function in patients with pulmonary hypertension associated with ARDS. *Intensive Care Medicine* **16:**227–232.
8. Falke K, Rossaint R, Pison U, Slama K, Lopez F, Santak B & Zapol WM (1991) Inhaled nitric oxide selectively reduces pulmonary hypertension in severe ARDS and improves gas exchange as well as right heart ejection fraction: A case report. *American Review of Respiratory Diseases* **143(Suppl):**A248.
9. Radermacher P, Santak B, Wust HJ, Tarnow J & Falke KJ (1990) Prostacyclin for the treatment of pulmonary hypertension in the adult respiratory distress syndrome: effects on pulmonary capillary pressure and ventilation–perfusion distributions (see comments). *Anesthesiology* **72:**238–244.
10. Melot C, Lejeune P, Leeman M, Moraine JJ & Naeije R (1989) Prostaglandin E_1 in the adult respiratory distress syndrome. Benefit for pulmonary hypertension and cost for pulmonary gas exchange. *American Review of Respiratory Disease* **139:**106–110.
11. Vlahakes GJ, Turley K & Hoffman JI (1981) The pathophysiology of failure in acute right ventricular hypertension: hemodynamic and biochemical correlations. *Circulation* **63:**87–95.
12. Frostell C, Fratacci MD, Wain JC, Jones R & Zapol WM (1991) Inhaled nitric oxide. A selective pulmonary vasodilator reversing hypoxic pulmonary vasoconstriction. *Circulation* **83:**2038–2047.

13. Pison U, Lopez FA, Heidelmeyer CF, Rossaint R & Falke K (1993) Inhaled nitric oxide selectively reverses hypoxic pulmonary vasoconstriction without impairing pulmonary gas exchange. *Journal of Applied Physiology* **74:**1287–1292.
14. Rossaint R, Falke KJ, Lopez F, Slama K, Pison U & Zapol WM (1993) Inhaled nitric oxide in adult respiratory distress syndrome. *New England Journal of Medicine* **328:**399–405.
15. Fierobe L, Brunet F, DHainaut JF, Monchi M, Belghith M, Mira JP, Dall'ava-Santucci J & Dinh-Xuan AT (1995) Effect of inhaled nitric oxide on right ventricular function in adult respiratory distress syndrome. *American Journal of Respiratory and Critical Care Medicine* **151:**1414–1419.
16. Rossaint R, Slama K, Steudel W, Gerlach H, Pappert D, Veit S & Falke K (1995) Effects of inhaled nitric oxide on right ventricular function in severe acute respiratory distress syndrome. *Intensive Care Medicine* **21:**197–203.
17. Sibbald WJ & Driedger AA (1983) Right ventricular function in acute disease states: pathophysiologic considerations. *Critical Care Medicine* **11:**339–345.
18. Wysocki M, Vignon P, Roupie E, Humbert M, Adnot S, Lemaire F & Brochard L (1993) Improvement in right ventricular function with inhaled nitric oxide in patients with the adult respiratory distress syndrome (ARDS) and permissive hypercapnia. *American Review of Respiratory Disease* **147:**A350.
19. Gerlach H, Rossaint R, Pappert D & Falke KJ (1993) Time-course and dose–response of nitric oxide inhalation for systemic oxygenation and pulmonary hypertension in patients with adult respiratory distress syndrome. *European Journal of Clinical Investigation* **23:**499–502.
20. Roberts JD, Lang P, Bigatello LM, Vlahakes GJ & Zapol WM (1993) Inhaled nitric oxide in congenital heart disease. *Circulation* **87:**447–453.
21. Schulze-Neick I, Rossaint R, Berger F, Werner H, Uhlemann F, Hausdorf G, Falke KJ & Lange Pe (1994) Inhaled nitric oxide and intravenous prostacyclin for preoperative evaluation of pulmonary vascular resistance in patients with congenital heart disease. *European Heart Journal* **15:**524.
22. Wessel DL, Adatia I, Giglia TM, Thompson JE & Kulik TJ (1993) Use of inhaled nitric oxide and acetylcholine in the evaluation of pulmonary hypertension and endothelial function after cardiopulmonary bypass. *Circulation* **88:**2128–2138.
23. Wessel DL (1993) Inhaled nitric oxide for the treatment of pulmonary hypertension before and after cardiopulmonary bypass. *Critical Care Medicine* **21:** S344–S345.
24. Beghetti M, Habre W, Friedli B & Berner M (1995) Continuous low dose inhaled nitric oxide for treatment of severe pulmonary hypertension after cardiac surgery in paediatric patients. *British Heart Journal* **73:**65–68.
25. Berner M, Beghetti M, Ricou B, Rouge JC, Pretre R & Friedli B (1993) Relief of severe pulmonary hypertension after closure of a large ventricular septal defect using low dose inhaled nitric oxide. *Intensive Care Medicine* **19:**75–77.
26. Schranz D, Huth R, Wippermann CF, Ritzerfeld S, Schmitt FX & Oelert H (1993) Nitric oxide and prostacyclin lower suprasystemic pulmonary hypertension after cardiopulmonary bypass. *European Journal of Pediatrics* **152:**793–796.
27. Girard C, Lehot JJ, Pannetier JC, Filley S, Ffrench P & Estanove S (1992) Inhaled nitric oxide after mitral valve replacement in patients with chronic pulmonary artery hypertension. *Anesthesiology* **77:**880–883.
28. Rich GF, Murphy GD Jr, Roos CM & Johns RA (1993) Inhaled nitric oxide. Selective pulmonary vasodilation in cardiac surgical patients. *Anesthesiology* **78:**1028–1035.
29. Rich GF, Lowson SM, Johns RA, Daugherty MO & Uncles DR (1994) Inhaled nitric oxide selectively decreases pulmonary vascular resistance without impairing oxygenation during one-lung ventilation in patients undergoing cardiac surgery. *Anesthesiology* **80:**57–62.
30. Pepke-Zaba J, Higenbottam TW, Dinh-Xuan AT, Stone D & Wallwork J (1991)

Inhaled nitric oxide as a cause of selective pulmonary vasodilatation in pulmonary hypertension. *Lancet* **338:**1173–1174.

31. Mertes PM, Pinelli G, Hubert T, Carteaux JP, Hottier E, Larcan A & Villemont JP (1995) Impact of nitric oxide inhalation on right ventricular failure after implantation of novacor left ventricular assist system. *Journal of Thoracic and Cardiovascular Surgery* **109:**1251.
32. Kieler-Jensen N, Ricksten SE, Stenqvist O, Bergh CH, Lindelöv B, Wennmalm Ä, Waagstein F & Lundin S (1995) Inhaled nitric oxide in the evaluation of heart transplant candidates with elevated pulmonary vascular resistance. *Journal of Heart and Lung Transplantation* **13:**366–375.
33. Snell GI, Salamonsen RF, Bergin P, Esmore DS, Zepp F & Williams TJ (1995) Inhaled nitric oxide used as a bridge to heart–lung transplantation in a patient with end-stage pulmonary hypertension. *American Journal of Respiratory Critical Care Medicine* **151:**1263–1266.
34. Girard C, Durand PG & Vedrinne C (1993) Inhaled nitric oxide for right ventricular failure after heart transplantation: case conference. *Journal of Cardiothoracic and Vascular Anesthesiology* **7:**481–485.
35. Williams TJ, Salamonsen RF, Snell G, Kaye D & Esmore DS (1995) Preliminary experience with inhaled nitric oxide for acute pulmonary hypertension after heart transplantation. *Journal of Heart and Lung Transplantation* **14:**419–423.
36. Kieler-Jensen N, Lundin S & Ricksten SE (1995) Vasodilator therapy after heart transplantation: Effects of inhaled nitric oxide and intravenous prostacyclin, prostaglandin E_1, and sodium nitroprusside. *Journal of Heart and Lung Transplantation* **14:**436–443.

10

Cardiopulmonary Response to Home Oxygen Therapy: Nasal Prongs Versus Oxygen-Saving Devices

Christian Domingo
Enric Domingo

INTRODUCTION

In 1974,[1] at a meeting of the American Thoracic Society, it was reported that the use of long-term oxygen therapy was steadily spreading around the USA and Europe, although it had not been conclusively demonstrated that this treatment contributed to lengthening patients' lives. Two major studies, the NOTT[2,3] and MRC,[4] were set up as a result, and as Flenley stated in his conclusion,[5] in patients with chronic obstructive pulmonary disease (COPD) and chronic hypoxemia, as far as survival is concerned, no oxygen is bad, oxygen for some of the time is better, but oxygen for most of the time is the best.

From a hemodynamic point of view, the results of the various studies are contradictory. Although in some cases the hemodynamic benefits derived from long-term oxygen therapy[2,3,6] have been demonstrated, in other cases the benefits are not so clear.[4,7]

In recent years, research has been aimed at improving the patient's quality of life by introducing portable sources of liquid oxygen and oxygen-saving systems (which can be combined) to allow patients greater outdoor activity while maintaining correct oxygenation 24 hours a day.[8–11]

The purpose of this study is to ascertain the acute and long-term hemodynamic response of two oxygen-saving devices, the oxymizer (O) and the transtracheal catheter (TTC), while maintaining the previously established oxygen-saving properties, in a group of patients with COPD, who had previously been treated with long-term oxygen therapy through nasal prongs (NP) 18 h a day.

MATERIALS AND METHODS

We studied a group of 14 severe COPD patients with chronic hypoxemia (13 males and one female), included in a long-term oxygen therapy program under the care of 'Germans Trias i Pujol' University Hospital, Badalona (Barcelona). Ten patients (nine males and one female, aged 59.9 ± 5.8 years) were able to reach the end of our follow-up (two died and two refused a second catheterization). Patients had received long-term oxygen therapy through nasal prongs 18 h a day, for a mean period of 26 ± 17 months previous to being included in this study and were considered to be reliable followers of their treatment. No patient presented with exclusion criteria for TTC insertion.[9]

PROTOCOL

Before their inclusion in the study, the patients followed a pulmonary rehabilitation program, with carefully adjusted medication. After the study procedures were started, patients were not allowed to participate in any other rehabilitation program[12] nor to alter the bronchodilating, cardiotonic, or diuretic medication they were given. The study was performed according to the following steps.

(I) At the beginning and at end of the follow-up, complete pulmonary function tests (PFTs) were carried out in our pulmonary function laboratory,[13] which is equipped with automated PFT equipment (Sensor Medics, Amehein, USA), for pulmonary volume, diffusion, and spirometric tests, with the following components: a dry-piston rolling-seal spirometer with horizontal displacement and potentiometer, a pulmonary volume module by helium dilution, an IBM XT personal computer and an automated plethysmographic cabin for pulmonary volume and airway resistance tests (Spectramed, Holland).

(II) The oxygen flow required for correct oxygenation with the O and TTC was determined during rest and during exercise in the following way.[14]

1. A minimum of three nocturnal pulse oximetries (Oxyshuttle, Sensor Medics) with oxygen administered through nasal prongs, O and TTC were performed which allowed us to calculate the minimum oxygen flow needed to keep oxygen saturation above 88% during 95% of the time measured with each device.
2. Arterial gasometries on room air and with oxygen flow through nasal prongs and TTC determined as described in the previous paragraph (Corning 178 gasometer, Izasa) while the patient was awake were obtained at the beginning and end of the study.[12]
3. Oximetric monitoring of patients was performed when they were examined as outpatients.
4. A 6-min walking test (6 WT) was carried out at the beginning and end of the follow-up with patients receiving liquid oxygen via TTC delivered by a stroller of liquid oxygen (Vital Aire-SEO) carried by themselves under oximetric control to ascertain that the administered oxygen flow allowed correct oxygenation. The walking distance was measured and dyspnea assessed by a visual analog scale (VAS). Moreover, we attempted a

correlation between these variables and pulmonary vascular resistance (PVR), pulmonary arteriolar vascular resistance (PAVR), right ventricular ejection fraction (RVEF), and left ventricular ejection fraction (LVEF).

(III) In-patients were fitted with a TTC (Oxycath, Smad-Proclinics), as described previously.[9] The first TTC was replaced before the patient was discharged, and from then on they were replaced in our center on a weekly basis for 8–10 weeks after discharge. Subsequently, after being trained in TTC replacement and the use of portable oxygen sources, patients were again included in the COPD-monitoring procedures of our department, and received no further special care.[15,16]

(IV) Physical activity was monitored. An anamnesis aiming to specify whether the patients stayed away from home for 4 h or more every day was performed by interviewing the relatives in the absence of the patient and the patient him/herself at every outpatient examination.

(V) Studies were performed to evaluate the acute hemodynamic response. Isotopic ventriculography (IV) with the equilibrium technique and the radiopharmaceutical metastable technetium-99 (^{99m}Tc), with a 6 h average life and a 140 keV photon activity, was used. This study was carried out with the patient in the decubitus position and perpendicular to the Picker 4/15 gamma camera. ^{99m}Tc, 20 mCi in 1 ml of blood, was injected through an antecubital vein. The ejection fraction (EF) in each beat was calculated by the formula:

$$\text{EF} = \frac{\text{Diastolic count} - \text{Systolic count}}{\text{Diastolic count}}$$

The isotopic ventriculography was performed on an ergonomic bicycle with the patient at rest, and during exercise at a subjective maximum rate, and receiving oxygen through nasal prongs, O and TTC. In each case, the oxygen flow used was that preset by nocturnal pulse oximetries. Blood pressure and heart rate were measured thus making it possible to calculate the cardiac work (systolic blood pressure × cardiac rate) at rest and exercise.

(VI) Studies were performed to evaluate the long-term hemodynamic response to 24 h oxygenation with liquid oxygen via TTC.

1. Doppler and bidimensional echocardiograms (Toshiba, Sonolayer SSH 65-A), were taken with the patient in the supine decubitus position and receiving the oxygen flow previously determined through TTC. As well as the right-side catheterization data obtained, a right ventricle free wall stress (RVFWS) index was determined according to the formula:

$$\text{RVFWS} = \frac{\text{RVFWT} \times \text{PAPs}}{\text{RV diastolic diameter}}$$

   where RVFWT is the right ventricle free wall thickness expressed in mm, PAPs is the systolic pulmonary arterial pressure in mmHg, and RV is the right ventricle.
2. Isotopic ventriculography with oxygen administered via TTC at rest and exercise was used to determine RVEF and LVEF ventricular volumes.

Once the end-diastolic volume (EDV) and EF were known, the beat volume (BV) could be calculated (BV = EF × EDV). The end-systolic volume (ESV) can be obtained by subtracting the BV from the EDV.

3. Right heart catheterization was performed through the subclavian vein with a Swan–Ganz catheter, using the Seldinger technique, after subcutaneous lidocaine anesthetic. The distal end position of the floating catheter in the pulmonary artery was continuously controlled by monitoring the pressure curve in a Space Lab 701 monitor (Edwards). Cardiac output was obtained by thermodilution. We carried out at least five measurements, discarding the two end ones, and calculated an average with the remaining three, provided there was no more than 10% variation between the three measurements. The pressure waves of right atrium (RA), right ventricle (RV), pulmonary artery (PA) and pulmonary capillary wedge pressure (PCWP) were recorded on graph paper, on which the initial study measurements had been recorded. During the initial hemodynamic study, a radial artery catheter was inserted, which permitted the monitoring of the systolic and diastolic blood pressure (SBP, DBP), and series determinations of arterial gasometry. During the final hemodynamic study, blood pressure (BP) was measured by a sphygmomanometer and an arterial gasometry was performed by puncture after lidocaine local anesthetic. Patients were monitored through digital oximetry at all times.

(VII) Statistical evaluation was carried out with Pearson's correlation, and Student's *t* test for paired data and two-way analysis of variance.

RESULTS

Nocturnal pulse oximetries were performed in 14 patients, but the right heart catheterization in only ten. Of these ten patients, isotopic ventriculography

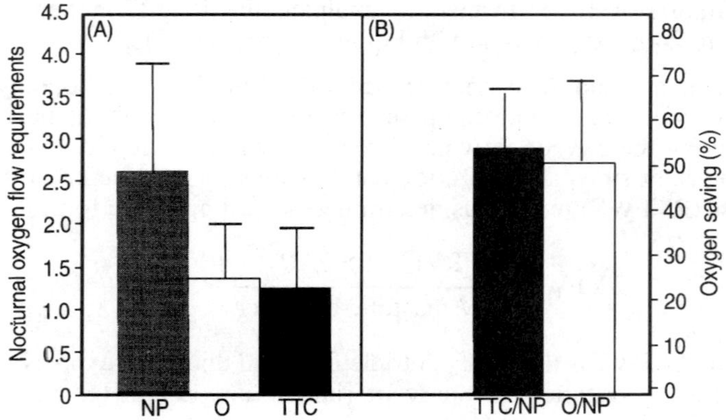

Figure 1. Mean nocturnal oxygen flow requirements (liters) with every device (A) and percentage of oxygen saving (B).

was performed in nine but ventricular volumes could be obtained in only five of them. The population studied was nine males and one female, average age 61.2 ± 5.6 years, weight 61.68 ± 8.7 kg, and height 162.8 ± 6.6 cm. The follow-up time was 11.4 ± 3.8 months. As observed elsewhere,[8] TTC insertion did not present any difficulties.[13,15]

The oxygen flow required to maintain oxygen saturation above 88% during 95% of the night time and percentage oxygen saving are shown in Figures 1(A) and 1(B).

The isotopic studies performed at the beginning of the study comparing the changes of the right and left ejection fractions (EF) at rest and during maximal exercise with the patients oxygenated via nasal prongs, O and TTC demonstrated that the LVEF and RVEF values during rest were similar with all three methods but during maximal exercise the EF increments of both ventricles were significantly higher with nasal prongs or TTC. In other words, at maximal exercise the LVEF increases less markedly and the RVEF decreases slightly more with O than with nasal prongs or TTC (Table 1 and Figure 2).

Table 1. Hemodynamic response to the three different oxygen-delivery devices evaluated by radionuclide ventriculography.

Device		RVEF		LVEF	
		Rest	Exercise	Rest	Exercise
NP	(T_0)	38 ± 9.7	42 ± 11.2	52.9 ± 9.4	61.5 ±11.1
O	(T_0)	39.6 ± 12.8	37.4 ± 7.5*	54.1 ± 7.4	56.2 ±9.5*
TTC	(T_0)	38.1 ± 12.2	42.6 ± 9.5	54.0 ± 11.5	59.8 ±15
	(T_1)	37.6 ± 9.8	44.4 ± 7.1	57.0 ± 7.46	58.7 ±10.6

Values are means ± S.D. * RVEF decreased slightly during exercise ($P = 0.06$) and LVEF increased less markedly during exercise with O than with NP or TTC ($P < 0.05$). Abbreviations: T_0, beginning of the study; T_1, end of the study.

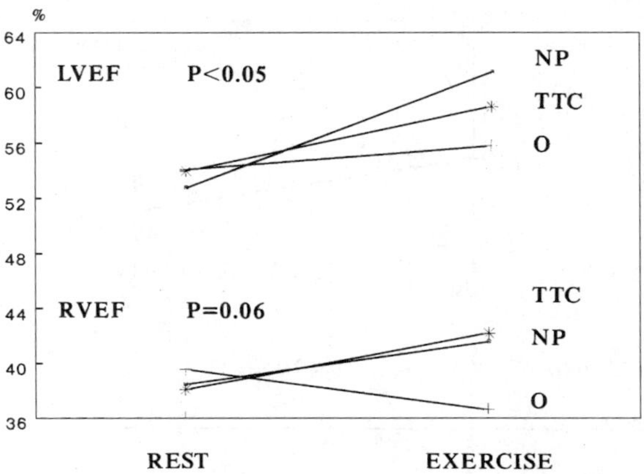

Figure 2. Mean values of RVEF and LVEF with the three different devices. At rest no differences were observed. During maximal exercise, the results when patients were oxygenated via O were less satisfactory than with NP or TTC.

The follow-up study showed that hemoglobin (Hb) values decreased from 15.21 ± 2.09 g/dl to 12.91 ± 1.48 g/dl ($P < 0.01$), the decrease being uniform (Figure 3A). The $Pa\text{O}_2$ at the beginning and end of the study with the patients oxygenated via TTC at the preset oxygen flow are shown in Figure 3(B). An increase is observed.

The initial PFTs are shown in Table 2. Only the FEV_1, the FEV_1/FVC quotient and DLCO (but not the KCO) deteriorated statistically significantly (Figure 3C).

The 6-min walking test did not deteriorate at the end of the follow-up (325 ± 134 m versus 327 ± 112 m), and there were no differences between the

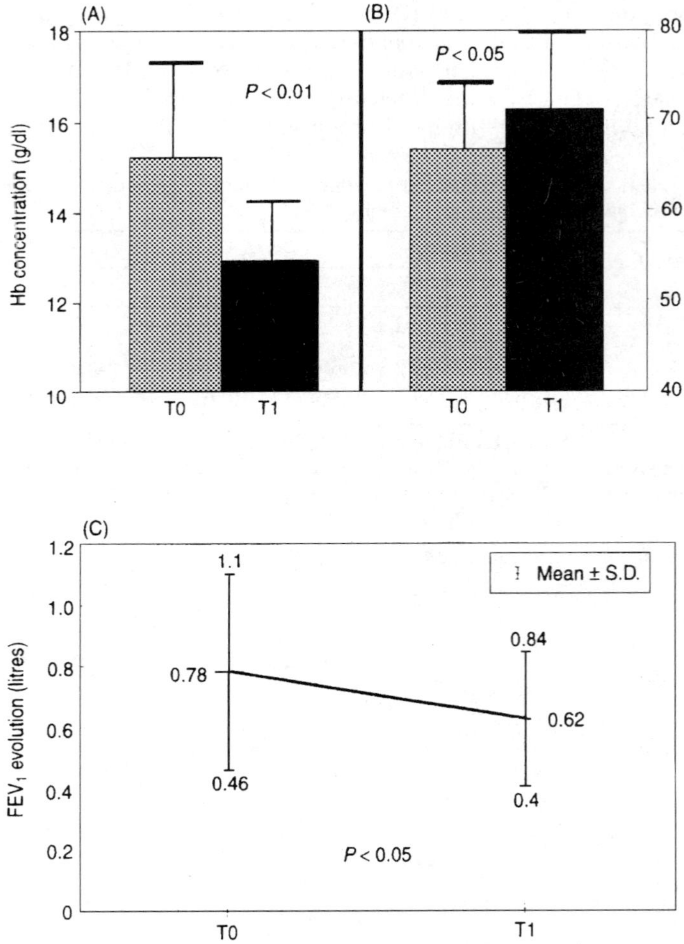

Figures 3. Hemoglobin (A), $Pa\text{O}_2$ (B) and FEV_1 evolution during oxygenation via TTC. An improvement in oxygenation (A and B) despite a deterioration in spirometric values (C) is observed.

Table 2. PFTs at the beginning (T_0) and end (T_1) of the study.

	T_0	T_1
FVC (liters)	1.68 ± 0.64	1.56 ± 0.65
FEV_1 (liters)	0.78 ± 0.32	0.62 ± 0.22*
FEV_1/FVC (%)	47 ± 9.9	34.7 ± 9.5*
RV (liters)	4.68 ± 1.61	4.55 ± 1.71
TLC (liters)	6.15 ± 3.02	6.84 ± 2.26
SG_{aw} (S^{-1} cmH_2O^{-1})	0.044 ± 0.039	0.037 ± 0.025
DLCO (%)	59.8 ± 28	51.2 ± 24*
KCO (%)	73.4 ± 39.2	68.2 ± 29.5
MVV (liters/min)	33.8 ± 12.7	32.8 ± 14.1

Values are means ± S.D. * $P < 0.05$ compared with the beginning of the study. Abbreviations: FVC, forced vital capacity; FEV_1, forced expiratory volume in the first second; RV, residual volume; TLC, total lung capacity; DLCO, diffusing lung capacity for CO; KCO, DLCO/alveolar volume; MVV, maximal voluntary ventilation; SG_{aw}, specific airways conductance.

cardiac rate (94 ± 11) and the VAS (3.5 ± 2.6) (Figure 4). There were only significant differences between heart rate and VAS at the beginning and end of each test, which indicates that patients made a considerable effort, causing an increase in heart rate as well as a feeling of dyspnea. No correlation was found with any of the hemodynamic parameters previously mentioned.

The anamnesis performed routinely showed that all the patients usually spent more than 4 h away from their homes, and three of them restarted work; the oximetric monitoring ruled out an inaccurate oxygen delivery as is sometimes the case with some portable liquid oxygen devices.[17]

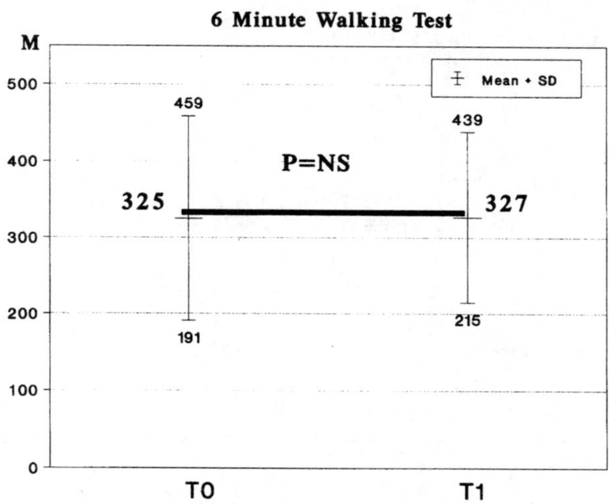

Figure 4. Mean values for the 6-min walking test at the beginning of the study (T_0) and at the end of the follow-up (T_1).

A comparison between RVEF and LVEF after 1 year of oxygenation via TTC and liquid oxygen 24 h a day showed no deterioration (Table 1). In five patients, reliable results for ventricular volumes were obtained. They showed that effort did not alter either RV or LV volumes, but at rest the ESV ($P = 0.05$) and EDV ($P = 0.06$) of the right ventricle showed a tendency to decrease (Figures 5A and 5B).

Data referring to right heart catheterization are shown in Table 3 and Figures 5(C) and 5(D). A sustained pulmonary arteriolar vascular resistance improvement was observed at the end of the follow-up. PAP, PVR, and cardiac output did not vary; PCWP was always within normal limits. Similarly, the cardiac work observed did not vary (9559 ± 1435 versus 9955 ± 1710).

The echocardiography evaluation showed that there was slight tricuspid regurgitation (TR) in six patients and moderate TR in two at the beginning and end of the follow-up. No differences were detected in the end-diastolic left ventricle diameter (41.7±9 mm), in the RV free wall (RVFW) thickness (8.6 ± 1.8 mm), or in the septum thickness (11.1 ± 1.16 mm). The end-diastolic right ventricle diameter showed a non-significant tendency to decrease (31.6 ± 8 versus 27.5 ± 4.5 mm) (Figure 6A). We also calculated a proportional right ventricle free wall stress (RVFWS) index which showed a decrease in post-load (134 ± 60 versus 105±39 mmHg; $P<0.05$) (Figure 6B).

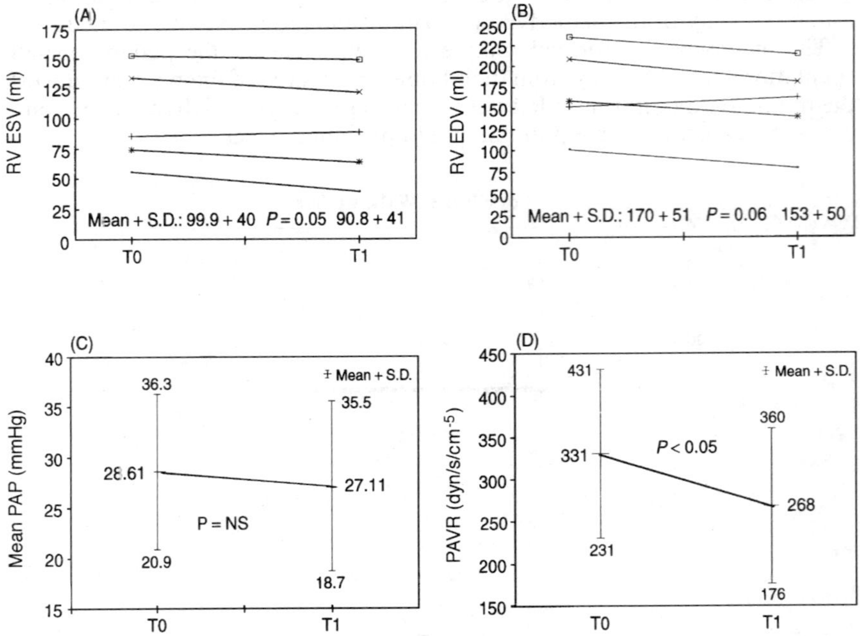

Figure 5. Evolution of RV end-systolic volume (A), end-diastolic volume (B), pulmonary arterial pressure (C) and pulmonary arteriolar vascular resistance (D) determined at rest after 1 year of oxygenation 24 h a day with liquid oxygen via TTC.

Table 3. Comparison of the hemodynamic data obtained after right heart catheterization at the beginning of the study (T_0) and after one year of oxygenation 24 h a day with liquid oxygen via transtracheal catheter T_1.

Parameter	T_0	T_1
Mean PAP (mmHg)	28.6 ± 7	27.1 ± 8.3
PVR (dyn/s/cm^{-5})	427 ± 120	390 ± 138
PAVR (dyn/s/cm^{-5})	331 ± 108	268 ± 92*
PCWP (mmHg)	6.0 ± 3.2	9.39 ± 3.5
CO (liters/min)	5.6 ± 0.9	5.67 ± 0.7
CI (liters/min/m^2)	3.35 ± 0.68	3.38 ± 0.49
SVRI (dyn/s/cm^{-5})	2111 ± 581	2138 ± 418
CW (mmHg-BPM)	9404 ± 1353	9559 ± 1435
IRVFWS (mmHg)	134 ± 60	105 ± 39*

Values are means ± S.D. * $P < 0.05$ compared with the beginning of the study. Abbreviations: CO, cardiac output; CI, cardiac index; SVRI, systemic vascular resistance index; CW, cardiac work (calculated as: systolic blood pressure × cardiac rate); BPM, beats per minute.

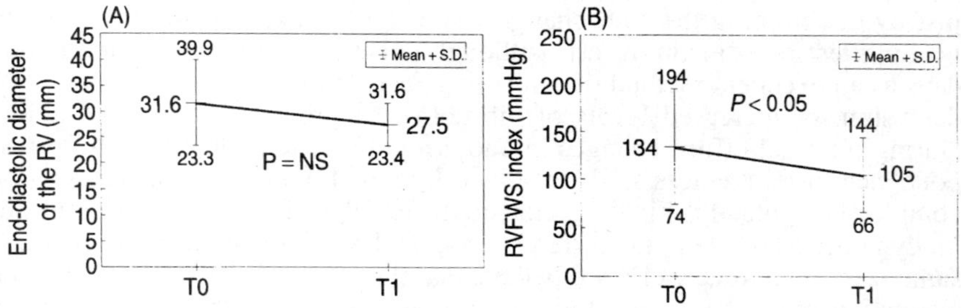

Figure 6. Tendency for the end-diastolic diameter of the right ventricle to decrease (A) and a significant decrease in RVFWS index (B), illustrating the better physiologic situation of the right ventricle after 1 year of oxygenation 24 h a day with liquid oxygen via TTC.

DISCUSSION

In this study we contrasted the hemodynamic responses to three different oxygen delivery devices in a group of patients suffering from very severe COPD, who had previously been receiving oxygen through nasal prongs 18 h a day. The patients were reliable followers of instructions, as was demonstrated by the continuous anamneses carried out with them and with their relatives, and the hemoglobin levels were in the normal upper range despite their baseline hypoxemia. The patients were in a stable situation since none had suffered a respiratory infection or a cor pulmonale decompensation during the 3 months previous to the beginning of the study, and the PFTs did not improve at the end of the study when compared with those at the beginning. Finally, cardiac output measured by thermodilution and average EF by isotopic ventriculography (both performed with oxygen) were within normal limits, and the PCWP ruled out the possibility of hyperhydration or left cardiac failure. Clinical data, anthropometric data and the morphology of desaturations ruled out the possibility of obstructive sleep apnea syndrome (OSAS), which could otherwise have been relieved with the insertion of a TTC. Clinical tolerance to TTC was good, in keeping with the literature on the subject.[18,19] The level of oxygen saving was as expected, with patients at rest (including sleep) or exercising.[14]

The evaluation of the acute response to the three different oxygen-delivery devices tested revealed that, with the patient at rest, the three methods are useful and that O and TTC save almost 50% of the oxygen consumption needed with nasal prongs. When patients performed maximal exercise, despite the fact they could reach the same level of cardiac work, the hemodynamic response of the right ventricle of the patients differed markedly depending on the oxygen device used. The clinical application of this observation is that, despite the use of O being a good method for oxygenating these patients at rest (including sleep) and despite the fact that it allows a 50% oxygen saving, in those patients who are keen to restart physical activity, the O is not the best oxygen-saving device. TTC, while maintaining the preset percentage of oxygen saving, allows a hemodynamic response as satisfactory as nasal prongs.

It may be that this different hemodynamic response could have been shown just by determining the $Sa\text{O}_2$ changes with a pulse oximeter during a 6-min walking test or a treadmill test. Although pulse oximetry is accepted nowadays as an excellent method of evaluating $Sa\text{O}_2$,[20] in some cases (patients with dark skin, or increased levels of bilirubin) the procedure is less reliable.[21] During physical effort, changes in $Sa\text{O}_2$ seem to be reliable but their correspondence to $Pa\text{O}_2$ is less so.[22] Moreover, light and motion artifacts cannot be completely avoided.[23] Finally, after observing that despite the different hemodynamic response to the different oxygen devices the patients reached the same level of cardiac work, we believe that the more reliable methods for the evaluation of the hemodynamic response are those tests that directly assess the hemodynamic function of the cardiac pump.

Since the O was not thought to be a good oxygenation device for patients undertaking considerable levels of physical activity, we performed a long-term evaluation only of patients oxygenated via TTC and liquid oxygen 24 h a day. Oxygenation in these patients improved, as demonstrated by the decrease in hemoglobin values, also noted by Christopher et al.[19] Attention should be drawn to the improvement observed in $Pa\text{O}_2$ at the end of follow-up, although the PFTs did not improve.[12] This has also been pointed out by O'Donohue,[24] who attributes it to the benefits of oxygen therapy.

The PFTs of our patients not only failed to improve, but some parameters, such as the FEV_1, worsened, thus ruling out the hypothesis that cardiopulmonary hemodynamic improvement might be due to an improvement in PFTs.[13] Christopher et al[25] suggested the possibility that the continuous oxygen flow may have a positive end-expiratory pressure effect. Couser & Make[26] demonstrated that TTC-delivered oxygen lowered the inspired minute/volume and that this was one of the mechanisms that improved the patient's clinical state.

VAS, 6-min walking test and maximum voluntary ventilation (MVV) did not worsen, possibly for the reasons stated in the theory of Couser & Make,[26] as much as the improvement in $Pa\text{O}_2$, but it is obvious that it was not due to PFT changes. Weitzemblum et al[27] observed that, although oxygen delivered via nasal prongs could partially reverse pulmonary arterial hypertension, it could not improve a patient's spirometry, nor could it be expected therefore to improve the spirometry of our group. Continuous oxygen delivered by TTC can slow down the deterioration in exercise capacity, but it does not improve static or dynamic PFT.[28] We could not relate 6-min walking test to any other hemodynamic parameter. Nevertheless, hemodynamic parameters are frequently not correlated to the patient's exercise capacity.

The echocardiography evaluation showed that the incidence of tricuspid regurgitation at the beginning and end of this study was practically identical, and never severe. Cardiac output calculated by thermodilution is therefore reliable.[29] Only the RV diameter showed a tendency to decrease, although it did not reach statistical significance.

According to some authors,[30] EF is a good noninvasive method of evaluating the function of both ventricles. MacKnee et al[31] studied the repercussion that oxygen administration could have on the ventricular function of patients with COPD without signs of cor pulmonale and on patients with decompensated cor pulmonale. He concluded that the RV and LV functions are normal in patients suffering from COPD without clinical signs of cor pulmonale, but they are diminished in patients with decompensated cor pulmonale. He also observed that mean PAP was not significantly different in the two groups, which led him to the conclusion that the lowering of contractility in patients with decompensated cor pulmonale was not due to a post-load increase. In other words, the worsening of pulmonary hypertension could not be the cause of right heart failure. Our results show that the RVEF is slightly lower in this group of patients than in the normal population and although RVEF and LVEF at rest were maintained, the response to exercise showed a deficit. Moreover, Weitzemblum et al[32] have recently observed in a longitudinal study that a hemodynamic worsening is observed in patients with COPD exhibiting both edema and an exacerbation of respiratory failure and could explain the development of right heart failure. Thus the lack of increase in mean PAP observed by Macknee could be due to the inability in their patients of the RV to generate a greater pressure and therefore to increase the EF or the cardiac output.

We observed a slight decrease in mean PAP at the end of the 1 year follow-up as well as a sustained increase in pulmonary arteriolar vasodilation. There was no deterioration in the EF of either ventricle; RV dilation tended to decrease when evaluated with two different techniques (isotopic ventriculography and echocardiogram), and there was also a fall in the proportional index of the RV wall stress. By oxygenating our patients in a more rational manner (reflected by a decrease in the hemoglobin values), we have achieved a long-term decrease in pulmonary arteriolar vascular resistance. This could possibly be attributed to several factors, such as decreasing blood viscosity secondary to a lower hematocrit and/or continuous capillary recruitment of the pulmonary vasculature. The long-term repercussion of this is demonstrated in the involution of RV dilation.

To summarize, we have shown that O and TTC are excellent methods for home oxygen therapy and that they allow a 50% oxygen saving, which is especially important when patients require high oxygen flows. In these cases, the oxygen-saving devices make the oxygen therapy more tolerable, allow the use of concentrators, and increase the autonomy of liquid oxygen strollers. If a patient intends to restart work or perform outdoor physical activity for very long, we believe that continuous 24 h a day oxygenation with liquid oxygen via TTC improves the hemodynamic situation of patients suffering from severe COPD and chronic hypoxemia although they were previously correctly oxygenated via nasal prongs for 18 h a day. Continuous oxygenation with TTC allows them to maintain the same exercise capacity and improve arterial blood gases. Therefore this confirms Flenley's point of view[5] that the more hours that oxygen is received by a patient the better, and it is obvious that, nowadays, the best method to achieve a 24 h oxygenation is via TTC. We have also been able to demonstrate that it is possible to intervene in the evolution of chronic cor pulmonale. Likewise, we should note that several studies carried out to date have evaluated patients applying only one technique, a situation that did not reliably reflect the effect that oxygen may have on pulmonary hemodynamics. In contrast, we have studied a series of patients by applying three different techniques simultaneously. Moreover, we have studied a number of parameters that have not been well studied in the literature published to date (pulmonary arteriolar vascular resistance, wall stress, ventricular volumes), and which may give a better reflection of the real evolution of chronic cor pulmonale treated by long-term oxygen therapy. Finally, our data confirm empirically clinical observations demonstrating the advantages of TTC-delivered oxygen, such as better tolerance to exercise,[28] improvement of cor pulmonale, and a lowering of the hematocrit.[19]

REFERENCES

1. American Thoracic Society (1974) Standards for the diagnosis and care of patients with chronic obstructive pulmonary disease (COPD) and asthma. *American Review of Respiratory Disease* **135:**225–243.
2. NOTT Study Group (1980) Is 12-hour oxygen as effective as 24-hour oxygen in advanced chronic obstructive pulmonary disease with hypoxemia? *Chest* **78:**419–420.
3. Nocturnal Oxygen Therapy Trial Group (NOTT) (1980) Continuous or nocturnal oxygen therapy in hypoxemic obstructive lung disease. A clinical trial. *Annals of Internal Medicine* **93:**391–398.
4. Report of the Medical Research Council Working Party (1981) Long term domiciliary oxygen therapy in chronic hypoxic cor pulmonale complicating chronic bronchitis and emphysema. *Lancet* **1:**681–686.
5. Flenley DC (1985) Long-term home oxygen therapy. *Chest* **87:**99–103.
6. Ashutosh K, Mead G & Dunsky M (1983) Early effects of oxygen administration and prognosis in chronic obstructive pulmonary disease and cor pulmonale. *American Review of Respiratory Disease* **127:**399–404.
7. MacKnee W, Morgan AD, Wathen CG, Muir AL & Flenley DC (1985) Right ventricular performance during exercise in chronic obstructive pulmonary disease. The effects of oxygen. *Respiration* **48:**206–215.
8. Heimlich HJ (1982) Respiratory rehabilitation with transtracheal oxygen system. *Annals of Otology, Rhinology and Laryngology* **91:**643–647.
9. Domingo CH, Léger P & Morera J (1990) Catéter transtraqueal: una puerta abierta a la oxigenoterapia moderna. *Medicina Clinica (Barcelona)* **94:**103–106.
10. Tiep BL, Nicotra B, Carter R, Belman MJ & Mittman C (1984) Evaluation of a

low-flow oxygen-conserving nasal cannula. *American Review of Respiratory Disease* **130:**500–502.

11. Tiep BL, Belman MJ, Mittman C, Phillips R & Otsap B (1985) A new pendant storage oxygen conserving nasal cannula. *Chest* **87:**381–383.
12. Domingo Ch, Domingo E, Coll R, Izquierdo J & Morera J (1992) Effect of oxygen therapy on increasing $Pa\text{O}_2$ in hypoxaemic patients with stable COPD while breathing ambient air. *Chest* **102:**1311.
13. Domingo Ch, Coll R, Izquierdo J, Roig J, Klamburg J, Domingo E, Moreno JA & Morera J (1995) Catéter transtraqueal y oxígeno líquido: 5 años de experiencia. *Archivos de Bronconeumologia* **31:**13–17.
14. Domingo CH, Roig J, Gallego M, Ruiz J, Izquierdo J & Morera J (1990) Oxygen saving during sleep with transtracheal catheter and oxymizer. *European Respiratory Journal* **3:**414s.
15. Domingo CH, Klamburg J, Coll, R, Izquierdo J, Torrabadella P & Tomasa A (1991) Catéter transtraqueal: complicaciones inmediatas. *Medicina Intensiva* **15:**123–126.
16. Domingo CH, Domingo E, Coll R, Roig J, Klamburg J & Morera J (1990) Transtracheal catheter and liquid oxygen: 2 years of experience in Spain. *European Respiratory Journal* **3:**414s.
17. Massey LW, Hussey JD & Albert RK (1988) Inacurate oxygen delivery in some portable liquid oxygen devices. *American Review of Respiratory Disease* **137:**204–205.
18. Heimlich HJ & Carr GC (1989) The micro-trach. A seven year experience with transtracheal oxygen therapy. *Chest* **95:**1008–1012.
19. Christopher KL, Spofford BT, Petrun M, McCarthy DC, Goodman JR & Petty TL (1987) A program for transtracheal oxygen delivery. *Annals of Internal Medicine* **107:**802–808.
20. Decker Mj, Hoekje PL & Strhl KP (1989) Ambulatory monitoring of arterial oxygen saturation. *Chest* **95:**717–722.
21. Ries Al, Prewitt LM & Johnson JJ (1989) Skin color and heart oximetry. *Chest* **96:**287–290.
22. Escourrou PJL, Delaperche MF & Visseaux A (1990) Reliability of pulse-oximetry during exercise in pulmonary patients. *Chest* **97:**635–638.
23. Tremper KK (1989) Pulse oximetry. *Chest* **95:**713–715.
24. O'Donohue WJ (1991) Effect of oxygen therapy on increasing arterial oxygen tension in hypoxaemic patients with stable chronic obstructive pulmonary disease while breathing ambient air. *Chest* **100:**968–972.
25. Christopher KL, Spofford BT, Brannin PK & Petty TL (1986) Transtracheal oxygen therapy for refractory hypoxemia. *Journal of the American Medical Association* **256:**494–7.
26. Couser JI & Make BJ (1989) Transtracheal oxygen decreases inspired minute ventilation. *American Review of Respiratory Disease* **139:**627–631.
27. Weitzenblum E, Sautegeau A, Ehrhart M, Mammosser M & Pelletier A (1985) Long-term oxygen therapy can reverse the progression of pulmonary hypertension in patients with chronic obstructive pulmonary disease. *American Review of Respiratory Disease* **131:**493–498.
28. Hoffman LA, Dauber JH, Ferson PF, Openbrier DR & Zullo TG (1987) Patient response to transtracheal oxygen delivery. *American Review of Respiratory Disease* **135:**153–156.
29. Cigarroa R, Lange RA, Williams RH, Bedotto JB & Hillis D (1989) Underestimation of cardiac output by thermodilution in patients with tricuspid regurgitation. *American Journal of Medicine* **86:**417–420.
30. Morrison DA, Henry R & Goldman S (1986) Preliminary study of the effects of low flow oxygen on oxygen delivery and right ventricular function in chronic lung disease. *American Review of Respiratory Disease* 1986; 133: 390–5.

31. MacKnee W, Wathen CG, Flenley DC & Muir AD (1988) The effects of controlled oxygen therapy on ventricular function in patients with stable and decompensated cor pulmonale. *American Review of Respiratory Disease* **137**:1289–1290.
32. Weitzemblum E, Apprill M, Oswald M, Chaouat A & Imbs JL (1994) Pulmonary haemodynamics in patients with chronic obstructive pulmonary disease before and during an episode of peripheral edema. *Chest* **105**:1377–1382.

11

Pulmonary Blood Flow in Lung Transplant Recipients

Kang H. Lee
Michael R. Pinsky
Arthur Boujoukos

INTRODUCTION

In our population of single lung transplant patients, we have been attempting to identify factors that determine their length of intensive care unit (ICU) stay after surgery.[1] It was reasoned that the ability to sustain spontaneous ventilation and having an adequate oxygenation level may be two such important factors. Oxygenation is dependent on the relative distributions of ventilation and perfusion to each lung (*V/Q* imbalances) which may be particularly disparate between the native and transplanted lung, especially in patients with pulmonary hypertension. The transplanted lung may also suffer from preservation injury contributing to overall hypoxemia.

Thus the ability to *quantify* individual lung function (transplant versus native lung) would aid better understanding of integrated lung physiology and allow the objective assessment of measures postulated to improve individual lung performance (e.g. nitric oxide, prostaglandins). We sought to quantify individual lung function by measuring each lung's venous admixture using the principle of conservation of mass, which first required a validation of a noninvasive method of assessing relative lung perfusion (right versus left).

ASSESSMENT OF RELATIVE LUNG PERFUSION

Total pulmonary blood flow can be estimated by thermodilution cardiac output measurements or by the Fick principle.[2] However, the noninvasive measurement of pulmonary blood flow to each lung separately is much more difficult.[3] Current techniques of quantifying differential lung blood flow involve radioactive material, xenon or technetium, which have inherent radioactive risks, are expensive, and are a single snapshot of the situation. We thus hypothesized that the much simpler technique of split-lung VCO_2 measurements by expiratory gas analysis would reflect relative lung perfusion.

In a canine model we measured VCO_2 from each lung separately with two metabolic monitors via a double-lumen endobronchial tube, and correlated this measurement with pulmonary artery flow measurements by ultrasonic flow probes placed via a left thoracotomy around the main and left pulmonary arteries. Correlation was sought under several different conditions: normal lungs, alterations in unilateral pulmonary blood flow, and after acute unilateral acid lung injury. The pooled results for all the conditions demonstrated that there was a significant linear relationship between percentage VCO_2 and percentage flow to that particular lung (Figure 1). We thus concluded that this was a valid method to assess changes in individual lung perfusion noninvasively even in situations where there was significant lung injury.

We then extended this finding to the clinical arena and studied four lung transplant patients after surgery. All the patients had double-lumen endotubes and had independent ventilation. VCO_2 was measured from each lung separately with a metabolic monitor, and technetium radionuclide perfusion scans were performed to quantify the relative perfusion between the two lungs. The results again confirm the linear relationship seen in the canine studies (Figure 2).

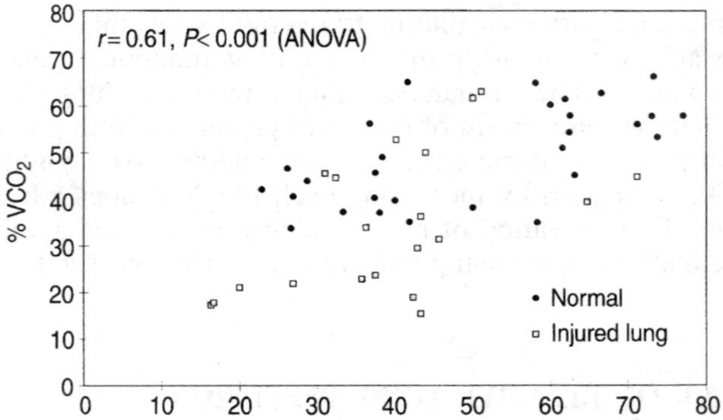

Figure 1. Relation between individual lung blood flow as a percentage of total blood flow (% Flow) and individual lung CO_2 production as a percentage of total CO_2 production (% VCO_2) in a canine model.

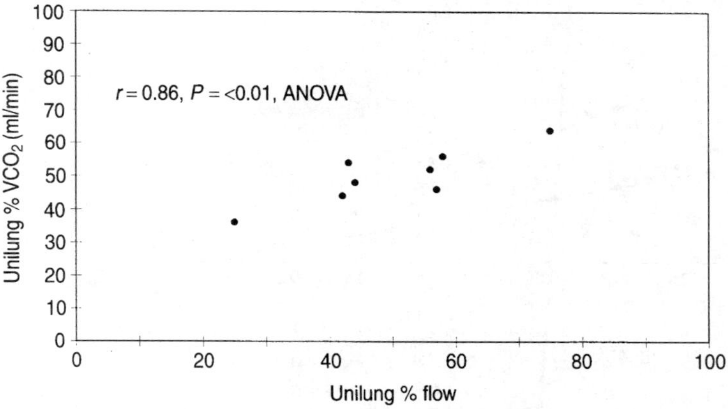

Figure 2. Relation between % blood flow and % CO2 production in a single lung from studies on humans.

CHARACTERIZATION OF UNILUNG VENOUS ADMIXTURE

Employing the principle of conservation of mass, one could create an equation where the total oxygen delivery is the sum of each lung's contribution. Each lung's contribution can be divided into a two-compartment model: one of perfect ventilation–perfusion matching and one of a shunt (venous admixture). Assuming no change in each lung's venous admixture, one can then either vary relative flow or vary the F_iO_2 to each lung separately to vary the oxygen content of capillarized blood in order to develop a set of simultaneous equations which can then be solved with unique solutions for each lung's venous admixture (Appendix 1). This equation requires the knowledge of relative lung perfusion (right versus left), which we deduced from measurements of VCO_2 from each lung.

We developed a computer program to solve the equation and applied this method in four single-lung transplant patients for the measurement of unilung venous admixture by varying the F_iO_2 to each lung (right lung 1.0, left lung 1.0; right lung 1.0, left lung 0.4; and right lung 0.4, left lung 1.0). This methodology shows early promise. Figure 3 demonstrates the graphical solution to the two simultaneous equations of one of the patients studied. Our initial results have suggested that alterations in F_iO_2 create only a small change in capillarized blood content, and this may thus lead to potential errors from the innate errors in blood gas measurements. Alteration of relative lung blood flow by changes in body position may allow a greater change that will allow for greater specificity. This has yet to be tested clinically.

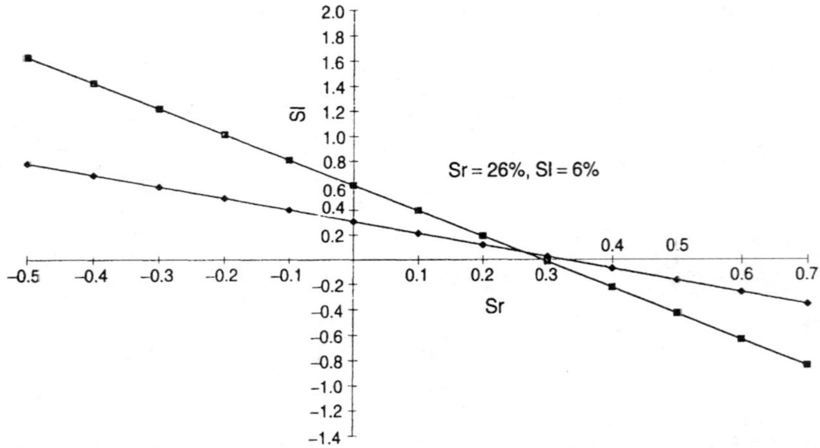

Figure 3. Graphical solution for the two simultaneous equations generated from applying the equation in Appendix 1. Sr, venous admixture for the right lung; Sl, venous admixture for the left lung.

SUMMARY

The percentage of unilung blood flow can be followed by the noninvasive method of percentage VCO_2 from each lung. Employing this method one can characterize unilung venous admixture. This will serve to improve our understanding of lung diseases with significant disparities between left and right lung function (e.g. after single-lung transplant) as well as providing the ability to document whether new therapeutic interventions have any beneficial effect on the transplanted lung.

REFERENCES

1. Lee KH, Martich GD, Bierman MI, Boujoukos AJ, Keenan RJ & Griffith BP (1994) Predictive indices for outcome following single lung transplantation (Abstract). *Chest* **106:**41S.
2. Gedeon A, Forslund L, Hedenstierna G & Romano E (1980) A new method for non-invasive bedside determination of pulmonary blood flow. *Medical and Biological Engineering and Computing* **18:**411–418.
3. Nunn JF (1993) *Applied Respiratory Physiology*, 4th edn. pp 193–194 London: Butterworth.

APPENDIX 1

$Q_T \times F_R\,[CcO_2^{R}\,(1 - S_R) + C\bar{v}O_2 \times S_R)] + Q_T \times F_2[CcO_2^{L}(1{-}S_L) + (C\bar{v}O_2 \times S_L)$ where Q_T = total cardiac output; F_R = fraction of blood flow to right lung; F_L = fraction of blood flow to left lung; CcO_2^{R} = capillary oxygen content on right; S_R fraction of stunt in right lung; $C\bar{v}O_2$ = mixed venous oxygen concentration; CaO_2 = arterial oxygen concentration.

Part III

Pulmonary Blood Flow

12

Acute Respiratory Failure: Pressure–Flow Relations and Nitric Oxide

Robert Naeije

PULMONARY HYPERTENSION IN ADULT (OR ACUTE) RESPIRATORY DISTRESS SYNDROME (ARDS)

The initial description of ARDS by Ashbaugh et al in 1967[1] did not include pulmonary hemodynamic measurements. This is not surprising since, at that time, invasive hemodynamic monitoring was not yet routine practice in the intensive care unit. The flow-directed thermodilution pulmonary artery catheter was reported by Swan, Ganz et al in 1970.[2] In 1977, Zapol and Snider demonstrated that pulmonary hypertension is a physiologic hallmark of ARDS, as are increased pulmonary shunt and decreased pulmonary compliance.[3] This pulmonary hypertension is seldom severe. In over 100 patients with ARDS studied between 1 and 30 days after the onset of symptoms while mechanically ventilated with 5–40 cmH_2O positive end-expiratory pressure (PEEP), Zapol and co-workers observed mean pulmonary arterial pressure (PAP) to be around 22–28 mmHg in the absence of severe hypoxemia, but higher, in the range of 28–35 mmHg and more in severe hypoxemia.[4] The highest PAPs were seen in patients with the most advanced ARDS and clinical signs of right heart failure. These observations have been repeatedly confirmed by others.[5–7] Thus a diagnosis of ARDS is very unlikely in patients with a PAP < 20 mmHg and a cardiac output (Q) above 2.5 liters/min per m^2. On the other hand, very high levels of PAP suggest the existence of other causes of pulmonary hypertension.

Zapol and co-workers described pulmonary hemodynamics in ARDS by pulmonary vascular resistance (PVR) calculations, and by PAP versus Q plots or PVR versus Q plots. In addition to constantly elevated PVR or PAP at given levels of Q, they found an apparent independence of PAP and Q, contrasting with a hyperbolic decrease in PVR with increasing Q. This striking behavior of the pulmonary circulation in ARDS was evident when data from a large group of patients were pooled, as well as when data were obtained from individual patients in whom pulmonary blood flow was altered either by vasoactive drugs or by a change in bypass flow during extracorporeal membrane oxygenation (ECMO) studies (Figure 1).[8] A proposed explanation for these PAP/Q and PVR/Q relationships was that pulmonary hypertension in ARDS would be accounted for by an increased pulmonary vascular closing pressure.[4,8,9]

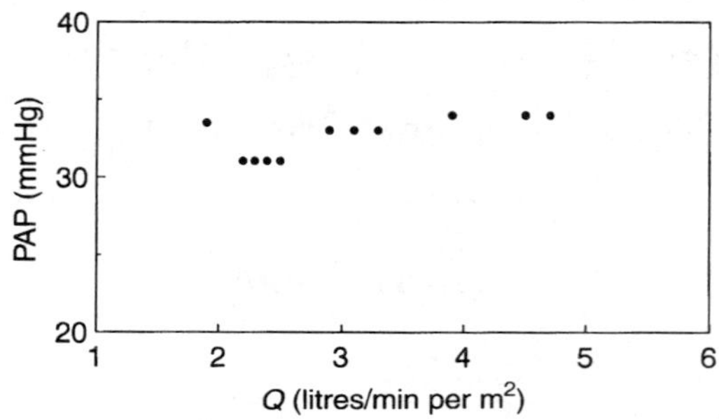

Figure 1. Absence of significant changes in mean PAP in a patient with ARDS whose pulmonary blood flow (Q) was altered by changes in bypass flow during ECMO and an infusion of isoproterenol.[8]

PULMONARY VASCULAR PRESSURE–FLOW RELATIONSHIPS

In pulmonary hemodynamic studies, PVR, calculated classically as PAP minus left atrial pressure (LAP) (estimated by pulmonary artery occluded pressure (PAOP)) divided by Q, is usually taken either as an index of the forces that oppose flow in the pulmonary circulation, or as an index of the pulmonary arteriolar cross-sectional area. In clinical practice, because of an often overlooked insufficient frequency response of fluid-filled catheters for the accurate measurement of instantaneous pressures, and because of the use of thermodilution cardiac output determinations, only valid numbers for mean PAP and for mean Q can be obtained. The calculation of PVR thus ignores the natural pulsatility of the pulmonary circulation. It has been shown that the 'steady-flow' hemodynamic approach underestimates right ventricular afterload by 30–50% in normal subjects, possibly more in patients with pulmonary hypertension.[10] Still, PVR can be used to estimate pulmonary arteriolar tone, by using a transposition of Poiseuille's law to the pulmonary circulation, provided that two major assumptions are made. The first is that PAP/Q or (PAP – PAOP)/Q plots are described by a linear approximation. The second is that the extrapolation of (PAP – PAOP)/Q plots crosses the origin.

Pulmonary vascular pressure versus flow plots have been found to be well described by a linear approximation over a physiological range of flows in healthy as well as in diseased lungs, *in vivo* as well as *in vitro*. In healthy well-oxygenated lungs perfused in zone 3, the extrapolation of a (PAP – PAOP)/*Q* plot crosses the origin. However, when lungs are perfused in zone 2, hypoxic or diseased, the extrapolated pressure intercept of (PAP – PAOP)/*Q* plots may become positive. This means that pulmonary blood flow stops when the inflow pressure (PAP) becomes equal to or lower than a closing pressure higher than LAP (estimated by PAOP). In these situations, PAOP becomes an apparent outflow pressure of the pulmonary circulation, of which the effective outflow pressure is the pulmonary vascular closing pressure, and PVR is no longer a constant value independent of the absolute levels of PAP or *Q*. Because blood vessels are collapsible and have tone, most vascular systems present with a closing pressure higher than their venous pressure. In the same way that the flow of a waterfall is unaffected by its height, the flow within a vascular system is unaffected by changes in its apparent venous outflow pressure as long as the latter remains lower than its closing pressure.[11]

An important consequence of the presence of an increased closing pressure within the pulmonary circulation is that PAP/*Q* plots are curvilinear, with a convexity to the pressure axis at low flow. The pulmonary circulation is then derecruited because of collapse of the vessels with the highest closing pressure. At higher rates of flow, all the pulmonary vessels are recruited, and an estimate of mean closing pressure can be obtained by extrapolation of the linear portion of the PAP/*Q* plots. When the extrapolation of the linear portion of (PAP – PAOP)/*Q* curves does not cross the origin, PVR calculations are misleading, as illustrated in Figure 2. The more the linear portion of a (PAP – PAOP)/*Q* curve is parallel to the flow axis, the more PVR passively decreases with the slightest increases in *Q*. Thus, when pulmonary hypertension is due to an increased closing pressure, PVR should not be calculated, and the functional state of the pulmonary circulation should be described by multipoint pulmonary vascular pressure versus flow curves.

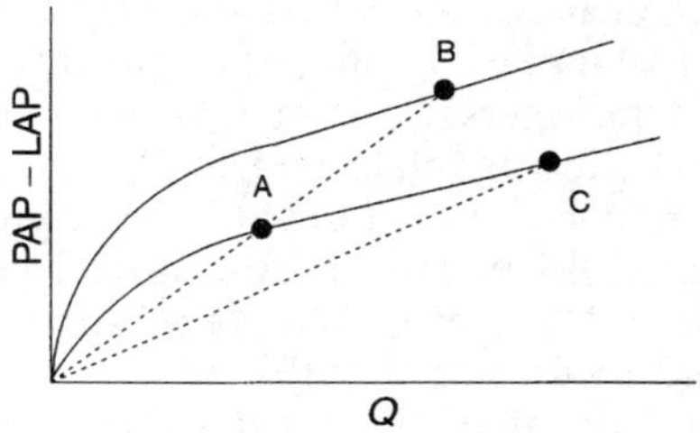

Figure 2. Misleading PVR calculations shown on hypothetical mean plots of PAP – LAP versus *Q* at two levels of pulmonary hypertension. A passive increase in PAP due to an increase in *Q* (from point A to C) is associated with a decrease in PVR, or slope of the dashed (PAP – LAP)/*Q* lines. An active pulmonary vasoconstriction (from point A to B) is associated with an unchanged PVR.

PULMONARY HYPERTENSION IN EXPERIMENTAL ARDS

Two methods can be used to show the presence of a closing pressure higher than the apparent outflow pressure within a vascular system.[12] The first is to measure vascular pressures at several rates of flow, preferably with the apparent outflow pressure kept low and constant, and to extrapolate the linear part of the pressure–flow curves obtained to the pressure axis. The linear part of these pressure–flow curves can be described by a slope, which is taken as the incremental PVR upstream to the site of vascular closure, and by an extrapolated pressure intercept, which is taken as the mean closing pressure of the pulmonary vessels. The second is to increase the apparent outflow pressure with the flow kept constant, and to record the level at which this maneuver results in an increase in the inflow pressure. Both methods are obviously technically difficult and would also be unethical in patients. We therefore went to the laboratory to investigate the pulmonary circulation in anesthetized dogs with oleic acid lung injury.[13] Oleic acid administration in dogs has been shown to induce a multifocal hemorrhagic pulmonary edema which bears close pathological and physiological similarities to the early stages of clinical ARDS.[14]

In a first series of experiments, we manipulated venous return, which was either decreased by stepwise inflations of a balloon in the inferior vena cava or increased by the opening of a femoral arteriovenous bypass, so as to measure PAP over a wide range of *Q*. LAP was kept constant by small inflations or deflations of a balloon inserted into the left atrium. PAP/*Q* plots thus obtained were linear before as well as after oleic acid administration. Before oleic acid, the extrapolated pressure intercept of the PAP/*Q* plots approximated LAP. Oleic acid administration shifted PAP/*Q* plots in parallel toward higher pressures (Figure 3). In a second series of experiments, *Q* was kept constant and LAP progressively increased. Before oleic acid, this induced a proportional increase in PAP. After oleic acid, only the highest LAP resulted in an increase in PAP (Figure 3). We concluded that in experimental ARDS, closing pressure exceeds LAP, becomes the effective outflow of the pulmonary circulation and is responsible for pulmonary hypertension.[13]

In order to get a deeper insight into the functional state of the pulmonary circulation in experimental ARDS, we studied the effects of an increased alveolar pressure (PEEP) on PAP/*Q* plots at constant transmural LAP and on PAP at constant *Q* and transmural LAP, in dogs before and after induction of oleic acid lung injury. Following oleic acid, PAP/*Q* plots were unaffected by a PEEP of 4 mmHg, but were shifted toward higher pressures by a PEEP of 10 mmHg. Increasing PEEP from 0 to 10 mmHg at constant *Q* led to an almost linear increase in PAP before oleic acid administration, but did not affect PAP after oleic acid until a PEEP of 8 mmHg. These functional dissociations between PAP and PEEP, illustrated in Figure 4, suggested to us that the site of vascular closure responsible for pulmonary hypertension in experimental ARDS would be extra-alveolar. If indeed the site of vascular closure had been alveolar, direct additive effects of PEEP and oleic acid lung injury would have been apparent on PAP/*Q* and PAP/PEEP plots at all levels of PEEP.[15] In all these canine studies, PAOP and LAP remained virtually

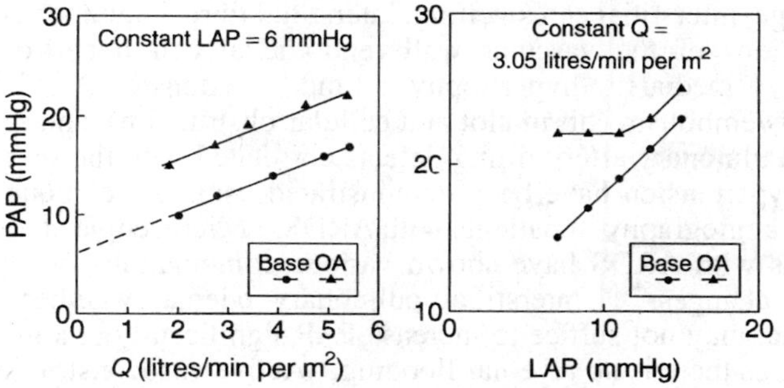

Figure 3. Mean PAP versus Q at constant LAP (left panel) and PAP versus LAP at constant Q (right panel) in a dog before and after induction of an acute oleic acid lung injury (OA). Oleic acid lung injury was associated with an increased extrapolated pressure intercept of the PAP/Q plot, and with a functional dissociation between PAP and LAP, both suggestive of an increased closing pressure accounting for pulmonary hypertension in this model of experimental ARDS.[13]

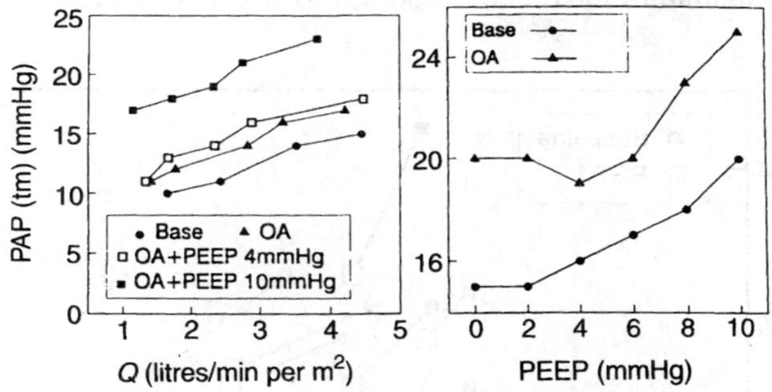

Figure 4. Transmural mean PAP (PAP (tm)) versus Q (left panel) and PAP (tm) versus PEEP at constant Q (right panel) in a dog before and after induction of an acute oleic acid lung injury (OA) and treated with progressively increased levels of PEEP. Only the highest level of PEEP shifted the PAP (tm)/Q plot to higher pressures. An increase in PAP (tm) occurred only after the highest levels of PEEP. This functional dissociation between PAP and PEEP suggests an extra-alveolar site for increased pulmonary vascular closing pressure in this model of experimental ARDS.[15]

identical in all experimental circumstances.[13,15] Zapol and co-workers had also noted that PEEP up to 20 cmH_2O affected PAP and PAOP little or not at all in patients with severe ARDS.[4]

MECHANISMS OF PULMONARY HYPERTENSION IN ARDS

Possible mechanisms for increased PAP in ARDS are active vasoconstriction, lumen compression by extravascular events (alveolar and interstitial hemorrhage, interstitial cell swelling, interstitial fibrosis), lumen compression by alterations of the vascular wall (endothelial cell hypertrophy and or swelling, medial hypertrophy and extension), intravascular thrombosis/embolism (fibrin clot and cellular obstruction), and reduced lung volume.[4] Pulmonary artery filling defects correlated with the severity of pulmonary hypertension have been demonstrated using a technique of balloon occlusion angiography in patients with ARDS.[16] Microscopic studies of lungs of patients with ARDS have shown various combinations of all the above structural changes.[17–19] Interstitial pulmonary edema, whether lesional or hydrostatic, may not suffice to increase PAP significantly at a given level of Q, as long as there is no alveolar flooding.[20] Active vasoconstriction has been demonstrated by a partial reversibility of pulmonary hypertension in patients with ARDS after the administration of vasodilators such as isoproterenol,[4] nitroprusside,[4,21] ketanserin,[21] diltiazem,[22] prostaglandin E_1[23] and nitric oxide (NO) or prostacyclin.[24] All these agents decreased PVR, but this was not only due to an increased Q. As illustrated in Figure 5, a reduction in pulmonary vascular tone is unequivocal when a decrease in PAP occurs in spite of an increase in Q.

Many vasodilators have been reported to decrease PVR in experimental

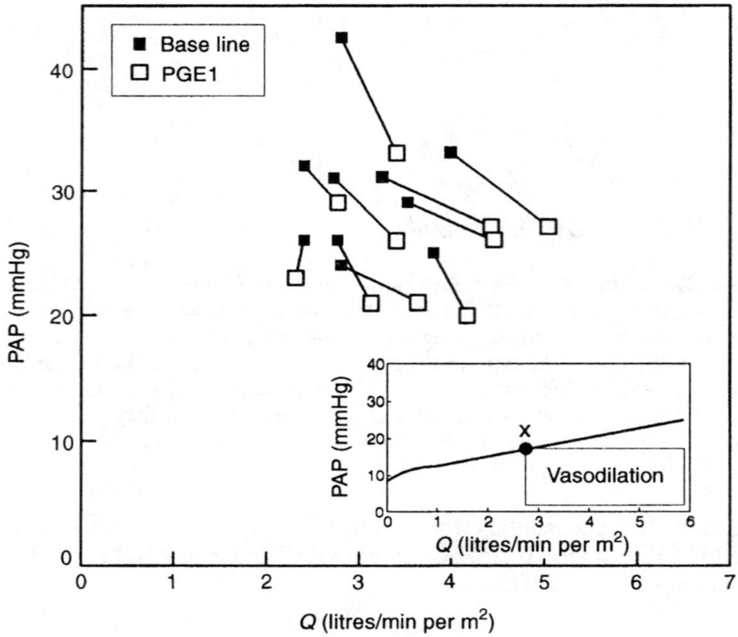

Figure 5. Mean PAP and Q in ten patients with ARDS before and after an infusion of prostaglandin E_1. Prostaglandin E_1 induced a pulmonary vasodilatation, as suggested by a decreased PAP in all the patients while Q increased in nine of them (six of these patients were reported by Mélot et al.)[23]

ARDS. We investigated the effects of prostaglandin E_1 and nitroprusside in dogs with oleic acid lung injury using the PAP/Q plot approach.[25] Nitroprusside was ineffective, while prostaglandin E_1 induced a 50% reversal of pulmonary hypertension (Figure 6). In studies on the acid–base status in canine oleic acid lung injury, we observed a quasi-complete reversal of pulmonary hypertension by severe metabolic alkalosis (arterial pH 7.6, arterial $P\text{CO}_2$ 40 mmHg).[26] Thus most of the increase in PAP in experimental ARDS appears to be reversible. Whether this finding might be transposed to early stages of clinical ARDS remains to be investigated.

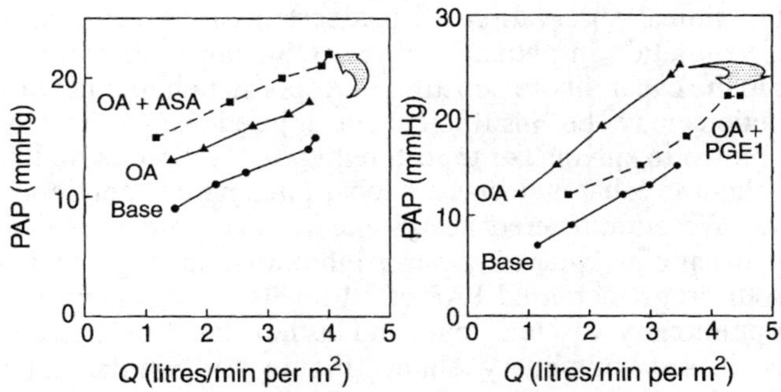

Figure 6. Mean PAP versus Q plots in a dog given successively oleic acid (OA) and acetylsalicylic acid (ASA) (left panel) and in another dog given successively OA and an infusion of prostaglandin E_1 (right panel). Pulmonary hypertension in this model of experimental ARDS is at least in part functional.[25,34]

PULMONARY VASCULAR TONE AND GAS EXCHANGE IN ARDS

Attempts at pharmacological pulmonary vasodilatation in ARDS have been justified by concern about a risk of excessively rapidly increasing right ventricular afterload in some patients,[4] and by the speculation that associated increased oxygen delivery (by means of an increased Q) and decreased pulmonary capillary pressures would be helpful.[27] Very often, intravenous vasodilators deteriorate gas exchange. More or less important increases in shunt have been reported in patients with ARDS after nitroprusside,[4,21] isoproterenol,[4] diltiazem,[22] prostaglandin E_1[23] and prostacyclin.[24] Postulated mechanisms of vasodilator-induced increases in pulmonary shunt are: (1) an increase in pulmonary blood flow, which promotes vascular recruitment in nonventilated lung units, increases alveolar edema, or blunts hypoxic vasoconstriction by means of an increased mixed venous $P\text{O}_2$, and (2) an altered distribution of pulmonary perfusion by direct inhibition of hypoxic vasoconstriction. In contrast, inhaled vasodilators improve gas exchange. Rossaint et al[24] reported a decrease in pulmonary shunt by inhaled NO at the doses of 18 or 36 ppm. Similar results were reported by Puybasset et al[28] with much lower doses of NO, in the range 100–2000 ppb, reducing the risk of NO toxicity.[28] Walmrath et al[29] reported that inhaled prostacyclin also reduces intrapulmonary shunt in patients with ARDS. These results are explained by a preferential vasodilation in the better aerated and less diseased lung areas, leading to improved ventilation/perfusion matching. It should be noted that the effect of inhaled NO or prostacyclin on pulmonary shunt in ARDS is variable, absent in some patients, and on average of not more than 5% of cardiac output. The decrease in PAP obtained is generally modest as well, in the range of a few mmHg. Whether these changes are important enough to improve outcome is not yet known. In a retrospective study on 87 patients with severe ARDS, survival was no different in the 30 treated with inhaled NO.[30]

Anecdotal clinical observations of inadvertent airway disconnection from mechanical ventilation in patients with ARDS suggest that their pulmonary vessels retain the capability to constrict in response to hypoxia.[4] Still, hypoxic vasoconstriction may be insufficient in injured lungs. Cyclooxygenase inhibitors, known to enhance or to restore hypoxic vasoconstriction, decrease pulmonary shunt in lobar atelectasis,[31] lobar pneumonia[32] and lobar oleic acid lung injury.[33] We administered acetylsalicylic acid and indomethacin, two structurally dissimilar cyclooxygenase inhibitors, in dogs with oleic acid ARDS.[34] Both drugs increased PAP at all levels of Q studied indicating an increase in pulmonary vascular tone, and at the same time increased arterial $P\text{O}_2$ and decreased pulmonary shunt (Figure 6). Similar findings were reported after the administration of meclofenamate, another cyclooxygenase inhibitor, also in dogs with oleic acid lung injury.[35] We compared the effects of aspirin and indomethacin with those of a placebo in 24 patients with severe ARDS.[36] While placebo had no effect, both cyclooxygenase inhibitors decreased pulmonary shunt by an average of 5%, interestingly without detectable effect on pulmonary hemodynamics.[36] Administration of L-arginine analogs, such as L-nitrosyl arginine (L-NA)[37] or *N*-monomethyl-L-arginine (L-NMMA)[38] in dogs with oleic acid lung injury increases pulmonary vascular tone, but does not improve gas exchange, leaving uncertainty as to the contribution of endogenous NO to abnormal gas exchange. However, a nonspecific (non $P\text{O}_2$-dependent) increase in pulmonary vascular tone enhances the beneficial effect of inhaled NO on gas exchange,[38] probably by an increased driving pressure to flow to the better ventilated lung regions.

Almitrine, a peripheral chemoreceptor agonist that has been shown to improve ventilation/perfusion matching in patients with chronic obstructive pulmonary disease, presumably through an enhancement of hypoxic pulmonary vasoconstriction (HPV),[39] has been reported to improve gas exchange in patients with ARDS.[40] We found that in dogs with oleic acid lung injury, almitrine increased pulmonary vascular tone to the same extent as cyclooxygenase inhibitors, but actually deteriorated gas exchange.[34] We interpreted these discrepant findings by the fact that in dogs the pulmonary vascular effects of almitrine may be dependent on preexisting tone as well on the dose administered.[41] Whether such dose- and tone-dependent effects of almitrine occur in patients with ARDS is not settled. To our knowledge, there has been no double-blind controlled study on the effects of almitrine on gas exchange and pulmonary hemodynamics in patients with ARDS. Recently, almitrine has been reported to enhance the beneficial effects of inhaled NO on gas exchange in patients with ARDS.[42]

Until now, no pharmacological manipulations of pulmonary vascular tone to improve gas exchange in ARDS has been proved to affect outcome. There certainly is a need here for placebo-controlled studies.

VENTRICULOVASCULAR COUPLING IN ARDS

Pulmonary arterial pulse pressure represents about half of mean PAP, in contrast with aortic pulse pressure, which represents only about 20% of mean aortic pressure. Pulsatile hydraulic power output is therefore a proportionally more important part of total hydraulic power output of the right ventricle than of the left ventricle, about 40% and 10% respectively.[10] If systolic pressure increases in the face of an unchanged mean pressure, which occurs for example because of a decreased vascular compliance or an increase in wave reflections, pulse pressure and ventricular afterload are increased. The forces that oppose ventricular ejection result from a dynamic interplay between arteriolar resistance, closing pressure, vascular compliance and reflected waves. All these determinants of total ventricular afterload can be quantified by an analysis of vascular pressure and flow waves in the frequency domain rather than in the time domain.[10]

For the study of pulsatile pulmonary hemodynamics, it is mandatory to measure instantaneous PAP (by a high-fidelity micromanometer-tipped catheter), and instantaneous Q (by an echographic or electromagnetic flow meter). Pulmonary arterial flow and pressure waves are separated into their respective sums of harmonics using a Fourier analysis, and pulmonary vascular impedance (PVZ) calculated. PVZ is defined as the ratio of pressure to flow oscillations.[10] The results are expressed as a spectrum of PVZ, which is the ratio of pressure and flow moduli versus frequency and the phase angle versus frequency (Figure 7). PVZ at 0 Hz (Z_o) corresponds to PVR calculated as PAP/Q ('total PVR'). It decreases rapidly to a first minimum at 2–3 Hz and increases again a little to a first maximum at 5–6 Hz. At low frequencies the phase angle is negative, which means that flow leads pressure.

Possible changes in an impedance spectrum are the following. An increase in the ratio of P and Q moduli at all frequencies is a sign of reduced distensibility, or stiffening of the large arteries. A shift of the frequency at which minima and maxima appear signals a change in either wave velocity or in the dominant reflection sites. A more negative phase angle at low frequencies indicates an increased influence of reflected pressure waves on systolic pressure. Flow normally leads pressure because of reflected pressure waves at the main site of increased pulmonary arteriolar resistance.

A useful number is characteristic impedance, Z_c, defined as the input impedance without wave reflection. Characteristic impedance can be visually estimated as PVZ averaged for the higher frequencies above the first minimum, or calculated as a PVZ at a frequency equal to the infinite. Characteristic impedance is dependent on the ratio of inertial elements to compliant elements of the pulmonary vascular system. The extent to which Z_o

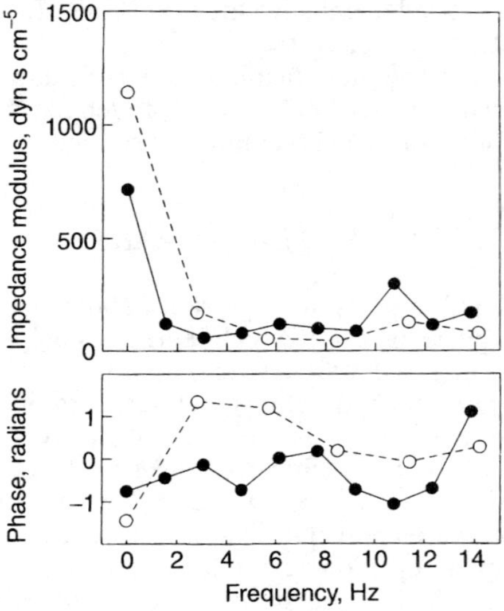

Figure 7. Spectrum of PVZ in a dog before (mean PAP 15 mmHg; ●) and after (PAP 35 mmHg; ○) induction of an acute microembolic lung injury by injection of 150 μm glass beads. Pulmonary hypertension in this model of experimental ARDS is characterized by an increased 0 Hz impedance, a shift of the first minimum and maximum of the impedance moduli to higher frequencies, a decrease in characteristic impedance and a more negative phase angle at the lowest frequencies.[43]

differs from Z_c can be used to quantify wave reflection. The proportion of forward wave that is reflected back is expressed as a reflection coefficient which can be estimated from the equation:

$$R_c = [1 - (Z_c/Z_o)]/[1 + (Z_c/Z_o)]$$

Changes in the spectrum of PVZ that occur in acute canine microembolic pulmonary hypertension, another experimental ARDS model characterized by more severe pulmonary hypertension than in oleic acid lung injury, are illustrated in Figure 7. An increase in PAP induced by the injection of 150 μm glass beads in dogs increased Z_o, indicating an increased pulmonary arteriolar resistance, shifted the first minima and maxima of the impedance moduli to higher frequencies, suggesting increased wave speed and wave reflections, increased the negativity of the phase angle at low frequencies, also suggesting increased wave reflections, and somewhat surprisingly decreased Z_c.[43] The latter was explained by a marked (possibly active) dilatation of the proximal pulmonary vascular tree in the face of unchanged or decreased pulmonary arterial compliance.

Previous studies have shown that a more proximal pulmonary vascular obstruction, induced by banding of the main pulmonary artery, increases both Z_o and Z_c.[44,45] A reduction in Z_c results in a decrease in the pulsatile component of the hydraulic load imposed upon the right ventricle, and, thereby, decreases right ventricular afterload. An intriguing hypothesis is that such vascular changes, obviously undetected by steady-flow hemodynamic studies, could be of adaptative value, and possibly amenable to pharmacological interventions.

Recent studies show that inhaled NO in patients with ARDS increases right ventricular ejection fraction without associated increase in stroke volume.[46,47] These results can be explained by the right ventricle operating on another part of its pressure–volume loop in relation to some decrease in afterload, rather than by an improved right ventricular function *per se*. Whether this is clinically relevant is at present unclear. More experimental and clinical studies on pulsatile pulmonary hemodynamics may show us to what extent right ventricular–vascular coupling can be improved, and whether this may prevent or treat right ventricular failure in patients with pulmonary hypertension secondary to ARDS.

REFERENCES

1. Ashbaugh DG, Bigelow DB, Petty TL & Levine BE (1967) Acute respiratory distress in adults. *Lancet* **2:**319–323.
2. Swan HJC, Ganz W, Forrester JS, Marcus H, Diamond G & Chonette D (1970) Catheterization of the heart in man with use of a flow-directed catheter. *New England Journal of Medicine* **283:**447–451.
3. Zapol WM & Snider MT (1977) Pulmonary hypertension in severe acute respiratory failure. *New England Journal of Medicine* **296:**476–480.
4. Zapol WM, Snider MT, Rie MA, Quinn DA & Fikker M (1986) Pulmonary circulation during adult pulmonary distress syndrome. In Zapol WM & Falke KJ (eds) *Acute Respiratory Failure*, vol 24, pp 241–273. New York: Marcel Dekker.
5. Bone RC, Maunder R, Slotman G et al (1989) An early test of survival in patients with the adult respiratory distress syndrome. *Chest* **96:**849–851.
6. Sloane PJ, Gee MH, Gottlieb JE et al (1992) A multicentre registry of patients with acute respiratory distress syndrome. *American Review of Respiratory Disease* **146:**419–426.
7. Suchyta MR, Clemmer TP, Elliott CG, Orme JF & Weaver LK (1992) The adult respiratory distress syndrome. A report of survival and modifying factors. *Chest* **101:**1074–1079.
8. Zapol WM, Snider M, Schneider RC, Rie M & Roth S (1978) Clinical pulmonary hemodynamics during severe acute respiratory failure: effect on venoarterial bypass. In Baan J, Noodergraaf A & Raines J (eds) *Cardiovascular System Dynamics*, pp 352–361. Cambridge, MA: MIT Press.
9. Naeije R (1993) Medical treatment of pulmonary hypertension in acute lung disease. *European Respiratory Journal* **6:**1521–1528.
10. Milnor WR (1982) *Hemodynamics*. Baltimore: Williams and Wilkins.
11. Permutt S & Riley RL (1963) Hemodynamics of collapsible vessels with tone: the vascular waterfall. *Journal of Applied Physiology* **18:**924–932.
12. Mitzner W & Chang HK (1989) Hemodynamics of the pulmonary circulation. In Chang HK & Paiva M (eds) *Respiratory Physiology. An Analytical Approach*, vol. 40, pp 561–631. New York: Marcel Dekker.
13. Leeman M, Lejeune P, Closset J, Vachiéry JL, Mélot C & Naeije R (1990) Nature of pulmonary hypertension in canine oleic acid pulmonary edema. *Journal of Applied Physiology* **69:**293–298.

14. Schuster DP (1994) ARDS: Clinical lessons from the oleic acid model of acute lung injury. *American Journal of Respiratory and Critical Care Medicine* **149:**245–260.
15. Leeman M, Lejeune P, Closset J, Vachiéry JL, Mélot C & Naeije R (1990) Effects of PEEP on pulmonary hemodynamics in intact dogs with oleic acid pulmonary edema. *Journal of Applied Physiology* **69:**2190–2196.
16. Greene R, Zapol WM, Snider MT et al (1981) Early bedside detection of pulmonary vascular occlusion during acute respiratory failure. *American Review of Respiratory Disease* **124:**593–601.
17. Tomashefski JF, Davies P, Boggis C, Greene R, Zapol WM & Reid LM (1983) The pulmonary vascular lesions of the adult respiratory distress syndrome. *American Journal of Pathology* **112:**112–126.
18. Bachofen M & Weibel E (1982) Structural alterations of lung parenchyma in the adult respiratory distress syndrome. *Clinical Chest Medicine* **3:**35–56.
19. Snow RL, Davies P, Pontoppidan H, Zapol WM & Reid L (1982) Pulmonary vascular remodeling in adult respiratory distress syndrome. *American Review of Respiratory Disease* **126:**887–892.
20. Michel RP, Zocchi L & Rossi A et al (1987) Does interstitial lung edema compress airways and arteries? A morphometric study. *Journal of Applied Physiology* **62:**108–115.
21. Radermacher P, Huet Y, Pluskwa F et al (1988) Comparison of ketanserin and sodium nitroprusside in patients with severe ARDS.*Anesthesiology* **68:**152–157.
22. Mélot C, Naeije R, Mols P, Hallemans R, Lejeune P & Jaspar N (1987) Pulmonary vascular tone improves gas exchange in the adult respiratory distress syndrome. *American Review of Respiratory Disease* **136:**1232–1236.
23. Mélot C, Lejeune P, Leeman M, Moraine JJ & Naeije R (1989) Prostaglandin E_1 in the adult respiratory distress syndrome. Benefit for pulmonary hypertension and cost for pulmonary gas exchange. *American Review of Respiratory Disease* **139:**106–110.
24. Rossaint R, Falke KJ, Lopez F, Slama K, Pison U & Zapol W (1993) Inhaled nitric oxide for the adult respiratory distress syndrome. *New England Journal of Medicine* **328:**399–405
25. Leeman M, Lejeune P, Mélot C & Naeije R (1988) Pulmonary vascular pressure: flow plots in canine oleic acid pulmonary edema. Effects of prostaglandin E_1 and nitroprusside. *American Review of Respiratory Disease* **138:**362–367.
26. Brimioulle S, Vachiéry JL, Lejeune P, Leeman M, Mélot C & Naeije R (1991) Acid-base status influences gas exchange in canine oleic acid lung injury. *American Journal of Physiology* (*Heart Circulation Physiology*) **29:**H1080–H1086.
27. Prewitt RM, McCarthy J & Wood LDH (1981) Treatment of acute low pressure pulmonary edema in dogs. Relative effects of hydrostatic and oncotic pressure, nitroprusside, and positive end-expiratory pressure. *Journal of Clinical Investigation* **67:**409–418.
28. Puybasset L, Rouby JJ, Mourgeon E et al (1994) Inhaled nitric oxide in acute respiratory failure: dose–response curves. *Intensive Care Medicine* **20:**319–327.
29. Walmrath D, Schneider T, Pilch J, Grimminger F & Seeger W (1993) Aerosolised prostacyclin in adult respiratory distress syndrome. *Lancet* **342:**961–962.
30. Rossaint R, Gerlach H, Schmidt-Ruhnke et al (1995) Efficacy of inhaled nitric oxide in patients with severe ARDS. *Chest* **107:**1107–1115.
31. Garrett RC & Thomas III HM (1984) Meclofenamate uniformly decreases shunt fraction in dogs with lobar atelectasis. *Journal of Applied Physiology* **54:**284–289.
32. Light RB (1986) Indomethacin and acetylsalicylic acid reduce intrapulmonary shunt in experimental pneumococcal pneumonia. *American Review of Respiratory Disease* **134:**520–525.
33. Ali J & Duke K (1987) Does indomethacin affect shunt and its response to PEEP in oleic acid pulmonary edema? *Journal of Applied Physiology* **62:**2187–2192.

34. Leeman M, Lejeune P, Hallemans R, Mélot C & Naeije R (1988) Effects of increased pulmonary vascular tone on gas exchange in canine oleic acid pulmonary edema. *Journal of Applied Physiology* **65:**662–668.
35. Schulman LL, Lennon PF, Ratner SJ & Enson Y (1988) Meclofenamate enhances blood oxygenation in acute oleic acid lung injury. *Journal of Applied Physiology* **64:**710–718.
36. Leeman M, Mélot C & Naeije R (1995) Cyclooxygenase inhibition acutely improves gas exchange in patients with ARDS (abstract). *American Journal of Respiratory and Critical Care Medicine* **151(Suppl):**A77.
37. Leeman M, Zegers de Beyl V, Gilbert E, Mélot C & Naeije R (1993) Is nitric oxide released in oleic acid lung injury? *Journal of Applied Physiology* **74:**650–654.
38. Putensen C, Räsänen J & Downs JB (1994) Effect of endogenous and inhaled nitric oxide on the ventilation–perfusion relationships in oleic acid lung injury. *American Journal of Respiratory and Critical Care Medicine* **150:**330–336.
39. Mélot C, Naeije R, Rothschild T, Mertens P, Mols P & Hallemans R (1983) Improvement in ventilation–perfusion matching by almitrine in COPD. *Chest* **83:**528–533.
40. Reyes A, Roca J, Rodriguez-Roisin R, Torres A, Ussetti P & Wagner PD (1988) Effect of almitrine on ventilation–perfusion distribution in adult respiratory distress syndrome. *American Review of Respiratory Disease* **137:**1062–1067.
41. Naeije R, Lejeune P, Vachiéry JL et al (1990) Restored hypoxic pulmonary vasoconstriction by peripheral chemoreceptor agonists in dogs. *American Review of Respiratory Disease* **142:**789–799.
42. Payen DM, Gatecel C & Plaisance P (1993) Almitrine effect on nitric oxide inhalation in adult respiratory distress syndrome (letter). *Lancet* **341:**1664.
43. Naeije R, Maarek JM & Chang HK (1990) Pulmonary vascular impedance in acute canine microembolic pulmonary hypertension. *Respiration Physiology* **79:**205–218.
44. Calvin JE Jr, Baer RW & Glantz SA (1985) Pulmonary artery constriction produces a greater right ventricular dynamic afterload than lung microvascular injury in the open chest dog. *Circulation Research* **56:**40–56.
45. Fitzpatrick JM & Grant BJB (1990) Effects of pulmonary vascular obstruction on right ventricular afterload. *American Review of Respiratory Disease* **141:**944–952.
46. Rossaint R, Slama K, Steudel W et al (1995) Effects of inhaled nitric oxide on right ventricular function in severe acute respiratory distress syndrome. *Intensive Care Medicine* **21:**197–203.
47. Fierobe L, Brunet F, Dhainaut JF et al (1995) Effect of inhaled nitric oxide on right ventricular function in adult respiratory distress syndrome. *American Journal of Respiratory and Critical Care Medicine* **151:**1414–1418.

13

Effect of Combined Inhaled Nitric Oxide and Pulmonary Vasoconstriction Enhancement

Sadek Beloucif
Didier M. Payen

INTRODUCTION

Despite recent therapeutic advances in modern intensive care, mortality and morbidity of patients with acute (or adult) lung injury secondary to acute respiratory distress syndrome (ARDS) or acute pneumonia remain high. Support of pulmonary function is based on mechanical ventilation which, although alleviating hypoxemia, may induce significant side effects such as lung distension, baro/volutrauma, alterations in alveolar permeability and tissue injury, especially when high levels of inspired oxygen concentrations (F_iO_2) and positive end-expiratory pressure (PEEP) are required.[1–4] Wagner et al[5] proposed that the lung might be viewed as the resultant of venous admixture, dead space, and ideal gas-exchange compartments. Hypoxemia would then result from an increased number of pulmonary compartments with abnormal ventilation/perfusion V_A/Q ratios. If mechanical ventilation with PEEP can recruit pulmonary parenchyma and improve gas exchange, theoretically, further improvement in $Pa O_2$ could be gained from therapies aimed at reducing pulmonary blood flow in shunting areas, while increasing flow in normally ventilated areas.[6] We thus hypothesized that: (1) co-administration of inhaled nitric oxide (NO) and intravenous administration of almitrine, a drug that enhances physiologic hypoxic pulmonary vasoconstriction, would significantly potentiate the increase in $Pa O_2$ observed with either drug; (2) this combined therapy might produce significant reduction in the level of PEEP and F_iO_2 in severely hypoxemic patients.

The beneficial effect of inhaled NO was first observed in 1988 by Higenbottam et al[7] with a significant pulmonary vasodilation in patients with chronic obstructive pulmonary disease. Inhaled NO being selectively delivered in ventilated alveoli, several authors,[6,8–10] and particularly Rossaint et al[11] demonstrated in ARDS patients a significant improvement in $Pa\text{O}_2$ and a reduction in pulmonary hypertension with no associated deleterious systemic hypotension. Furthermore, the exclusive delivery of NO to ventilated alveoli would preserve hypoxic pulmonary vasoconstriction (HPV) present in atelectatic areas. Accordingly, a reduction in flow to low V_A/Q regions and a significant reduction in right to left shunting was demonstrated using the six inert gas technique.[11]

When resistance in normal lung areas has been reduced by inhaled NO, diverting blood flow from atelectatic regions and reducing the oxygen shunt, variable effects have also been reported in terms of $Pa\text{O}_2$ responses. Theoretically, $Pa\text{O}_2$ can increase with NO inhalation only when some constriction in addition to HPV is present in small arteries or veins.[12] Based on this rationale, NO should selectively reduce vascular resistance in normally ventilated lung regions to decrease shunt flow, but should not access poorly ventilated lung regions, precluding an effect on end capillary oxygen content that might offset the benefit to gas exchange.[13] Therefore, the gain in $Pa\text{O}_2$ observed with NO should be enhanced when combined with an infused vasoconstrictor.[13]

The vasoconstrictor used in combination with NO should mimic or enhance HPV, since Marshall et al[14] using the nonselective vasoconstrictor norepinephrine failed to observe beneficial effects on hypoxemia. Almitrine bimesylate[15] was chosen since numerous experimental and clinical studies have shown that its action may mimic HPV. This drug has negligible direct effects on the systemic circulation and acts preferentially on vessels supplying poorly/unventilated lung areas, potentiating or restoring HPV. Finally, its action is predominant on prealveolar vessels, thus avoiding any pulmonary venous hypertension and edema. The maintenance of a gradient of vascular resistance between ventilated regions receiving NO, and regions where perfusion is reduced by HPV would be particularly advantageous during the early stages of ARDS, in the presence of situations characterized by a reduced or abolished HPV response such as pulmonary infection,[16] septicemia,[17] direct lung trauma and septic shock.[18] However, the combined therapy is unlikely to be as effective in the late stages of ARDS when small pulmonary vessels are not actively constricted, but fibrotic or irreversibly narrowed.[19]

In addition to these situations, endogenous release of NO can also modulate HPV.[20,21] Administration of NO-synthesis inhibitors to isolated perfused lungs ventilated with a hypoxic gas mixture further increased pulmonary arterial pressure, suggesting the existence of a previous attenuation of HPV by NO. Sprague et al[21] also demonstrated in rabbits that endogenous NO release by the lung might oppose regional HPV and support blood flow to hypoxic lung units, thereby decreasing $Pa\text{O}_2$. Lungs were separately ventilated with unilateral alveolar hypoxia. This resulted in a significant intrapulmonary redistribution of blood flow (as flow to the hypoxic lung was reduced), without any change in pulmonary artery pressure. The administration of an NO synthase inhibitor further reduced blood flow to the hypoxic alveoli with a corresponding increase in $Pa\text{O}_2$. This effect was also reversed by an infusion of L-arginine (the NO synthase substrate), suggesting that endogenous NO synthesis is present in the lung during alveolar hypoxia and acts to oppose HPV.

HPV is a physiologic adaptation that contributes to gas exchange efficiency by reducing blood flow to lung regions with low V_A/Q ratios,[22,23] improving the match between gas exchange and blood flow distribution of the lung. The stimulus of HPV seems to be a function of both mixed venous[24] and alveolar[25] oxygen tension, through a complex cellular mechanism. The vasoconstrictive response of pulmonary vascular smooth muscle cells during hypoxic alveolar gas ventilation is amplified in the presence of a low mixed venous O_2 tension. HPV concerns basically all the pulmonary vessels which respond to hypoxia by vasoconstriction,[23,26] although *in vivo* the HPV response predominates in small arteries of less than 500 μm in diameter. Many substances and circumstances can alter the HPV response, and the role of endogenous release of NO in HPV has been recently demonstrated.[22,23] In isolated perfused lungs, the administration of NO synthesis inhibitors during ventilation with a hypoxic gas mixture enhanced the increase in pulmonary arterial pressure, suggesting an attenuation of HPV by NO release. In an anesthetized rabbit model, an impact of endogenous NO on V_A/Q matching has been hypothesized by opposing regional HPV thus supporting blood flow to hypoxic lung units, thereby decreasing $Pa\text{O}_2$.[23] In rabbit lungs separately ventilated *in vivo* with unilateral alveolar hypoxia, the administration of an NO inhibitor resulted in a dose-dependent reduction in the intrapulmonary distribution of the blood flow to hypoxic alveoli with a concomitant increase in $Pa\text{O}_2$. This effect was reversed by L-arginine infusion, confirming the NO implication. In large pulmonary vessels, HPV is less profound than in small vessels (because of the presence of vasa vasorum deriving from bronchial arteries), and is observed only when systemic hypoxemia is present,[23] although a biphasic response with further dilation is observed when $Pa\text{O}_2$ further decreases below 50 mmHg.[23]

Almitrine bimesylate is an agonist of the peripheral arterial chemoreceptors that increases discharge in the carotid sinus nerve[27] through an unknown mechanism. The acute effects on ventilation, pulmonary hemodynamics and gas exchange have been studied after oral[28–30] and intravenous[31–33] administration. Plasma concentrations peak 1.5–2.4 h after an oral dose with a wide interindividual variation, not related to body weight. Optimal therapeutic plasma concentration is 200–300 μg/ml. Almitrine binds tightly (>99%) to low-density lipoprotein, but not to hemoglobin or carbonic anhydrase. It is distributed throughout the body with high levels found in liver, small intestine and stomach, with time-dependent elimination. Plasma concentrations decrease biexponentially after a bolus intravenous dose, with an initial plasma half-life of 2.5 h. Terminal half-life is much longer and can range from 27 h in rats to 25 days in man. Human tissue levels peak 6–24 h after the intravenous dose and decline over the subsequent 96 h with a mean tissue half-life of 12 h. The total elimination of the drug and its metabolites (one of them showing some almitrine-like activity) takes more than 900 h. They are excreted either in the bile, or directly into the intestines from the gut circulation. Urinary elimination is low because of its high molecular weight. Finally, although slow, the elimination is complete, without irreversible retention.

The only significant side effect is a sensory peripheral neuropathy, usually affecting lower limbs,[34] reported in some patients after prolonged (9–25 months) oral treatment.[35] Its incidence (around 30%) is higher when defined by electrophysiological changes rather than clinically. Recovery can take from 3 to more than 12 months after discontinuation of the drug. As the incidence of this complication is considerably reduced with lower oral doses, one might reasonably expect that low intravenous doses for short periods of time (few days) as an associated therapy for ARDS would have limited consequences.

Several experimental studies have confirmed that almitrine improves $Pa\text{O}_2$, possibly because of a redistribution of blood flow away from poorly ventilated areas without stimulating ventilation.[36–38] In isolated perfused lungs, almitrine caused a constriction of relaxed vessels of normoxic and chronic hypoxic rats.[39] Gottschall et al[40] have verified that almitrine mimics HPV. Based on the hypothesis that almitrine has a similar impact to hypoxia on the pulmonary circulation, one would anticipate that almitrine would: (1) produce a pulmonary vasoconstriction; (2) potentiate or enhance HPV; (3) enhance HPV induced by other agents (such as catecholamines, $PGF_{2\alpha}$, and nonsteroid antiinflammatory drugs); (4) be inhibited by agents inhibiting HPV; (5) act at the precapillary level, implying that the drug is not predominantly a pulmonary venoconstrictor; (6) have little or no effect on systemic vessels.

Most of these actions of almitrine have been described. Addition of almitrine to the reservoir of blood-perfused rat lungs induced a dose-dependent increase in vascular resistance, with no effect on microvascular pressure, accounting for a precapillary vasoconstriction. Moreover, almitrine potentiated the subsequent hypoxic pressure response, but had no effect on established hypoxic vasoconstriction. The latter observation was not related to the elevated pulmonary vascular tone before almitrine *per se*, since almitrine further increased pressure after KCl-induced contraction.[40] Agents known to enhance or inhibit HPV had similar effects on almitrine-induced vasoconstriction. Finally almitrine had no effect on pulmonary conduit arteries.

Although the mechanism by which hypoxia is detected remains uncertain, it has been suggested that O_2 tension is detected in the vasculature through its effects on energy status, as reflected by the level of high-energy phosphates such as ATP.[41,42] It has been shown in bovine heart and rat liver mitochondria[43] that almitrine may affect energy metabolism such as oxidative phosphorylation. In aerobic organisms, this process is the major source of ATP formed, as electrons are transferred from NADH to O_2 through a series of electron carriers. It is carried out by respiratory assemblies that are located in the inner membrane of mitochondria. Almitrine inhibits ATP synthesis or impairs electron transport downstream from the rotenone-blocking site, localized in the NADH–cytochrome Q reductase complex. These actions may correspond to the locus of hypoxic sensing[36] where the signal may be generated by ATP reduction in a distinct cellular compartment, as recently shown by Archer et al[42] in the pulmonary vasculature.

Some *in vivo* studies, particularly in dog models, have reported conflicting results on the pulmonary vascular effects of almitrine. Hughes et al[44] showed that an intravenous bolus of 10 μg/kg almitrine vasoconstricted pulmonary vessels specifically in normoxic but not in hypoxic conditions. This vasoconstriction was not abolished by α- or β-blockade, indomethacin, vagotomy, or bilateral common carotid artery clamping. The potential enhancement of HPV by almitrine has also been tested in dogs with normal lungs.[36] Using the multiple inert gas technique, almitrine was found to increase pulmonary vascular resistance by 60% during hypoxic ventilation, but it did not change pulmonary vascular resistance during ventilation with 100% O_2. These results suggest a direct pulmonary vascular effect, since systemic hemodynamics, blood gases and other parameters of oxygenation remained unchanged. Almitrine thus enhanced hypoxic vasoconstriction in the lung, an effect that may explain the observed $Pa\text{O}_2$ increase in hypoxic patients.

In a normal dog separately ventilated with hyperoxic gas on one side and hypoxic mixture on the other, Chen et al[37] tested the impact of almitrine on HPV at increasing doses from 0.003 to 3 μg/kg per min. Significant reduction in flow to the hypoxic lung (with a concomitant increase in $Pa\text{O}_2$) occurred only at 3 μg/kg per min. Naieje et al[45] pointed out contradictory results published in the literature: in healthy dogs[36] and humans,[33] the increase in pulmonary vascular resistance induced by hypoxia is enhanced by almitrine, whereas in isolated canine lungs, almitrine constricted hyperoxic pulmonary lung vessels, but had no effect on preconstricted hypoxic vessels.[44] These observations suggest that the pulmonary vasoconstricting activity of almitrine may inhibit the function of HPV. Accordingly, in a pulmonary oleic acid injury model, the increase in pulmonary vascular tone induced by a high dose of almitrine worsened gas exchange.[46] Expecting a dose-dependent biphasic effect of almitrine, these authors tested the effect on pulmonary pressure–flow relationship of lower doses of almitrine (2 and 4 μg/kg per min) than those used in their previous studies. In dogs exhibiting a HPV response, 2 μg/kg per min had no vascular effect, whereas 4 μg/kg per min inhibited HPV. In dogs exhibiting no HPV response to a hypoxic gas mixture, almitrine at 2 and 4 μg/kg per min restored HPV, as did the intravenous administration of the chemoreceptor agonist doxapram. The authors concluded that a low dose of almitrine restores HPV in dogs, probably by a direct effect on the pulmonary vessels.

In parallel to these experimental studies, almitrine has been studied in humans. An improvement in hypoxia with a reduction in V_A/Q mismatching was demonstrated using radionuclide and multiple inert gas techniques[28] in patients with chronic pulmonary disease and ARDS in whom both shunt and V_A/Q mismatching explained severe hypoxia.[38] In patients with severe acute respiratory failure secondary to shock or sepsis, intravenous almitrine significantly improved $Pa\text{O}_2$ with negligible pulmonary and systemic hemodynamic changes.[47] Using the multiple inert gas technique, Reyes et al[38] have shown in nine ARDS patients ventilated at constant $F_i\text{O}_2$ an 80% increase in $Pa\text{O}_2$ during infusion of 16 μg/kg per min almitrine. The multiple inert gas technique showed a redistribution of pulmonary blood flow from shunt areas to lung units with normal V_A/Q ratio, while pulmonary artery pressure increased from 26 ± 5 to 30 ± 5 mmHg. These changes returned to baseline 30 min after cessation of the infusion of the drug.

Almitrine was also tested in severe hypoxemia caused by shunting through a unilateral pneumonia.[48] A positive effect of the drug would be expected since redistribution of pulmonary flow might reduce V_A/Q inequalities. Using a high dose of almitrine (17 μg/kg per min), the authors failed to find any increase in pulmonary vascular resistance or $P\text{aO}_2$. These surprising negative results may have resulted from the use of a high dose of almitrine as suggested by canine studies, or may reflect the particular lung disease, since HPV has been shown to be abolished in acute unilateral bacterial pneumonia.[16,17]

In summary, the observed strong similarities between the effects of almitrine and hypoxia suggest a similar mechanism of action, possibly through oxidative phosphorylation at the mitochondrial level. The observed benefit on $P\text{aO}_2$ has been related to the pulmonary vasoconstrictor effect of the drug. The dose range seems to be crucial since low doses (<10 μg/kg per min) reinforce or restore HPV, whereas higher doses have no effects. Interindividual differences in the magnitude of HPV response exist in humans, and minimal or no response could have been evidenced in selected patients. The use of almitrine is thus extremely attractive to improve V_A/Q inequalities via restoration of HPV. However, the benefit/risk ratio has to be considered. In the acute situation in which we propose to use almitrine, short-term intravenous administration of low doses would probably limit the risk of sensory peripheral neuropathy.

Based on the previously described rationale, we hypothesized that the ability of NO in improving oxygenation should be enhanced when combined with almitrine. Accordingly, in mechanically ventilated patients suffering from ARDS or severe acute pneumonia, co-administration of inhaled NO and pulmonary vasoconstriction enhancement with almitrine augmented the improvement in $P\text{aO}_2$ observed with NO or almitrine alone.

The investigation was carried out after informed consent had been obtained from the patient's closest relatives. Eighteen consecutive patients suffering from severe acute lung injury based on a $P\text{aO}_2/F_\text{i}\text{O}_2$ value of less than 150 mmHg were prospectively studied. Eight patients (ARDS group) carried the diagnosis of acute respiratory distress syndrome (Murray Score: 3.1±0.2) based on classical criteria including a compatible underlying disease, a pulmonary artery occlusion pressure lower than 20 mmHg during mechanical ventilation, and bilateral lung infiltrates on chest X-ray. The etiology of ARDS was in 62% a direct lung injury and in 38% an indirect lung injury. Ten patients (ALI group) had a severe but non-diffuse acute pneumopathy assessed by chest X ray and thoracic computed tomography (CT) scan.

Mechanical ventilation ($F_\text{i}\text{O}_2$=1) was achieved by a Servo ventilator Siemens 900 C or 300 (Elema Siemens, Solna, Sweden). PEEP level averaged 12 ± 2 cmH_2O (ranging from 3 to 21) in the ARDS group and 6 ± 1.1 cmH_2O (ranging from 0 to 10) in the ALI group. Patients were sedated and paralyzed; when a pharmacologic cardiovascular support was needed, it was maintained throughout the study period.

NO (15 ppm) was continuously administered through a fenestrated silicone catheter positioned in the tracheal tube 2 cm above the tip. NO concentration administered was sequentially verified on the ventilator expiratory limb by chemiluminescence (Eco Physics, Massy, France). The accuracy of the flow meter delivering NO was further assessed by verifying that the difference between expiratory and inspiratory minute ventilation measured by the ventilator corresponded to the value of the added gas flow.

An oxymetric thermodilution pulmonary artery catheter (Abbott Laboratories, Chicago, IL, USA) was inserted in all patients (except four in the ALI group), to measure mean pulmonary artery (PAP), right atrial (Pra), and pulmonary artery occlusion (PAOP) pressures. Pressure values were the average over the respiratory cycle, except for PAOP which was measured at end expiration. Cardiac output (CO) was measured in triplicate by the thermodilution technique when available (n = 14). Systemic (Rsv) and pulmonary (Rpv) vascular resistances were calculated according to standard formulae in IU.

Arterial and mixed-venous blood gases were measured with standard blood gas electrodes (ABL 300, Radiometer, Copenhagen, Denmark) and total hemoglobin concentration, hemoglobin oxygen saturation, and methemoglobin levels were measured by spectrophotometry (OSM 2 Hemoximeter, Radiometer, Copenhagen, Denmark). Q_s/Q_t, oxygen consumption (VO_2 in ml O_2/min) and oxygen delivery (DO_2 in ml O_2/min) were calculated using standard formulae. Ventilatory parameters including peak inspiratory pressure (Ppi) and quasi-static compliance (Cqs) were continuously monitored by a ventilatory module (Siemens).

To analyze the impact of NO inhalation on arterial oxygenation, the data analyzed before and after NO had to be obtained at a similar F_iO_2. Since the addition of NO in N_2 modifies F_iO_2 which is difficult to measure accurately, the control point was an inhalation of pure N_2 at the same flow rate as that used for NO in N_2. Thus, we successively studied in all patients, after a control point (O_2+N_2), the effects of inhaled NO (NO), intravenous almitrine added to NO (NO + Alm), and finally the effects of almitrine alone (Alm).

Hemodynamic and gasometric parameters were recorded: (1) after 30 min in the control situation; (2) after 60 min of NO inhalation; (3) 60 min after intravenous almitrine (Servier, Suresnes, France) (titrated from 8 to 16 μg/kg per min in the ARDS group[38] and from 4 to 8 μg/kg per min in the ALI group to achieve the best $Pa O_2/F_iO_2$); and (4) since NO inhalation acts as an 'on-off' phenomenon,[49] the impact of almitrine alone was verified 60 min after withdrawal of NO inhalation and replacement by pure nitrogen when it was possible. This last step of the protocol was not performed in three patients from the ARDS group and three patients from the ALI group because of severe hypoxia.

After completing the protocol described above, co-administration of NO and almitrine was continued and F_iO_2 was then reduced to a level which ensured a $Pa O_2$ between 75 and 120 mmHg. When F_iO_2 was reduced to 0.4, PEEP level reduction was performed according to the defined ranges of $Pa O_2$. Finally, criteria for weaning of almitrine were a stable $Pa O_2$ higher than 200 mmHg at F_iO_2=1. Then a day by day test of NO weaning was performed, and NO was discontinued when $Pa O_2$ was close to 100 mmHg at an $F_iO_2 \leq 0.50$ during 4 h after NO withdrawal.

Except for the type of lung disease, the clinical characteristics of the two groups were similar in terms of age, gravity score, previous duration of mechanical ventilation, lung quasi static compliance and outcome. However, for a similar level of $Pa{O_2}/F_i{O_2}$, the levels of $Pa{O_2}$ (since permissive hypercapnia was used) and PEEP were higher in ARDS patients.

HEMODYNAMIC PARAMETERS (Table 1)

Cardiac output and mean arterial pressure did not change throughout the study, either in the ARDS or ALI group.

In the ARDS group, NO decreased pulmonary artery pressure by 3±1.5 mmHg ($P<0.02$), which returned to baseline levels (O_2+N_2) when NO inhalation was combined with almitrine infusion (NO + Alm). NO withdrawal during almitrine infusion (Alm) led to a significant increase in pulmonary artery pressure (+5 mmHg; $P<0.02$).

In the ALI group, pulmonary artery pressure increased only during almitrine infusion without NO. Pulmonary vascular resistances during NO plus almitrine did not differ from control (O_2+N_2), while they were higher than those during NO alone.

In both groups, $Pa{O_2}$ increased during NO inhalation and further increased when almitrine was infused (Table 1). This effect was associated with a parallel decrease in Q_s/Q_t. NO and almitrine administered separately improved $Pa{O_2}$ to a similar extent. $Pa{CO_2}$, oxygen consumption and lung mechanics parameters did not change throughout the protocol.

After these measurements were completed, co-administration of NO inhalation and almitrine infusion in both groups of patients permitted a significant reduction in $F_i{O_2}$ required to maintain $Pa{O_2}$ between 75 and 100 mmHg (Figure 1). $F_i{O_2}$ reduction was more pronounced in the ALI group than in the ARDS group (−59% versus −31%; $P < 0.001$), and allowed reduction of the PEEP level from 6±1 to 4±1 cmH_2O ($P < 0.05$) in five out of ten patients. Causes of death in the non-survivors were multiple organ failure (one), severe sepsis (two), brain failure (three), cardiogenic shock (one), and terminal cancer (one).

Since CO and PAP values did not change during administration of NO plus almitrine, improvements in gas exchange reflect modifications of V_A/Q mismatching. Compared with controls, PAP decreased with NO, and increased by 3 and 6 mmHg in ALI and ARDS groups respectively when almitrine was infused without NO. In the presence of NO, infusion of almitrine induced a 2–3 mmHg increase in PAP. Although statistically significant, this increase may be of limited clinical relevance because the resulting PAP values were not significantly different from control (O_2+N_2) measurements. Changes in pulmonary vascular resistance, a weak indicator of the modifications of the vasoactive status of the pulmonary circulation following pharmacologic interventions, paralleled changes in PAP (i.e. it decreased with NO and increased with almitrine).

$Pa{O_2}$ values under control conditions and after NO inhalation did not differ between the two groups. However, with the combination of NO plus almitrine, the improvement in $Pa{O_2}$ was more prominent in the ALI group

Table 1. Hemodynamic, gazometric, ventilatory and metabolic parameters in ARDS and ALI groups for the four conditions of the protocol.

Parameter	N_2	NO	NO + Alm	Almitrine	ANOVA
ARDS group					
HR (beats/min)	99.2 ± 9.3	105.8 ± 6.1	111.8 ± 7.2	105.5 ± 5.3	ns
Pra (mmHg)	11 ± 0.6	10.3 ± 0.8	11.9 ± 0.8	11.8 ± 1.4	ns
PAOP (mmHg)	11.1 ± 0.5	10.7 ± 0.5	12.6 ± 1	15 ± 2.7	ns
PAP (mmHg)	31.1 ± 1.6	28 ± 1.4*	31.4 ± 1.7 †	37 ± 3.9	*P*<0.02
Psa (mmHg)	71.1 ± 4.1	67 ± 4.1	74.5 ± 4.6	70.8 ± 5.9	ns
CO (liters/min)	7.2 ± 0.8	7.2 ± 0.7	7.9 ± 0.6	7.8 ± 0.5	ns
Rpv (IU)	5.2 ± 0.7	4.3 ± 0.6*	4.4 ± 0.5 †	4.9 ± 1.3	*P*<0.002
Rsv (IU)	15.8 ± 1.1	15.2 ± 1.3	12.9 ± 1.4	13.4 ± 1.7	ns
$Pa{O_2}$ (mmHg)	88 ± 7.1	137 ± 12*	238 ± 31*†	102 ± 15.4*‡	*P*<0.006
$Sa{O_2}$ (%)	94 ± 0.6	98 ± 0.7*	99 ± 0.4*†	97 ± 1.2*	*P*<0.02
$Pv{O_2}$ (mmHg)	37 ± 0.7	40 ± 1*	43 ± 2*†	40 ± 1.2*‡	*P*<0.002
$Sv{O_2}$ (%)	65 ± 0.9	69 ± 1.4*	74 ± 2.5*†	68 ± 3 ‡	*P*<0.02
Q_s/Q_t (%)	37 ± 1.8	30 ± 1.4*	25 ± 1.3*†	33 ± 1.7*‡	*P*<0.02
$Pa{CO_2}$ (mmHg)	47 ± 2.1	49 ± 2.7	47 ± 2.6	49 ± 3	ns
$Ca{O_2}$ (ml O_2/min)	12.6 ± 1.6	13.1 ± 1.5	13.6 ± 1.8*	12.7 ± 1.8	*P*<0.03
DO_2 (ml O_2/min)	864 ± 81	907 ± 71	1041 ± 79*†	972 ± 51	*P*<0.004
VO2 (ml O_2/min)	265 ± 23	270 ± 23	287 ± 22	290 ± 22	ns
Ppi (cmH_2O)	33.1 ± 2.2	33 ± 2	33.2 ± 1.8	32 ± 1.8	ns
Cqs (ml/cmH_2O)	40.7 ± 7	40.5 ± 6.4	39.8 ± 6.3	38.8 ± 5.9	ns
ALI group					
HR (beats/min)	91.9 ± 5.8	90.3 ± 4.2	88.3 ± 4.9	98.5 ± 5.8	ns
Pra (mmHg)	10.0 ± 1.2	10.3 ± 1.4	9.6 ± 0.5	11.7 ± 0.7	ns
PAOP (mmHg)	12.7 ± 2.8	12.2 ± 2.5	11.3 ± 1.8	14.2 ± 1.5	ns
PAP (mmHg)	25.7 ± 2.9	23.3 ± 2.6	25.3 ± 2.1	28.5 ± 3.1†	*P*<0.03
Psa (mmHg)	73.7 ± 2.9	75.3 ± 3.5	69.5 ± 2.4	68.3 ± 4.9	ns
CO (liters/min)	6.1 ± 0.7	5.9 ± 0.8	5.9 ± 0.7	5.5 ± 1.1	ns
Rpv (IU)	3.7 ± 0.6	3.2 ± 0.4	4.0 ± 0.6†	5.8 ± 0.7†	*P*<0.002
Rsv (IU)	16.8 ± 2.5	17.7 ± 2.9	15.2 ± 2.4	18.3 ± 2.9	ns
$Pa{O_2}$ (mmHg)	89.0 ± 7.6	196 ± 23*	366 ± 32*†	251 ± 51*‡	*P*<0.0001
$Sa{O_2}$ (%)	96 ± 1	99 ± 1*	100*†	99 ± 1*	*P*<0.0003
$Pv{O_2}$ (mmHg)	36.0 ± 1.0	40.0 ± 1.8*	43.0 ± 2.1*	43.0 ± 3.2	*P*<0.007
$Sv{O_2}$ (%)	70 ± 3	77 ± 2*	81 ± 2*	79 ± 4	*P*<0.001
Q_s/Q_t (%)	31 ± 4	22 ± 3*	15 ± 3*†	17 ± 4*	*P*<0.0002
$Pa{CO_2}$ (mmHg)	38.0 ± 1.0	36.0 ± 1.3	36.0 ± 1.5	38.0 ± 2.6	ns
$Ca{O_2}$ (ml O_2/min)	12.6 ± 0.9	13.4 ± 0.9*	14.1 ± 0.9*†	14.4 ± 1.7	*P*<0.008
DO_2 (ml O_2/min)	729 ± 65	765 ± 82	822 ± 89	725 ± 114	ns
VO_2 (ml O_2/min)	218 ± 19	215 ± 24	226 ± 30	195 ± 39	ns
Ppi (cmH_2O)	23.0 ± 0.7	24.0 ± 0.7	23.0 ± 0.8	23.0 ± 1.1	ns
Cqs (ml/cmH_2O)	39.0 ± 3.8	40.0 ± 3.9	40.0 ± 3.4	39.0 ± 4.5	ns

N_2, nitrogen control situation; NO, 60 min after 15 ppm continuous NO inhalation; Alm, intravenous almitrine infusion; HR, heart rate; Psa, mean systemic arterial pressure; $Sa{O_2}$, arterial hemoglobin oxygen saturation; $Pv{O_2}$, partial mixed venous oxygen pressure; $Sv{O_2}$, mixed venous hemoglobin oxygen saturation; Q_s/Q_t, calculated intrapulmonary shunt; $Ca{O_2}$, arterial oxygen content. Results are expressed as means ± SEM. All measurements were performed at a similar $F_i{O_2}$ (see the text for explanations). * $P < 0.05$, compared with N_2; † $P < 0.05$ compared with NO; ‡ $P < 0.05$, compared with NO + Alm. ns, not significant.

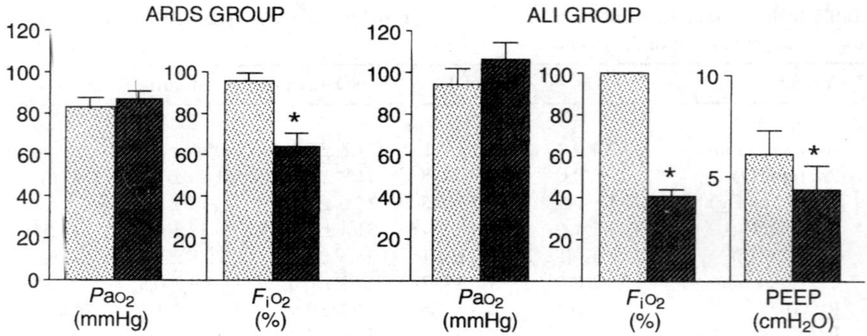

Figure 1. In both ARDS and ALI groups, compared with control, the combination therapy of NO and almitrine produced significant reduction in F_iO_2 while maintaining PaO_2. In the ALI group, NO + almitrine therapy produced a further reduction in the level of PEEP. Dotted bars, control; hatched bars, continuous treatment by NO inhalation + almitrine infusion. * $P < 0.001$, compared with control.

($P < 0.001$). This could be related to a more pronounced effect of almitrine on HPV in this group, consistent with previous reports of an impairment of HPV during unilateral pneumonia.[16] Thereby, in light of the supposedly important areas with normal V_A/Q ratios, a reinforcement of HPV would divert a large proportion of blood from the shunting areas, explaining the large increase in PaO_2 observed. An alternate hypothesis would be that, even if baseline and post-NO levels of PaO_2 were similar in ARDS and ALI patients, one might reasonably assume that the extent of the alteration of the lung parenchyma was quantitatively more important in the former. Therefore, following almitrine, the pulmonary blood diverted from non- or poorly ventilated areas to normally ventilated areas would flow in a relatively small fraction of the remaining lung parenchyma responsible for normal gas exchange, resulting in a smaller increase in PaO_2 in ARDS patients.

Finally, the combination of NO and almitrine reduced F_iO_2 in all patients, while maintaining a similar PaO_2. This beneficial effect on gas exchange might have important therapeutic and prognostic implications since it might reduce hyperoxic-induced lung injury, and limit the pulmonary baro-/volutrauma associated with 'aggressive' modes of mechanical ventilation.

In conclusion, the co-administration of inhaled NO with almitrine infusion resulted in a vasodilation of normally ventilated areas, and a further constriction of shunting zones, thus markedly improving arterial oxygenation. Although NO inhalation alone significantly increased PaO_2, the enhancement of pulmonary vasoconstriction with almitrine magnified this improvement in PaO_2 and allowed the levels of F_iO_2 and PEEP required for adequate gas exchange to be reduced. Finally, the proportion of shunting zones and the pulmonary vascular reactivity of the underlying lung disease was a determinant of the level of PaO_2 achieved with this co-administration. Further studies are needed to quantify the benefit of this co-administration in terms of decreased baro/volutraumatic complications.

ACKNOWLEDGEMENTS

This work was supported in part by Grants from University Paris VII 1994, Délégation à la Recherche Clinique AP-HP 1993, and Direction de la Recherche et de l'Enseignement Doctoral (D.R.E.D.) 1994.

REFERENCES

1. Dreyfuss D & Saumon G (1994) Ventilator-induced lung injury. In Tobin MJ (ed) *Principles and Practice of Mechanical Ventilation*, pp 793–811. New York: McGraw-Hill.
2. Payen D, Brun Buisson C, Carli P et al (1987) Hemodynamic, gas exchange and hormonal consequences of LBPP during PEEP ventilation. *Journal of Applied Physiology* **62:**61–70.
3. Payen D, Farge D, Beloucif S et al (1987) No involvment of ADH in acute anti-diuresis during PEEP ventilation in human. *Anesthesiology* **66:**17–23.
4. Rouby J, Lherm T, Martin de Lassale E et al (1993) Histologic aspects of pulmonary barotrauma in critically ill patients with acute respiratory failure. *Intensive Care Medicine* **19:**383–389.
5. Wagner P, Saltzman H & West J (1974) Measurement of continuous distribution of ventilation–perfusion ratios: theory. *Journal of Applied Physiology* **36:**588–599.
6. Payen D, Gatecel C & Plaisance P (1993) Almitrine effect on nitric oxide inhalation in adult respiratory distress syndrome. *Lancet* **341:**1664.
7. Higenbottam T, Pepke-Zaba J, Scott J, Woolman P, Coutts C & Wallwork J (1988) Inhaled endothelium-derived relaxing factor in primary pulmonary hypertension. *American Review of Respiratory Disease* **137(Suppl):**107(Abstr).
8. Payen D, Gatecel C & Guinard N (1993) Inhalation of low dose of nitric oxide (NO) and IV L-Arg in ARDS patients: effect on pulmonary hemodynamic, gas exchange and NO metabolites. *American Review of Respiratory Disease* **147:**A720 (Abstr).
9. Puybasset L, Rouby J, Mourgeon E et al (1994) Inhaled nitric oxide in acute respiratory failure: dose–response curves. *Intensive Care Medicine* **20:**319–327.
10. Wysocki M, Delclaux C, Roupie E et al (1994) Additive effect on gas exchange of inhaled nitric oxide and intravenous almitrine bismesylate in the adult respiratory distress syndrome. *Intensive Care Medicine* **20:**254–259.
11. Rossaint R, Falke K, Lopez F, Slama K, Pison U & Zapol W (1993) Inhaled nitric oxide for the adult respiratory distress syndrome. *New England Journal of Medicine* **328:**399–405.
12. Zapol W, Rimar S, Gillis N, Marletta M & Bosken C (1994) Nitric oxide and the lung. *American Journal of Respiratory Critical Care Medicine* **149:**1375–1380.
13. Marshall B, Hanson C, Frasch F & Marshall C (1994) Role of hypoxic pulmonary vasoconstriction in pulmonary gas exchange and blood flow distribution. *Intensive Care Medicine* **20:**379–389.
14. Doering EB, Hanson CW, Reily DJ, Marshall C & Marshall BE (1995) Improvement in oxygenation by both nitric oxide and phenylephrine in ARDS patients. *Anesthesiology* **83; 3A**:A77 (Abstr).
15. Laubie M & Diot F (1972) A pharmacological study of the respiratory stimulant action of S 2620. *Journal of Pharmacology* **3:**363–374.
16. Graham L, Vasil A, Vasil M, Voelkel N & Stenmark K (1990) Decreased pulmonary vasoreactivity in an animal model of chronic *Pseudomonas* pneumonia. *American Review of Respiratory Disease* **142:**221–229.
17. Spaden H & Vincken W (1987) Pulmonary arterial hypertension in sepsis and the adult respiratory distress syndrome. *Acta Clinica Belgica* **47:**30–40.

18. Reeves J & Grover R (1974) Blockade of acute hypoxic pulmonary hypertension by endotoxin. *Journal of Applied Physiology* **36:**328–332.
19. Jones R, Reid L, Zapol W et al (1985) Pulmonary vascular pathology. In Zapol W & Falke K (eds), *Acute Respiratory Failure*, pp 23–160. New York: Dekker.
20. Persson MG, Gustafsson LE, Wiklund NP, Moncada S & Hedqvist P (1990) Endogenous nitric oxide as a probable modulator of pulmonary circulation and hypoxic pressor response in vivo. *Acta Physiologica Scandinavica* **140:**449–457.
21. Sprague R, Thiemermann C & Vane J (1992) Endogenous endothelium-derived relaxing factor opposes hypoxic pulmonary vasoconstriction and supports blood flow to hypoxic alveoli in anesthetized rabbits. *Proceedings of the National Academy of Sciences USA* **89:**8711–8715.
22. Voelkel N (1986) Mechanisms of hypoxic pulmonary vasoconstriction. *American Review of Respiratory Disease* **133:**1186–1195.
23. Marshall B, Marshall C, Frasch F & Hanson C (1994) Role of hypoxic pulmonary vasoconstriction in pulmonary gas exchange and blood flow distribution. *Intensive Care Medicine* **20:**291–297.
24. Payen D, Carli P, Brun-Buisson C et al (1985) Lower body positive pressure versus dopamine during PEEP ventilation. *Journal of Applied Physiology* **58:**77–82.
25. Marshall C & Marshall B (1983) Site and sensitivity for stimulation of hypoxic pulmonary vasoconstriction. *Journal of Applied Physiology* **55:**711–716.
26. Marshall B, Marshall C, Magno M, Lilagan P & Pietra G (1991) Influence of bronchial arterial Po_2 on pulmonary vascular resistance. *Journal of Applied Physiology* **70:**405–415.
27. Laubie M & Schmitt H (1980) Long-lasting hyperventilation induced by almitrine: evidence for a specific effect on carotid and thoracic chemoreceptors. *European Journal of Pharmacology* **61:**125–136.
28. Melot C, Naieje R, Rotschild T et al. (1983) Improvement in ventilation-perfusion matching by almitrine in COPD. *Chest* **83:**528–533.
29. Georgopoulos D, Walker S & Anthonisen A (1989) Increased chemoreceptor output and ventilatory response to sustained hypoxia. *Journal of Applied Physiology* **67:**1157–1163.
30. Castaing Y, Manier G & Guenard H (1986) Improvement in ventilation-perfusion relationships by almitrine in patients with chronic obstructive pulmonary disease during mechanical ventilation. *American Review of Respiratory Disease* **143:**910–916.
31. Herve P, Musset D, Simmoneau G, Wagner Jr W & Duroux P (1989) Almitrine decreases the distensibility of the large pulmonary arteries in man. *Chest* **96:**572–577.
32. Clergue F, Ecoffey C, Derenne J & Viars P (1984) Oxygen drive to breathing during halothane anesthesia: effects of almitrine bismesylate. *Anesthesiology* **61:**627–628.
33. Melot C, Dechamps P, Hallemans R, Decroly P & Mols P (1989) Enhancement of hypoxic pulmonary vasoconstriction by low dose almitrine bismesylate in normal humans. *American Review of Respiratory Disease* **139:**111–119.
34. Gherardi R, Louarn F, Benvenuti C et al (1985) Peripheral neuropathy in patients treated with almitrine bismesylate. *Lancet* **2:**1247–1250.
35. Voisin C, Howard P & Ansquer J (1987) Almitrine bismesylate. A long term placebo controlled double blind study in COPD. Vectarion international multicentre study group. *Bulletin Européen de Physiopathologie Respiratoire* **23(Suppl 11):**169–182.
36. Romaldini H, Rodriguez-Roisin R, Wagner P & West J (1983) Enhancement of hypoxic pulmonary vasoconstriction by almitrine in the dog. *American Review of Respiratory Disease* **128:**288–293.
37. Chen L, Miller F, Clarke W et al (1990) Low-dose almitrine bismesylate enhances hypoxic pulmonary vasoconstriction in closed chest dogs. *Anesthesia and Analgesia* **71:**475–483.

38. Reyes R, Roca J, Rodriguez-Roisin R et al (1988) Effect of almitrine on ventilation–perfusion distribution in adult respiratory distress syndrome. *American Review of Respiratory Disease* **137:**1062–1067.
39. Bee D, Gill G, Emery C et al Action of almitrine on the pulmonary vasculature in ferrets and rats. *Bull Europ Physiopath Resp* **19:**539–545.
40. Gottschall EB, Fernyak S, Wuertemberger G & Voelkel N (1992) Almitrine mimics hypoxic vasoconstriction in isolated rat lungs. *American Journal of Physiology* **263:**H383–H391.
41. Rounds S & McMurtry I (1981) Inhibitors of oxidative ATP production cause transient vasoconstriction and block subsequent pressor responses in rat lungs. *Circulation Research* **48:**393–400.
42. Archer S, Huang J, Henry T, Peterson D & Weir E (1993) A redox-based O_2 sensor in rat pulmonary vasculature. *Circulation Research* **73:**1100–1112.
43. Rigoulet M, Fraisse L, Ouhabi R et al (1990) Flux-dependent increase in the stoichiometry of charge translocation by mitochondrial ATPase/ATP synthase induced by almitrine. *Biochimica Biophysica Acta* **1018:**91–97.
44. Hughes J, Allison D, Goatcher A & Tripathi A (1986) Influence of alveolar hypoxia on pulmonary vasomotor responses to almitrine in the dog. *Clinical Sciences* **70:**555–564.
45. Naeije R, Lejeune P, Vachiéry J et al (1990) Restored hypoxic pulmonary vasoconstriction by peripheral chemoreceptor agonists in dogs. *American Review of Respiratory Disease* **142:**789–795.
46. Leeman M, Lejeune P, Hallemans R, Melot C & Naieje R (1988) Effects of increased pulmonary vascular tone on gas exchange in canine oleic acid pulmonary edema. *Journal of Applied Physiology* **65:**662–668.
47. Reyes A, Lopes-Messa J & Alonso P (1987) Almitrine in acute respiratory failure. Effects on pulmonary gas exchange and circulation. *Chest* **91:**388–393.
48. Dreyfuss D, Djedaini K, Lanore J et al (1992) A comparative study of the effects of almitrine bismesylate and lateral position during unilateral bacterial pneumonia with severe hypoxemia. *American Review of Respiratory Disease* **146:**295–299.
49. Frostell C, Fratacci MD, Wain J, Jones R & Zapol W (1991) Inhaled nitric oxide, a selective pulmonary vasodilator reversing hypoxic pulmonary vasoconstriction. *Circulation* **83:**2038–2047.

14

Factors Predicting the Response to Inhaled Nitric Oxide in Acute Respiratory Failure

J. J. Rouby

INTRODUCTION

Gaseous nitric oxide (NO) and nitrogen dioxide (NO_2) are well known atmospheric outdoor pollutants the toxicity of which was extensively studied in the 1970s. In the 1980s, inhaled NO was used in humans as an alternative to CO to measure the oxygen-diffusing capacity of the lungs.[1,2] In 1987, one of the endothelium-derived relaxing factors was identified as NO.[3,4] It was then demonstrated that NO was continuously released by the endothelial cells after activation of the constitutive NO synthase in response to shear stress. Later, NO was found to be involved in a large number of physiological systems[5,6] such as coagulation,[7,8] neuronal transmission and inflammation.

The first description of inhaled NO as a therapeutic agent in humans was published in 1988 in an abstract form by Higenbottam's group.[9] Inhaled NO was shown to reduce pulmonary pressure, without any systemic effect, in seven patients with severe primary pulmonary hypertension. This work was published as a full paper in 1991.[10] Inhaled NO-induced selective pulmonary vasodilation was later confirmed in different experimental models of pulmonary hypertension: injection of an analog of thromboxane A_2 or injection of heparin-protamine,[11] hypoxic pulmonary vasoconstriction,[12–14] lipopolysaccharide or streptococcal intravenous infusion.[15–17] Concomitant with reduction in pulmonary artery pressure, a sustained inhaled NO-induced improvement in arterial oxygenation was described in patients with respiratory distress syndrome (ARDS) by Falke's group in 1993[18] and then confirmed by other studies.[19–21] In addition, pulmonary hypertension secondary to cardiac surgery[22,23] or chronic obstructive pulmonary disease (COPD)[24,25] was shown to be also responsive to inhaled NO. However, some patients with ARDS or perioperative pulmonary hypertension do not respond to inhaled NO and a good knowledge of factors predicting the response to NO is of critical importance for the physician at the bedside.

MONITORING AND TOXICITY

Methods of monitoring

Owing to the potential toxicity of NO itself and of its oxidative derivatives NO_x, it is recommended that NO and NO_x concentrations be measured during long-term administration of inhaled NO in humans with acute respiratory failure. Because measurements are performed on gases saturated in humidity, only two methods of monitoring appear to be adequate: chemiluminescence and the electrochemical method. The infrared method requires analysis of dry gas and therefore the interposition of a humidity absorber on the suctioning circuit is necessary. However, NO_2 is absorbed together with water and thus can no longer be measured when using the infrared method. The electrochemical method is less expensive than chemiluminescence but has some disadvantages: frequent recalibrations are necessary, the electrochemical cells themselves have to be replaced regularly and the precision of the method is low for NO and NO_2 concentrations below 2 ppm. As far as NO is concerned, the concentration of 2 ppm is precisely the optimum concentration to be used in nonseptic shock patients.[20] Concerning NO_2, 2 ppm is far greater than the acceptable threshold in humans. A bronchoconstrictor effect of NO_2 has been described for a concentration of 0.3 ppm[26] and a pro-inflammatory pulmonary effect for a concentration of 2.25 ppm.[27] Thus the electrochemical method appears less appropriate than chemiluminescence for clinical monitoring of NO concentrations during long-term administration of inhaled NO in humans.

The reference method, chemiluminescence, allows measurements of very low NO and NO_2 concentrations with a precision in the ppb range. When designed for measuring atmospheric pollution, the time to response of chemiluminescence apparatus used in industry is low, around 40 s (NOX 2000, Sérès, Aix-en-Provence, France). However the intrinsic time to response of chemiluminescence itself is high, in the millisecond range. In fact, the observed time to response depends mainly on the aspirative flow and on the dead space of connecting and internal circuits. As recently demonstrated,[28] chemiluminescence apparatus designed for medical use has a fast time to response of around 1 s (NOX 4000) and allows the accurate measurement of inspired and expired concentrations of NO if a high aspirative flow is selected (1 liter/min). Inspiratory NO concentration is the 'effective' dose delivered to pulmonary vessels via alveolar spaces and should be monitored (Figure 1).

It should be emphasized that mean NO concentrations measured within the inspiratory limb of the ventilator using a chemiluminescence device with a slow response time are representative of 'true' inspiratory tracheal concentrations only when NO is uniformly distributed within the tubing. This is not true when the gas is continuously administered into the inspiratory limb before the Y piece: each tidal volume 'pushes' into the tracheobronchial tree

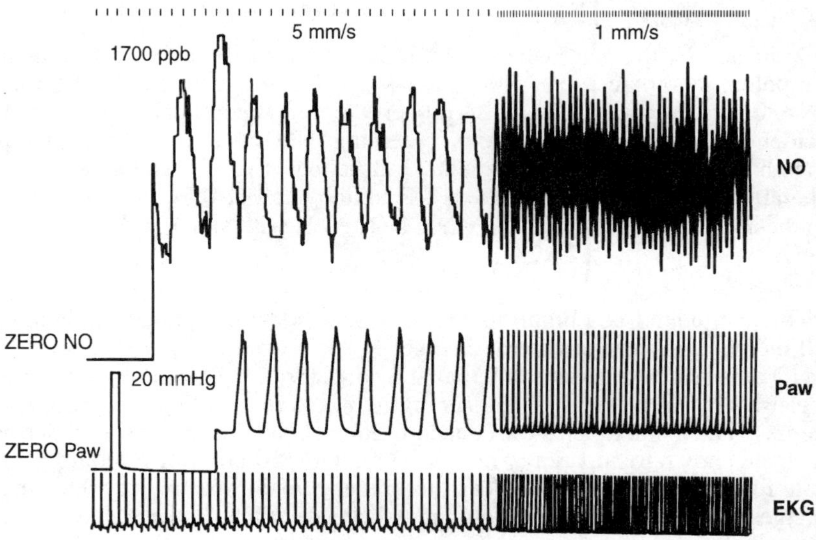

Figure 1. Continuous recordings of inspiratory and expiratory concentrations of NO measured using a chemiluminescence apparatus NOX 4000, airway pressure (Paw) and electrocardiogram (EKG) in a patient with ARDS. Two different paper speeds (5 mm/s and 1 mm/s) are used. The patient is ventilated using a respiratory frequency of 20 b/min, an inspiratory time of 30% and a positive end-expiratory pressure (PEEP) of 10 cmH_2O and receives an inspiratory intratracheal concentration of NO of 1.5 ppm (1500 ppb). The delay between peak inspiratory pressure and inspiratory NO concentration is 1.6 s and is related to the transit time of tracheal gas from the endotracheal tube to the chemiluminescence apparatus, the aspiration flow rate being set at 1 liter/min. At the 5 mm/s paper speed (left part of the Figure) it can be seen that five measurements of NO concentration are performed during 1 s, thus determining a response time of the NOX 4000 of 200 ms. Inspiratory NO concentrations are fluctuating around a value of 1.5 ppm (1500 ppb), whereas expiratory NO concentrations are fluctuating around 0.6 ppm. (Taken from reference[28]).

a bolus of NO incompletely mixed by the inspiratory flow. In contrast, when NO is mixed with nitrogen and oxygen before the ventilator or administered exclusively during the inspiratory phase, the inspiratory concentration is constant throughout inspiration, the ventilator or the inspiratory limb serving as mixing chambers. The same inspiratory concentration administered either throughout the entire inspiration or during only a fraction of inspiration could have different cardiorespiratory effects.[28]

Toxicity of inhaled NO

Inhaled NO toxicity, apart from the generation of high levels of methemoglobin, can be due to NO itself and to its oxidative derivative, NO_2.

Toxicity of NO

NO released by the macrophage after induction of the inducible NO synthase is a potent cytotoxic agent. NO also has a high mutagenic potential through DNA deamination.[29–32] This last property could theoretically increase the incidence of cancers in patients receiving NO as a long-term therapy. Thereby, the registration of patients and neonates receiving long-term NO inhalation should be implemented. NO toxicity can also be the result of the synthesis of peroxynitrite anion when NO reacts with superoxide anion:

$$NO + O_2^{-\bullet} \rightarrow ONOO^-$$

This compound is a highly potent oxidant, inducing lipid peroxidation of cell membranes[33] and structural changes in surfarctant.[34]

NO administered in dogs is lethal at a concentration of 20 000 ppm. Death is caused by high levels of methemoglobin and noncardiogenic pulmonary edema.[35] The inhalation of low concentrations of NO during very long periods has been shown to apparently not cause toxicity: 10 ppm for 6 months[36] or 2 ppm for 2 years in mice[37] does not induce major pulmonary histologic changes. Emphysema-like lesions have been described in one study of rats after inhalation of 20 ppm of NO for 6 weeks.[38]

Toxicity of NO_2

The amount of NO_2 generated when NO is in the presence of oxygen depends on the contact time (k.t.), the F_iO_2 and the NO concentration according to the equation:[39]

$$[NO_2] = \text{k.t.}\ (F_iO_2)\ [NO]^2$$

Figure 2 shows mean intratracheal NO_2 concentrations measured by chemiluminescence at steady state in ten patients with acute respiratory failure inhaling pure oxygen and increasing concentrations of NO in the range 0.1–100 ppm. At an NO concentration of 10 ppm, the observed NO_2 concentration is above the toxic threshold of 0.3 ppm. Toxicity of NO_2 is different whether it is administered acutely or chronically.

Toxicity of inhaled NO_2 administered acutely. Inhalation of NO_2 induces acute lung injury, increases bronchial reactivity and enhances the development of lung viral infections. NO_2 inhaled at a concentration of 400 ppm for 1 h in dogs induces interstitial and alveolar edema.[41] Similar results have been described in other species such as guinea-pigs[42] and rats.[43,44] In the human, inflammatory cell responses in bronchoalveolar lavage fluid have been observed after inhalation of NO_2 at concentrations as low as 2.25 ppm.[27]

NO_2 increases the bronchomotor tone of isolated human bronchi.[45] In asthmatics, inhaled NO_2 at a concentration of 0.3 ppm potentiates exercise-induced bronchospasm.[26] NO_2 can also increase the bronchial reactivity of healthy volunteers if inhaled at a concentration of 1.5 ppm for 3 h.[46]

Mice inhaling NO_2 show a concentration-dependent increase in the incidence of lung pneumonia after intratracheal instillation of a normally

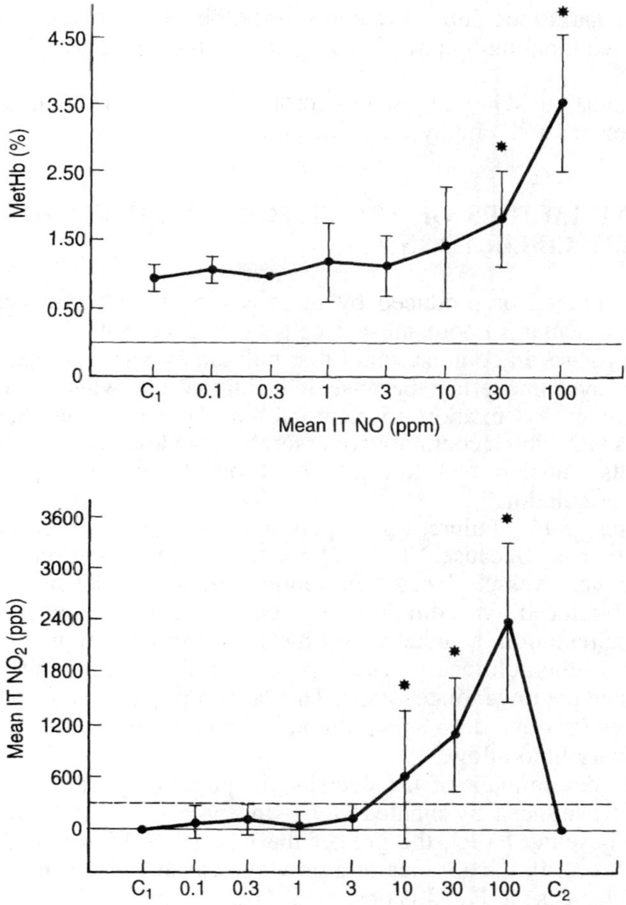

Figure 2. Acute toxicity of inhaled NO in ARDS. The figure represents methemoglobin (MetHb) concentrations (upper panel) and mean intratracheal (IT) NO_2 concentrations (lower panel) measured in ten patients inhaling increasing concentrations of NO. The x-axis is in a log scale. The measured NO concentration is a mean concentration of expired and inspired gas. The F_iO_2 was maintained at 100% and the temperature at 37 °C throughout the procedure. Measurements were performed after a steady state of 20 min. A significant increase in methemoglobin concentration was observed when mean NO concentrations delivered to the patient were above 10 ppm. Mean NO_2 concentrations are above the toxicity threshold of 300 ppb as soon as mean NO concentrations delivered to the patient are higher or equal to 10 ppm. *Significantly different from control ($P < 0.05$). (Taken from reference[40]).

noninfectant viral inoculum. It requires 100 times less virus to induce pneumonia in mice inhaling 5 ppm of NO_2 than in control animals.[47]

Toxicity of inhaled NO_2 administered chronically. It is very similar to that of oxygen or ozone with emphysema-like pulmonary lesions.[48]

PREDICTIVE FACTORS OF THE EFFECTS OF NO ON THE PULMONARY CIRCULATION

NO, either inhaled or produced by the vascular endothelium, relaxes the pulmonary vascular smooth muscle cell through activation of the soluble guanylate cyclase. In contrast with other pulmonary vasodilators,[49,50] inhaled NO has no systemic effect because it is inactivated when it reaches the vascular lumen by fixation to hemoglobin. However, in contrast with endogenous NO, which continuously vasorelaxes pulmonary vascular smooth muscle cells, inhaled NO has no effect on the normal nonconstricted pulmonary circulation.[51]

In acute respiratory failure, a large part of the lung parenchyma is no longer accessible to gas. Because NO is administered via inhalation, it can only reach pulmonary vessels located in ventilated parts of the lung. Therefore inhaled-NO-induced vasodilation is doubly specific: specific to the pulmonary circulation, as inhaled NO has no effect on systemic circulation, and specific to the pulmonary vessels of the ventilated part of the lung, as it does not reach the unventilated zone. This last property explains why inhaled NO increases $Pa\text{O}_2$ and decreases pulmonary shunt through a redistribution of intrapulmonary blood flow.

The main determinant of the decrease in pulmonary vascular resistance index (PVRI) induced by inhaled NO is the basal level of PVRI.[19,23,52] The greater the baseline PVRI, the greater the inhaled NO-induced decrease in PVRI (Figure 3). In the absence of a previous constriction of the pulmonary vessels, no decrease in PVRI is observed. The NO-induced decrease in PVRI varies from 0% in the case of normal basal PVRI to 50% for PVRI of around 2000 dyn s cm^{-5} m^2.

The increase in PVRI characterizing acute respiratory failure is partly related to the presence of circulatory inflammatory mediators such as thromboxane A_2, platelet activating factor or endothelin[53] and partly related to fixed nonreversible mechanisms such as microthrombosis or increase in vascular thickness secondary to smooth muscle proliferation.[54] The so-called 'NO-responders' are patients with an increase in PVRI related to vasoconstriction (> 200 dyn s cm^{-5} m^2). 'NO-nonresponders' are either patients with normal pulmonary vascular tone or patients with an increase in PVRI mainly related to thrombosis or to anatomical remodeling of the pulmonary vessels. The correlation between the basal level of PVRI and the NO-induced decrease in PVRI observed during ARDS[19,52] has also been described for pulmonary hypertensions complicating cardiac surgery.[23]

The correlation between inhaled-NO-induced decrease in mean pulmonary artery pressure (MPAP) and baseline MPAP, although stastistically

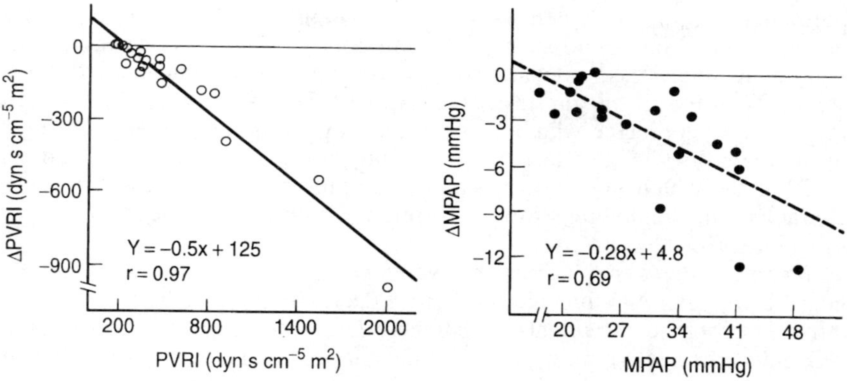

Figure 3. Pulmonary vascular effects of inhaled NO: predictive factors. Regression lines between basal PVRI and inhaled-NO-induced decrease in PVRI (ΔPVRI) and between basal mean pulmonary arterial pressure (MPAP) and inhaled-NO-induced decrease in MPAP (ΔMPAP) are shown. Each point is representative of a patient with severe ARDS, and inhaled NO was administered to each patient at a concentration of 2 ppm. (Taken from reference[52]).

significant, appears less tight than the correlation between NO-induced decrease in PVRI and baseline PVRI (Figure 3). At least two reasons can be given to explain this result. First, pulmonary hypertension can be mainly flow-dependent with a tiny increase in PVRI. As a consequence, NO will not reduce MPAP even if the baseline MPAP is elevated. Secondly, the inhalation of NO can indirectly increase cardiac output, for instance by unloading a failing right ventricle, and thus, despite a decrease in PVRI, MPAP will not decrease or will decrease only slightly. Such an inhaled-NO-induced increase in cardiac output is observed in the presence of right heart failure due to either acute respiratory failure or another cause.

If NO normalizes an initially low cardiac output, the observed decrease in MPAP will be proportionally less than the decrease in PVRI because the pressure–flow relationship of the pulmonary circulation is curvilinear for low cardiac output.[55,56] NO is a pharmacologic tool which can be used to test the vasodilation reserve of the pulmonary circulation during acute respiratory failure. The correlation shown in Figure 3 was obtained in patients during the early phase of their ARDS. However, patients in whom a decrease in PVRI was observed during this early phase continued to show decreased PVRI after NO inhalation during the entire course of their disease, as long as their basal PVRI remained elevated. This result supports the hypothesis that a vasodilation reserve persists during the course of ARDS and that the fixed part of elevated pulmonary pressure does not increase with time. In fact, initially 'NO-responder' patients become 'NO-nonresponder' patients when their basal PVRI values return to normal in the recovery phase of acute lung injury. There is no real tachyphylaxia to inhaled NO.[19] Inhaled-NO-induced decrease in PVRI does not seem to be correlated to the initial degree of hypoxemia and pulmonary shunt.[52] This is due to the fact that in ARDS, arterial hypoxemia depends on many factors: hypoxic pulmonary vasoconstriction in non-ventilated lung areas, extension of the alveolar disease and hemodynamic status. Therefore it has no direct link with PVRI. This also applies to static respiratory compliance which is considered a good index of the extension of the alveolar disease[57] but does not predict the pulmonary effect of inhaled NO. PVRI alone, which can be seen as an index of the pulmonary vascular disease characterizing acute lung injury, is predictive of NO-induced pulmonary vascular effect.

In some patients, no decrease or even a paradoxical increase in MPAP can be observed after NO inhalation despite a decrease in PVRI. This unexpected effect is observed in patients with severe left ventricular failure: following NO-induced selective pulmonary vasodilatation, venous return to the failing left ventricle increases, inducing a marked increase in left ventricular end-diastolic pressure, pulmonary wedge pressure and PAP.[58–61] As a consequence, MPAP does not decrease despite the marked reduction in PVRI, and pulmonary edema may follow the inhalation of NO.

The diameter of resistive arteries of the human pulmonary circulation varies from 200 to 500 μm. The muscular coat of the arteries is initially circular, and becomes partially muscular before it disappears at the capillary level. 'Intermediate cells' located in partially muscular arteries can change their phenotype during acute lung injury or chronic exposition to hypoxia and can be transformed into muscular cells. This mechanism partially explains the observed increase in PVRI during ARDS.[62] A recent experimental study has suggested that prolonged inhalation of NO might attenuate pulmonary vascular smooth muscle hypertrophy in newborn rats submitted to chronic hypoxia.[63]

Inhaled NO is potentially both an arterial and a venous vasodilator. Arteries and veins have different pathways inside the secondary pulmonary lobule: arteries follow the bronchovascular axis of the lobule whereas veins go back to the left atrium with the lymphatics within the interlobular septa. As a consequence, arteries and veins are in contact with alveoli and therefore can be reached by NO administered via inhalation. Part of the increase in PVRI during ARDS is due to venous constriction and should be reversed after NO inhalation. Experimental and clinical arguments in favor of inhaled-NO-induced venodilation have been recently presented.[64,65]

PREDICTIVE FACTORS OF THE EFFECTS ON GAS EXCHANGE

Inhaled NO improves arterial oxygenation by diverting pulmonary blood flow away from nonventilated toward ventilated lung areas:[18] inhaled-NO-induced pulmonary vasodilation involves selectively ventilated lung territories and does not inhibit hypoxic pulmonary vasoconstriction characterizing non-ventilated lung areas. In contrast with intravenous vasodilators,[49,50] inhaled NO usually has no effect on cardiac output and does not induce any vaso-dilation in pulmonary vessels irrigating nonventilated lung areas. As a consequence, pulmonary shunt does not increase and $Pa\text{O}_2$ does not deteriorate following NO inhalation.[18] Inhaled-NO-induced increases in $Pa\text{O}_2$ and decreases in pulmonary shunt depend on the initial level of PVRI.[52] The greater the baseline PVRI, the greater the inhaled NO-induced increase in $Pa\text{O}_2$ and the greater the inhaled NO-induced decrease in pulmonary shunt (Figure 4). The correlation between baseline PVRI and inhaled-NO-induced increase in $Pa\text{O}_2$, although statistically significant, is weak because $Pa\text{O}_2$ is a complex parameter depending on many factors such as ventilation/perfusion V_A/Q at the alveolar level, cardiac output and oxygen consumption. Inhaled-NO-induced increase in $Pa\text{O}_2$ depends on baseline $Pa\text{O}_2$ only when the most hypoxemic patients are those who have the greatest pulmonary vascular resistance.[19,52]

Alveolar recruitment resulting from the application of PEEP potentiates inhaled NO-induced improvement in arterial oxygenation.[52] This beneficial effect of PEEP is observed only when it is associated with alveolar recruitment (Figure 5). When PEEP induces lung overdistension, the effect of inhaled NO on arterial oxygenation does not differ in PEEP and zero end-expiratory pressure (ZEEP) conditions. As a consequence, the effect of

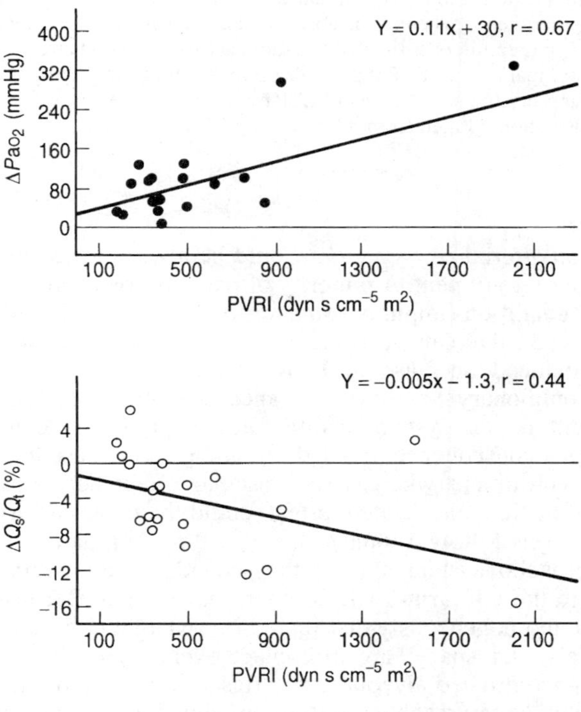

Figure 4. Effects of inhaled NO on arterial oxygenation: predictive factors. Regression lines between basal PVRI and inhaled-NO-induced increase in $Pa\text{O}_2$ and inhaled-NO-induced decrease in Q_s/Q_t are represented. Each point is representative of a patient with severe ARDS, and inhaled NO was administered to each patient at a concentration of 2 ppm. (Taken from reference[52]).

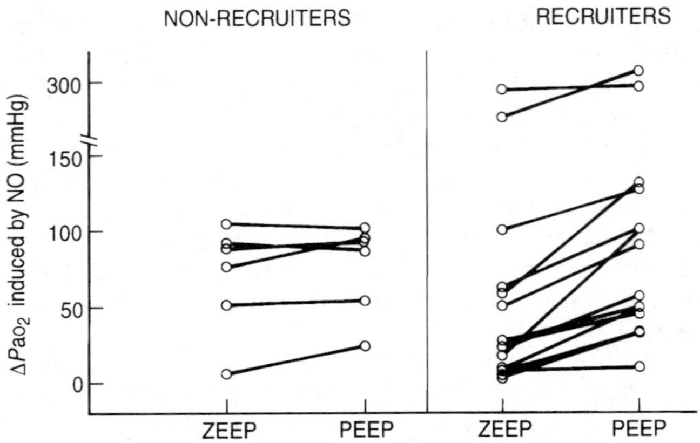

Figure 5. Influence of PEEP and alveolar recruitment on inhaled-NO-induced improvement in arterial oxygenation. In 20 critically ill patients with severe ARDS, PEEP-induced alveolar recruitment was assessed using a high-resolution thoracic computed tomography (CT) scan. A significant alveolar recruitment was evidenced following PEEP of 10 cmH_2O in 14 patients ('recruiters') whereas the absence of any alveolar recruitment was observed in six patients ('nonrecruiters'). Inhaled-NO-induced individual changes in $Pa\text{O}_2$ ($\Delta Pa\text{O}_2$, $F_i\text{O}_2 = 1$) are more marked in PEEP than in ZEEP in recruiters only, suggesting that PEEP-induced alveolar recruitment rather than PEEP by itself enhances the effect of inhaled NO on arterial oxygenation. (Taken from reference[52]).

inhaled NO on arterial oxygenation should be always tested after optimization of alveolar recruitment. A minority of patients considered as nonresponders in ZEEP conditions might become responders after PEEP administration.

PEEP-induced alveolar recruitment has an unforeseeable effect on inhaled-NO-induced decrease in PVRI. As a mean, inhaled-NO-induced decrease in pulmonary vascular resistance is similar in ZEEP and PEEP conditions and is not systematically potentiated by alveolar recruitment (Figure 6). As a consequence, inhaled-NO-induced increase in $Pa\text{O}_2$ depends on alveolar recruitment whereas the vascular effect does not. A possible explanation for this dissociated effect could have an anatomical basis. Pulmonary vessels follow a long pathway within lung parenchyma: arteries follow the bronchovascular axis of the secondary pulmonary lobules and veins return to the left atrium within interlobular septa. Because pulmonary lesions are nonhomogeneously distributed in ARDS, and because pulmonary vessels and alveolar spaces are in contact over a long distance, there are always enough ventilated alveolar territories surrounding pulmonary vessels to allow inhaled NO to reach and relax constricted vascular smooth muscles. The primary effect of inhaled-NO-induced arteriolar vasodilation is to increase pulmonary blood flow within the corresponding capillary network, the effect on gas exchange then depending on the V_A/Q ratio at the alveolar level. For a given secondary pulmonary lobule, V_A/Q and $Pa\text{O}_2$ will remain

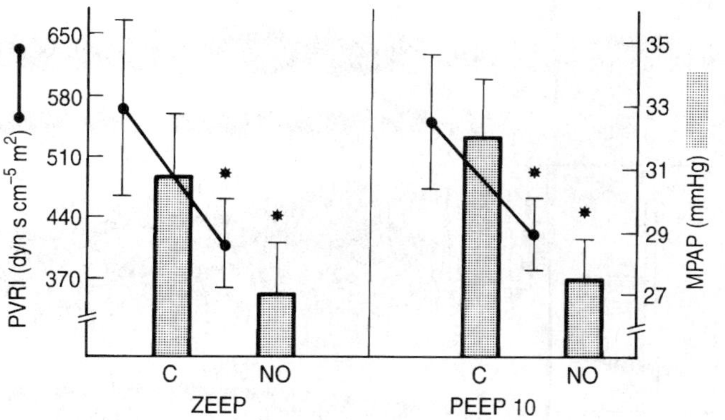

Figure 6. Influence of PEEP and alveolar recruitment on inhaled NO-induced pulmonary vascular effects. In the 20 patients of Figure 3, inhaled NO-induced changes in PVRI and MPAP are similar in ZEEP (zero end-expiratory pressure) and PEEP conditions suggesting that alveolar recruitment does not potentiate the pulmonary vascular effect of inhaled NO. (Taken from reference[52]). *Significantly different from control, $P < 0.05$.

unchanged if the increased pulmonary blood flow is equally distributed among ventilated and nonventilated acini. V_A/Q and $Pa{O_2}$ will increase if the increased pulmonary blood flow is preferentially distributed to ventilated acini. The resulting effect on systemic arterial oxygenation will depend on the sum of each local effect. If this hypothesis is valid, inhaled NO should be associated in a small number of patients with a worsening of arterial oxygenation. It is also easy to explain why PEEP potentiates inhaled-NO-induced improvement in arterial oxygenation: by inducing alveolar recruitment, PEEP reduces the proportion of nonventilated alveolar territories, and inhaled NO, by dilating pulmonary arterioles, increases pulmonary blood flow in these newly aerated alveoli.

Most often NO inhalation induces an increase in end-tidal carbon dioxide tension ($Pet{CO_2}$) simultaneously with the decrease in pulmonary arterial pressure (Figure 7). These changes are observed independently of any change in minute ventilation and cardiac output and are generally associated with a small but significant reduction in alveolo–arterial CO_2 gradient corresponding to a marked decrease in alveolar dead space.[20,21,52] The reduction in lung area characterized by high V_A/Q ratio, which is likely related to the re-opening of constricted pulmonary arteries in ventilated lung regions, contributes to increased alveolar ventilation. The effect on alveolar dead space is independent of alveolar recruitment (Figure 8) and has a large interpatient variability. In a minority of patients, the decrease in $Pa{CO_2}$ induced by the reduction in alveolar dead space can reach 10 mmHg and gives the possibility of reducing tidal volume and peak airway pressure.

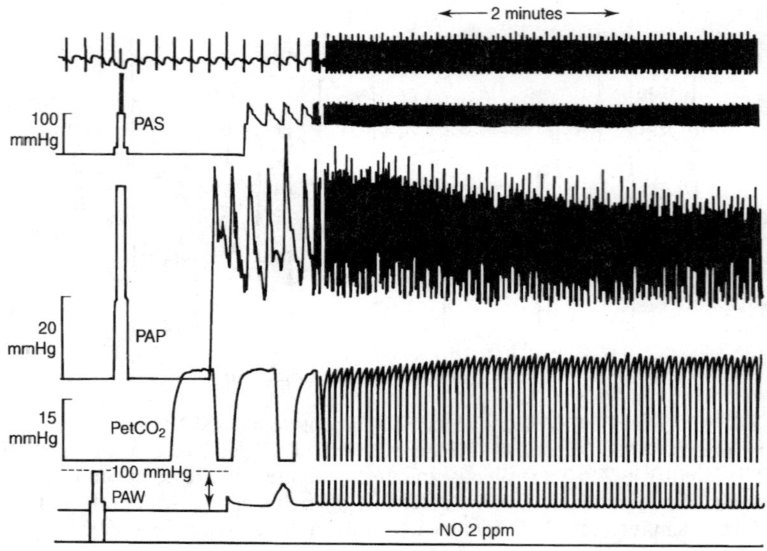

Figure 7. Effect of inhaled NO on end-tidal CO_2. Continuous recording of EKG, arterial pressure (PAS), pulmonary arterial pressure (PAP), end-tidal CO_2 (Petco$_2$, measured using a nonaspirative infrared capnometer) and airway pressure (PAW) was obtained in a critically ill patient with a severe ARDS. A few seconds after the inhalation of 2 ppm of NO (black line), a rise in Petco$_2$ is observed simultaneously with the decrease in PAP. In this patient, inhaled NO increased Pao$_2$ from 184 to 324 mmHg (F_io$_2$ = 1) and decreased alveolar dead space from 42 to 37%. (Taken from reference[20]).

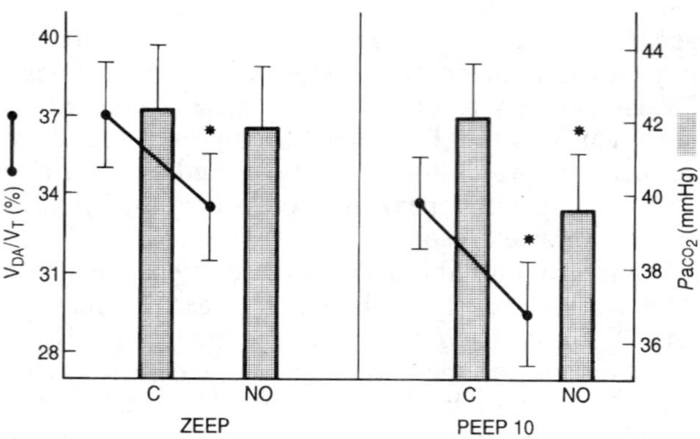

Figure 8. Influence of PEEP and alveolar recruitment on inhaled-NO-induced decrease in Paco$_2$ and alveolar dead space (V_{DA}/V_T). In 15 patients with severe ARDS, V_{DA}/V_T and Paco$_2$ were measured before and after the administration of PEEP 10 cmH_2O. The inhaled NO-induced decrease in V_{DA}/V_T and Paco$_2$ is similar in ZEEP and PEEP conditions and is not potentiated by PEEP-induced alveolar recruitment. The presentation of the figure is similar to Figures 5 and 6. *Significantly different from control, $P < 0.05$. (Taken from reference[52]).

PREDICTIVE FACTORS OF OTHER EFFECTS OF POTENTIAL BENEFIT

Mechanisms other than the diversion of pulmonary blood flow induced by arterial and venous vasodilation can be invoked to explain inhaled-NO-induced improvement in gas exchange. Because inhaled NO likely dilates both sides of the pulmonary circulation (arteries and veins), the reduction in pulmonary arterial pressure is associated with a reduction in hydrostatic capillary pulmonary pressure, which, in turn, could reduce the amount of pulmonary edema and improve arterial oxygenation. Because inhaled NO is a bronchodilator,[66] it could decrease venous admixture and reduce hypoxemia.

Inhaled NO could also limit the remodeling of the pulmonary circulation which occurs following lung injury.[62] In response to various types of lung injury, vascular smooth muscle rapidly appears in distal units of the pulmonary bed, increasing the proportion of vessels that are completely muscular. This anatomical remodeling of the pulmonary circulation forms the basis of the increase in pulmonary arterial pressure and pulmonary vascular resistance in ARDS. Endogenous NO released by pulmonary endothelial cells seems to exert a permanent antitrophic effect on adjacent vascular smooth muscle fibers.[67] Endothelial lesions observed in acute lung injury could annihilate NO-induced antiproliferative effects and enhance proliferation of vascular smooth muscle distally in the pulmonary vascular bed. Chronic inhalation of small concentrations of NO could reestablish the antiproliferative effect and prevent structural remodeling of the pulmonary circulation during the course of ARDS thus reducing pulmonary arterial hypertension.

Because inhaled NO inhibits platelet aggregation in patients with acute lung injury (Figure 9), it could prevent the formation of pulmonary thromboemboli which is observed at the early stage of ARDS and, consequently, reduce alveolar dead space and pulmonary hypertension. The antiplatelet effect observed in patients with ARDS consists of 50% each inhibition of platelet adhesion and platelet aggregation and does not appear to be dose-dependent in the range 1–100 ppm.[68] In patients with ARDS this potent antithrombotic effect is not associated with a lengthening of bleeding time (Figure 10). Surprisingly, the potent antiplatelet effect of inhaled NO observed in ARDS cannot be evidenced in healthy volunteers (personal communication). The reason for this discrepancy is not yet elucidated.

Inhaled NO has also been shown to inhibit polymorphonuclear activation which seems to be a key point in the pathophysiology of ARDS.[69] Experimentally, inhaled NO appears to either enhance or attenuate oxidant-induced acute lung injury. In isolated rabbit lungs submitted to oxidative stress, inhaled NO partially prevents the development of increased capillary permeability and pulmonary arterial hypertension[70] and dilates constricted pulmonary vessels in the presence of pulmonary endothelial injury.[71] On the other hand, it has been shown that endogenous NO likely mediates hyperoxia-induced damage of human lung cells[72] and is an essential intermediary in the production of acute lung injury due to Paraquat in guinea-pigs.[73] NO synthase inhibitors totally prevent lung injury caused by Paraquat and xanthine

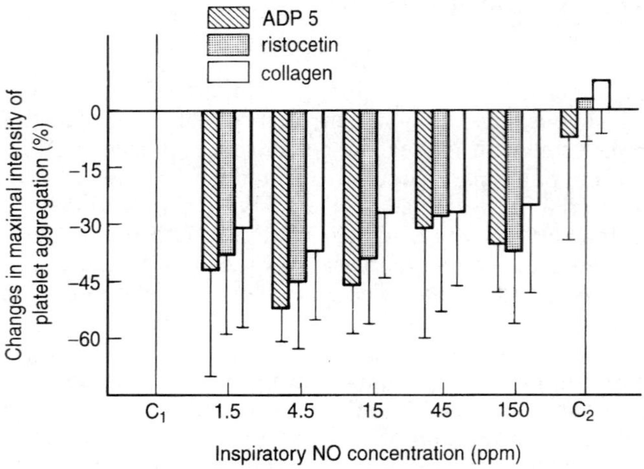

Figure 9. Changes in maximal intensity of platelet aggregation induced by five randomized incremental concentrations of NO administered to six patients with ARDS. Changes are expressed in percentage of variation from the first control value (C_1), which is by definition equal to 0%. Inhaled NO induced a significant and non-dose-dependent decrease in maximal intensity of platelet aggregation induced by three aggregating agents: 5 μm ADP, ristocetin, and collagen ($P < 0.01$). (Taken from reference[68]).

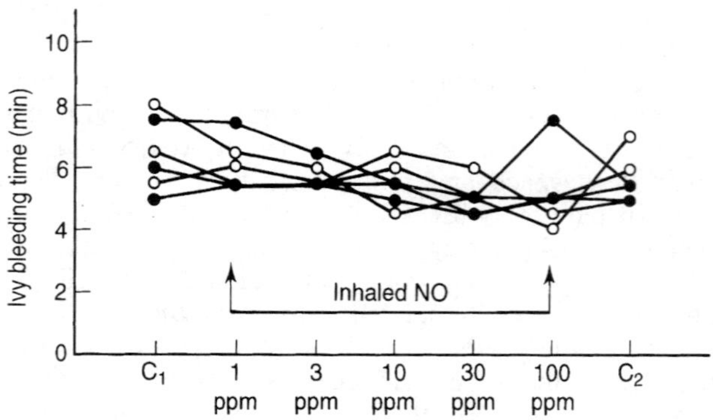

Figure 10. Changes in Ivy incision bleeding time induced by five randomized concentrations of NO administered to six patients with ARDS. (Taken from reference[68]).

oxidase. Therefore the administration of inhaled NO for treatment of patients with Paraquat-induced lung injury could be potentially harmful.

Inhaled NO inhibits metacholine-induced bronchoconstriction in guinea-pigs[66] and rabbits:[74] the bronchodilating effect is dose-dependent in the range 5–150 ppm. Acute lung injury is most often associated with increased respiratory resistance which can be caused by two different mechanisms: a part of the increased respiratory resistance is fixed, resulting from the external compression of bronchioles by the surrounding pulmonary edema; another part is reversible, resulting from the bronchoconstriction induced by circulating inflammatory mediators such as thromboxane A_2 and leukotrienes. In a recent study, inhaled NO-induced decrease in respiratory resistance could not be evidenced in patients with ARDS for NO concentrations ranging from 10 to 80 ppm (Figure 11).[75] Reasons for this lack of bronchodilating effect remain speculative. In patients with ARDS, the increased respiratory resistance might be entirely due to the reduction in lung volume, the specific bronchial resistance remaining normal. Therefore, the absence of true bronchoconstriction could explain the lack of inhaled-NO-induced bronchodilator effect. Another possibility could be that the inhaled-NO-induced bronchodilator effect is offset by an NO_2-induced bronchoconstrictive effect.[26,46] When NO concentrations greater than 10 ppm and F_iO_2 of 0.6 or above are used, NO_2 concentrations might be above 300 ppb[40] and could induce bronchoconstriction.[26] In spontaneously breathing asthmatic patients, inhaled NO at a concentration of 80 ppm exerts a bronchodilating effect that is much smaller than that produced by β_2-agonists.[76] Therefore, in humans with increased bronchial reactivity, inhaled NO appears to be a poorly effective bronchodilating agent.

INFLUENCE OF THE NO CONCENTRATION ADMINISTERED: DOSE–RESPONSE CURVES

As previously demonstrated in animals,[12] dose–response curves of inhaled NO in humans depend on the pathophysiology of the pulmonary arterial

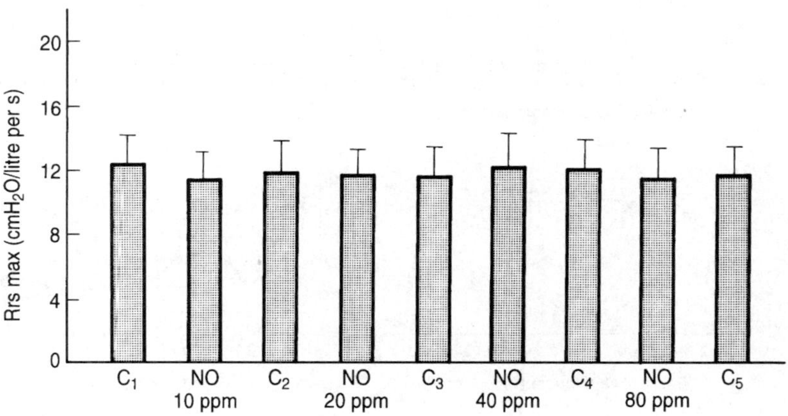

Figure 11. Effects of inhaled NO on respiratory resistance in patients with ARDS. Respiratory resistance (Rrs max) was measured using the end-inspiratory clamping technique in 11 patients with severe ARDS. Four different concentrations of inhaled NO were administered: 10, 20, 40 and 80 ppm. Control measurements were performed before NO administration (C_1) and between each concentration (C_2–C_5). No bronchodilating effect is observed despite the increased basal respiratory resistance (normal values for respiratory resistance: 3–5 cmH_2O/liter/s). Results are means ±SEM (Taken from reference[75]).

hypertension. An example is provided by the different dose–response curves obtained for patients with ARDS according to the presence or absence of associated septic shock. During septic shock, the inducible NO synthase is activated leading to the release by macrophages and vascular smooth muscles of endogenous NO which, in turn, contributes to the reduction in blood pressure.[77–79] Despite the excess endogenous NO production, critically ill patients with ARDS and septic shock still have pulmonary arterial hypertension. The presence of a septic shock associated with ARDS modifies the dose–response curve of inhaled NO.[80]

ARDS without septic shock

Minimal mean intratracheal concentrations of inhaled NO required to obtain the maximum effect on the pulmonary circulation and on arterial oxygenation are respectively around 2 and 1 ppm.[20,28] Dose–response curves for pulmonary arterial pressure, pulmonary vascular resistance, PaO_2, pulmonary shunt and SvO_2 are shown in Figures 12 and 13. In patients with ARDS treated by extracorporeal membrane oxygenation (ECMO), dose–response curves for systemic oxygenation and pulmonary hypertension are in the range 0.1–100 ppm.[81] This different dose–response curve could be related to a permanent

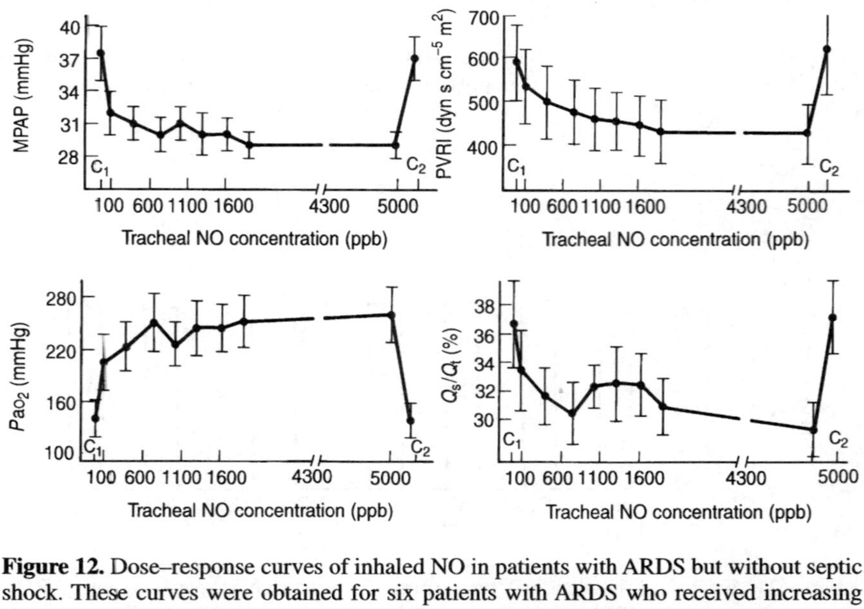

Figure 12. Dose–response curves of inhaled NO in patients with ARDS but without septic shock. These curves were obtained for six patients with ARDS who received increasing concentrations of inhaled NO in random order: 100, 400, 700, 1000, 1300, 1600, 1900, and 5000 ppb. The maximum effect on MPAP and PVRI is obtained for a mean intratracheal NO concentration of 1900 ppb. The maximum effect on PaO_2 ($F_iO_2 = 1$) and pulmonary shunt (Q_s/Q_t) is observed for a mean intratracheal NO concentration of 900 ppb. Control measurements were obtained before (C_1) and after (C_2) NO administration. (Taken from reference[20]).

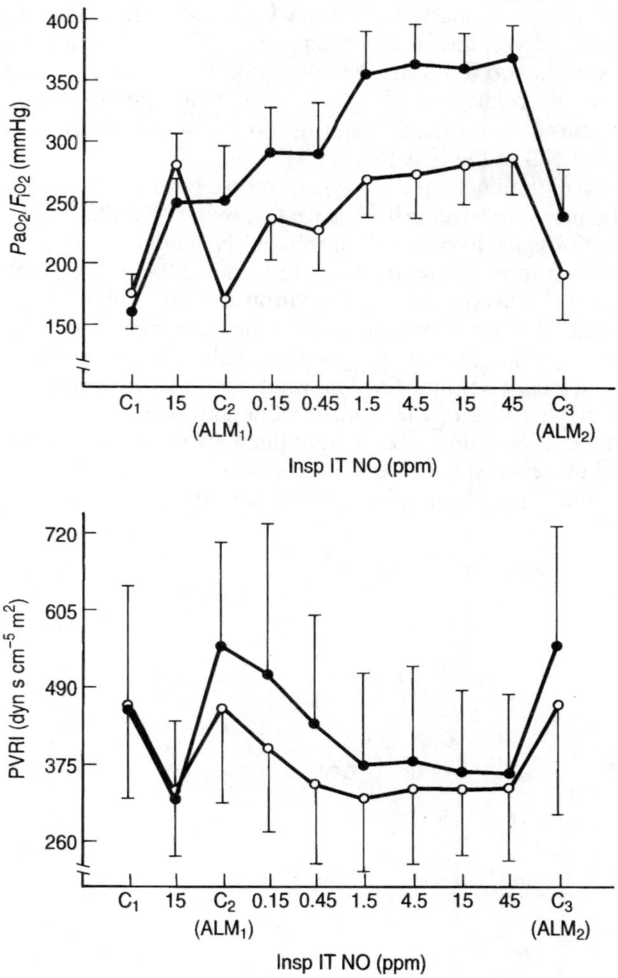

Figure 13. Changes in PaO_2/F_iO_2) ratio and PVRI induced by increasing inspiratory concentrations of inhaled NO (Insp IT NO) in the presence (●) or absence (○) of a continuous intravenous infusion of 16 µg/kg per min of almitrine in six patients with ARDS. PaO_2/F_iO_2 was measured: (1) before NO administration (C_1), (2) after the administration of 15 ppm of NO, (3) after the cessation of NO, with (ALM_1) or without (C_2) almitrine, (4) after six randomized concentrations of NO between 0.15 and 45 ppm, with or without almitrine and (5) after cessation of NO, with (ALM_2) or without (C_3) almitrine. Both conditions, NO alone and almitrine/NO, induce a significant and dose-dependent increase in PaO_2/F_iO_2 in the range 0.15–4.5 ppm ($P < 0.01$). However, there is no interaction between the factors almitrine and NO suggesting that the profile of the NO dose–response curve is not affected by the presence of almitrine. PaO_2/F_iO_2 ratio was significantly greater during almitrine/NO than during NO alone ($P < 0.001$). (Taken from reference[28]).

activation of the pulmonary circulation by ECMO. In some other patients, dose–response curves are in the range 20–100 ppb.[20,82] In a patient under general anesthesia and if inhaled NO does not change cardiac output, changes in Svo_2 are tightly related to changes in Sao_2. Consequently, continuous Svo_2 monitoring is an easy means of determining the minimal efficient concentration of inhaled NO at the bedside.

In critically ill patients with acute respiratory failure, systolic, diastolic and mean arterial pressures decrease by 25% following NO inhalation. In neonates with acute pulmonary hypertension, inhaled-NO-induced decrease in arterial pressure is much more pronounced and reaches 34% of the control value.[83,84] Dose–response curves for both oxygenation and pulmonary hypertension are between 0 and 5 ppm.[85] Systolic, diastolic and mean pulmonary arterial pressures decrease in the same proportion, excluding a predominant effect on pulmonary arterial compliance. Maximal increase in arterial oxygenation varies from 30 to 100% of the control value and is obtained for NO concentrations around 1 ppm in patients ventilated using conventional ventilatory support. For these very low NO concentrations, NO_2 concentrations remain low even if pure oxygen is administered and the risk of toxicity is limited (Figure 14).

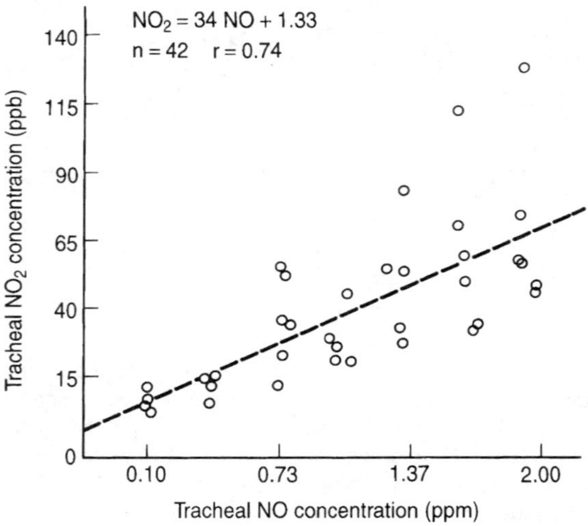

Figure 14. Mean intratracheal concentrations of NO_2 following the administration of increasing concentrations of NO in the range 0.1–2 ppm in six patients with ARDS ventilated using pure oxygen. There is a linear and significant relationship between NO_2 and NO concentrations. At 2 ppm NO, the maximum NO_2 concentration was 125 ppb. (Taken from reference[20]).

ARDS associated with septic shock

Dose–response curves of inhaled NO for arterial oxygenation in patients with ARDS are modified by the presence of septic shock (Figure 15). The maximum increase in Pao_2 is obtained at NO concentrations around 1 ppm in patients without septic shock and at NO concentrations around 100 ppm in patients with septic shock. However, the dose–response curves for pulmonary arterial hypertension and pulmonary vascular resistance are not different in

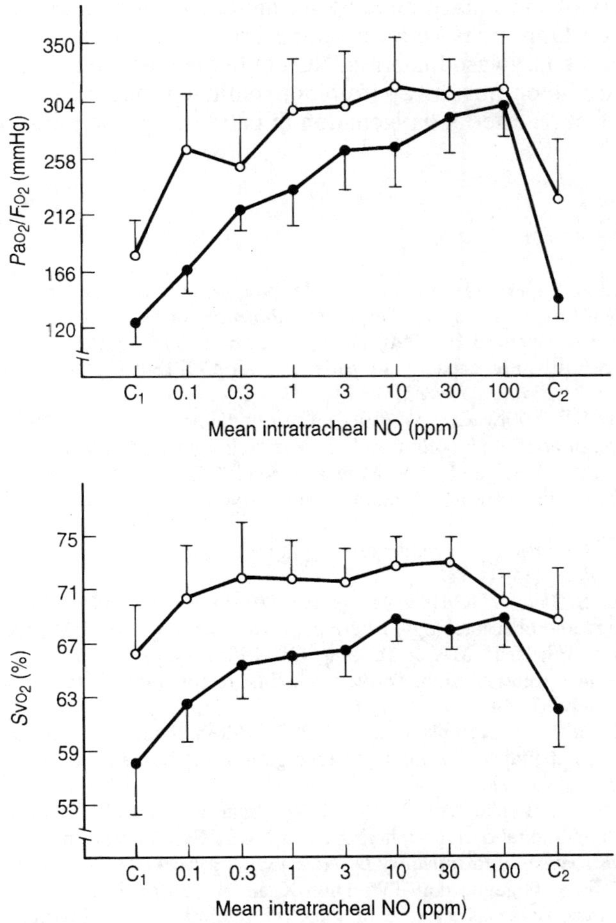

Figure 15. Dose–response curve of inhaled NO on Pao_2 ($F_iO_2 = 0.85$) and on mixed venous oxygen saturation (Svo_2) in patients with ARDS according to the absence or presence of septic shock. In patients with septic shock (●), the maximum effect on Pao_2 is obtained at NO concentrations of 100 ppm whereas in patients without septic shock (○) the maximum effect is obtained at concentrations around 1 ppm. Results are means ± SEM. (Taken from reference[80]).

patients with and without septic shock. In fact, dose–response curves in patients with septic shock or treated by ECMO are very similar.[80,81] The reasons for these differences between patients with and without septic shock remain unknown. The coexistence of septic shock with pulmonary arterial constriction implies the existence of circulating vasoactive mediators which constrict pulmonary vessels. Exogenous catecholamines administered to support blood pressure and circulating vasoconstrictors such as endothelin[53] could play a role in this pulmonary arterial constriction. Simultaneously, there might be a massive release of endogenous NO predominantly in inflammatory parts of the lung producing an increased pulmonary blood flow in nonventilated lung areas and worsening arterial hypoxemia. For the same selective pulmonary vasodilatation, NO could then induce a greater diversion of pulmonary blood flow away from nonventilated lung areas, thus inducing a greater effect on arterial oxygenation in patients with septic shock.

REFERENCES

1. Meyer M & Piiper J (1989) Nitric oxide (NO), a new test gas for study of alveolar capillary diffusion. *European Respiratory Journal* **2:**494–496.
2. Moinard J & Guenard H (1990) Determination of lung capillary blood volume and membrane diffusing capacity in patients with COPD using the NO-CO method. *European Respiratory Journal* **3:**318–322.
3. Furchgott RF & Zawadski JV (1980) The obligatory role of endothelial cells in the relaxation of arterial smooth muscle by acetylcholine. *Nature* **288:**373–376.
4. Palmer RMJ, Ferrige AG & Moncada S (1987) Nitric oxide release accounts for the biological activity of endothelium-derived relaxing factor. *Nature* **327:**524–526.
5. Berdeaux A (1993) Nitric oxide: an ubiquitous messenger. *Fundamental and Clinical Pharmacology* **7:**401–411.
6. Moncada S, Palmer RMJ & Higgs EA (1991) Nitric oxide: physiology, pathophysiology and pharmacology. *Pharmacological Reviews* **43:**109–142.
7. Macdonald PS, Read MA & Dushing GJ (1988) Synergistic inhibition of platelet aggregation by endothelium-derived relaxing factor and prostacyclin. *Thrombosis Research* **49:**437–449.
8. Alheid U, Frolich JC & Fosterman U (1987) Endothelial derived relaxing factor from human endothelial cells inhibits aggregation of human platelets. *Thrombosis Research* **47:**561–571.
9. Higenbottam T, Pepke-Zaba J, Scott J, Woolman P, Coutts C & Wallwork J (1988) Inhaled 'endothelial derived-relaxing factor' (EDRF) in primary hypertension (PPH). *American Review of Respiratory Disease* **137(Suppl):**A107 (Abstr).
10. Pepke-Zaba J, Higenbottam TW, Dinh-Xuan AT, Stone D & Wallwork J (1991) Inhaled nitric oxide as a cause of selective pulmonary vasodilation in pulmonary hypertension. *Lancet* **338:**1173–1174.
11. Fratacci MD, Frostell CG, Chen TY, Wain JC, Robinson DR & Zapol WM (1991) Inhaled nitric oxide: a selective pulmonary vasodilator of heparin–protamine vasoconstriction in sheep. *Anesthesiology* **75:**990–999.
12. Frostell C, Fratacci MD, Wain JC, Jones R & Zapol WM (1991) Inhaled nitric oxide: a selective pulmonary vasodilator reversing hypoxic pulmonary vasoconstriction. *Circulation* **83:**2038–2047.

13. Pison U, Lopez FA, Heidelmeyer CF, Rossaint R & Falke K (1993) Inhaled nitric oxide reverses hypoxic pulmonary vasoconstriction without impairing gas exchange. *Journal of Applied Physiology* **74:**1287–1292.
14. Roberts JD, Polaner DM, Lang P & Zapol WM (1992) Inhaled nitric oxide in persistent pulmonary hypertension of the newborn. *Lancet* **340:**818–819.
15. Weitzberg E, Rudehill A, Alving K & Lundberg JM (1991) Nitric oxide inhalation selectively attenuates pulmonary hypertension and arterial hypoxia in porcine endotoxin shock. *Acta Physiological Scandinavica* **143:**451–452.
16. Dyar O, Young JD, Xiong L & John S (1993) Dose–response relationship for inhaled nitric oxide in experimental pulmonary hypertension in sheep. *British Journal of Anaesthesiology* **71:**702–708.
17. Berger JI, Gibson RL, Redding GJ, Standaert TA, Clarke WR & Truog WE (1993) Effect of inhaled nitric oxide during group B streptococcal sepsis in piglets. *American Review of Respiratory Disease* **147:**1080–1086.
18. Rossaint R, Falke KJ, Lopez F, Slama K, Pison U & Zapol WM (1993) Inhaled nitric oxide for the adult respiratory distress syndrome. *New England Journal of Medicine* **328:**399–405.
19. Bigatello LM, Hurford WE, Kacmarek RM, Roberts JD & Zapol WM (1994) Prolonged inhalation of low concentrations of nitric oxide in patients with severe adult respiratory distress syndrome. *Anesthesiology* **80:**761–770.
20. Puybasset L, Rouby JJ, Mourgeon E, Stewart TE, Cluzel P, Belin MF, Grenier P, Arthaud M, Poète P, Bodin L, Korinek AM & Viars P (1994) Inhaled nitric oxide in acute respiratory failure: dose–response curves. *Intensive Care Medicine* **20:**319–327.
21. Puybasset L, Stewart TE, Rouby JJ, Cluzel P, Mourgeon E, Belin MF, Arthaud M, Landault C & Viars P (1994) Inhaled nitric oxide reverses the increase in pulmonary vascular resistance induced by permissive hypercapnia in patients with ARDS. *Anesthesiology* **80:**1254–1267.
22. Girard C, Lehot J, Pannetier J, Filley S, French P & Estanove S (1992) Inhaled nitric oxide after mitral valve replacement in patients with chronic pulmonary hypertension. *Anesthesiology* **77:**880–883.
23. Rich FR, Murphy GD, Roos CM & Johns RA (1993) Inhaled nitric oxide: Selective pulmonary vasodilation in cardiac surgical patients. *Anesthesiology* **78:**1028–1035.
24. Adnot S, Kouyoumdjian C, Defouilloy C, Andrivet P, Sediame S, Herigauklt R & Fratacci MD (1993) Hemodynamic and gas exchange responses to infusion of acetylcholine and inhalation of nitric oxide in patients with chronic obstructive lung disease and pulmonary hypertension. *American Review of Respiratory Disease* **148:**310–316.
25. Moinard J, Manier G, Pillet O & Castaing Y (1994) Effect of inhaled nitric oxide on hemodynamics and VA/Q inequalities in patients with chronic obstructive pulmonary disease. *American Journal of Respiratory and Critical Care Medicine* **149:**1482–1487.
26. Bauer MA, Utell MJ, Morrow PE, Speers DM & Gibb FR (1986) Inhalation of 0.30 ppm nitrogen dioxide potentiates exercise-induced bronchospasm in asthmatics. *American Review of Respiratory Disease* **134:**1203–1208.
27. Sandström T, Stjernberg N, Eklund A, Ledin M-C, Bjermer L, Kolmodin-Hedman B, Lindström K, Rosenhall L & Angström T (1991) Inflammatory cell response in bronchoalveolar lavage fluid after nitrogen dioxide exposure of healthy subjects: a dose–response study. *European Respiratory Journal* **3:**332–339.
28. Lu Q, Mourgeon E, Law-Koune JD, Roche S, Vézinet C, Abdennour L, Vicaut E, Puybasset L, Diaby M, Coriat P & Rouby JJ (1995) Dose–response curves of inhaled nitric oxide with and without intravenous almitrine in nitric oxide-responding patients with acute respiratory distress syndrome. *Anesthesiology* **83:**929–943.

29. Isomura K, Chikahira M, Terashini K & Hamada K (1984) Induction of mutations and chromosome aberrations in lung cells following *in vivo* exposures to nitrogen oxides. *Mutation Research* **136:**119–125.
30. Arroyo PL, Hatch-Pigott V, Mower HF & Cooney RV (1992) Mutagenicity of nitric oxide and its inhibition by antioxidants. *Mutation Research* **281:**193–202.
31. Nguyen T, Brunson D, Crospi CL, Penman BW, Wishnok JS & Tannenbaum SR (1992) DNA damage and mutation in human cells exposed to nitric oxide *in vitro*. *Proceedings of the National Academy of Sciences USA* **89:**3030–3034.
32. Wink DA, Kasprzak KS, Maragos CM, Elespuru RK, Misra M, Dunams TM, Cebula TA, Koch WH, Andrews AW, Allen JS & Keefer LK (1991) DNA deaminating ability and genotoxicity of nitric oxide and its progenitors. *Science* **254:**1001–1003.
33. Beckman JS, Beckman TW, Marshall PA & Freeman BA (1990) Apparent hydroxyl radical production by peroxynitrite: implications for endothelial injury from nitric oxide and superoxide. *Proceedings of the National Academy of Sciences USA* **87:**1620–1624.
34. Haddad LY, Crow JP, Yaozu Y, Beckman J & Matalon S (1994) Concurrent generation of nitric oxide and superoxide damages surfactant protein A (SP-A). *American Journal of Respiratory and Critical Care Medicine* **149(Suppl):**A549 (Abstr).
35. Greenbaum R, Bay J, Hargreaves MD, Kain ML, Kelman GR, Nunn JF, Prys-Roberts C & Siebold K (1967) Effects of higher oxides of nitrogen in the anaesthetized dog. *British Journal of Anaesthesiology* **39:**393–404.
36. Oda H, Nogami H, Kusumotos S, Nakajima T, Kurata A & Imai K (1976) Long-term exposure to nitric oxide in mice. *Journal of the Japanese Society of Air Pollution* **11:**150–160.
37. Oda H, Nogami H, Kusumoto S, Nakajima T & Kurata A (1980) Lifetime exposure to 2.4 ppm nitric oxide in mice. *Environmental Research* **22:**254–263.
38. Azoulay E, Soler P, Blayo MC & Basset F (1977) Nitric oxide effects on lung structure and blood oxygen affinity in rats. *Bulletin Européen de Physiopathologie Respiratoire* **13:**629–644.
39. Foubert L, Fleming B, Latimer R, Jonas M, Oduro A, Borland C & Higenbottam T (1992) Safety guidelines for use of nitric oxide. *Lancet* **339:**1615–1616.
40. Law-Koune JD, Roche S, Mourgeon E, Lu Q, Puybasset L, Kalfon P, Rouby JJ & Viars P (1994) Acute toxicity of inhaled NO in ARDS. *Anesthesiology* **81:**A263 (Abstr).
41. Man SFP, Williams DJ, Amy GC, Man GCW & Lien DC (1990) Sequential changes in canine pulmonary epithelial and endothelial cell functions after nitrogen dioxide. *American Review of Respiratory Disease* **142:**199–205.
42. Ranga V, Kleinerman J, Ip MPC & Collins AM (1980) The effect of nitrogen dioxide on tracheal uptake and transport of horseradish peroxidase in the guinea pig. *American Review of Respiratory Disease* **122:**483–490.
43. Guth DJ & Mavis RD (1985) Biochemical assessment of acute nitrogen dioxide toxicity in rat lung. *Toxicology Applied Pharmacology* **81:**128–138.
44. Stavert DM & Lehnert BE (1990) Nitrogen oxide and nitrogen dioxide as inducers of acute pulmonary injury when inhaled at relatively high concentrations for brief periods. *Inhalational Toxicology* **2:**53–57.
45. Ben-Jebria A, Marthan R & Savineau JP (1992) Effect of *in vitro* nitrogen dioxide exposure on human bronchial smooth muscle response. *American Review of Respiratory Disease* **146:**378–382.
46. Frampton MW, Morrow PE, Cox C, Gibb FR, Speers DM & Utell MJ (1991) Effects of nitrogen dioxide exposure on pulmonary function and airway reactivity in normal humans. *American Review of Respiratory Disease* **143:**522–527.
47. Rose RM, Fuglestad JM, Skornik WA, Hammer SM, Wolfhal SF, Beck BD & Brain JD (1988) The pathophysiology of enhanced susceptibility to murine cytomegalovirus respiratory infection during short-term exposure to 5 ppm nitrogen dioxide. *American Review of Respiratory Disease* **137:**912–917.

48. Mustafa MG & Tierney DF (1978) Biochemical and metabolic changes in the lung with oxygen, ozone, and nitrogen dioxide toxicity. *American Review of Respiratory Disease* **118:**1061–1088.
49. Radermacher P, Santak B, Wüst HJ, Tarnow J & Falke KJ (1990) Prostacyclin for the treatment of pulmonary hypertension in patients with acute respiratory distress syndrome: effects on pulmonary capillary pressure and ventilation–perfusion distributions. *Anesthesiology* **72:**238–244.
50. Radermacher P, Santak B, Becker H & Falke KJ (1989) Prostaglandin E_1 and nitroglycerin reduce pulmonary capillary pressure but worsen ventilation–perfusion distributions in patients with adult respiratory distress syndrome. *Anesthesiology* **70:**601–606.
51. Frostell CG, Blomqvist H, Hedenstierna G, Lundberg J & Zapol WM (1993) Inhaled nitric oxide selectively reverses human hypoxic pulmonary vasoconstriction without causing systemic vasodilation. *Anesthesiology* **78:**427–435.
52. Puybasset L, Rouby JJ, Mourgeon E, Cluzel P, Souhil Z, Law-Koune JD, Stewart TE, Devilliers C, Lu Q, Roche S, Kalfon P, Vicaut E & Viars P (1995) Factors influencing cardiopulmonary effects of inhaled nitric oxide in acute respiratory failure. *American Journal of Respiratory and Critical Care Medicine* **152:**318–328.
53. Langleben D, Demarchie M, Laporta D, Spanier AH, Schlesinger RD, & Stewart DJ (1993) Endothelin-1 in acute lung injury and the adult respiratory distress syndrome. *American Review of Respiratory Disease* **148:**1646–1650.
54. Zapol WM, Snider MT, Rie MA, Quinn DA & Frikker M (1985) Pulmonary circulation during adult respiratory distress syndrome. In Zapol WM & Falke KJ (eds) *Acute Respiratory Failure*, pp 209–226. New York: Dekker.
55. Mc Gregor M & Sniderman A (1985) On pulmonary vascular resistance: the need for more precise definition. *American Journal of Cardiology* **55:**217–227.
56. Bshouty Z & Younes M (1990) Distensibility and pressure flow relationships of the pulmonary circulation. II. Multibranched model. *Journal of Applied Physiology* **68:**1514–1527.
57. Gattinoni L, Pesenti A, Avalli L, Rossi F & Bombino M (1987) Pressure–volume curve of total respiratory system in acute respiratory failure. Computed tomographic scan study. *American Review of Respiratory Disease* **136:**730–736.
58. Kieler-Jensen N, Rieksten SE, Stenqvist O, Bergh CH, Lindelöv B, Wennmaln A, Waagstein F & Lundin S (1994) Inhaled nitric oxide in the evaluation of heart transplant candidates with elevated pulmonary vascular resistance. *Journal of Heart and Lung Transplantation* **13:**366–375.
59. Bocchi EA, Bacal F, Auler JOC, Josse de Carvalho Carmone M, Bellotti G & Pileggi F (1994) Inhaled nitric oxide leading to pulmonary edema in stable severe heart failure. *American Journal of Cardiology* **74:**70–72.
60. Semigran RCJ, Cockrill BA, Kacmarek R, Thompson T, Zapol WM, Dec W & Fifer HA (1994) Hemodynamic effects of inhaled nitric oxide in heart failure. *Journal of the American College of Cardiology* **24:**982–988.
61. Loh E, Stamler JS, Hare JM, Loscalzo J & Colucci WS (1994) Cardiovascular effects of inhaled nitric oxide in patients with left ventricular dysfunction. *Circulation* **90:**2780–2785.
62. Jones R, Langleben D & Reid LM (1991) Patterns and mechanisms of remodeling of the pulmonary circulation in acute and subacute lung injury. In Said SI (ed). *The Pulmonary Circulation and Acute Lung Injury*, pp 179–242. Mount Kisko, NY: Futura Publishing Company, Inc.
63. Roberts JD, Roberts CT, Jones RC, Zapol WM & Bloch KD (1995) Continuous nitric oxide inhalation reduces pulmonary arterial structural changes, right ventricular hypertrophy, and growth retardation in the hypoxic newborn rat. *Circulation Research* **76:**215–222.

64. Lindeborg DM, Kavanagh BP, Meurs KV & Pearl RG (1995) Inhaled nitric oxide does not alter the longitudinal distribution of pulmonary vascular resistance. *Journal of Applied Physiology* **78:**341–348.
65. Benzing A & Geiger K (1994) Inhaled nitric oxide lowers capillary pressure and changes longitudinal distribution of pulmonary vascular resistance in patients with acute lung injury. *Acta Anaesthesiologica Scandinavica* **38:**640–645.
66. Dupuy PM, Shore SA, Drazen JM, Frostell C, Hill WA & Zapol WM (1992) Bronchodilator action of inhaled nitric oxide in guinea pigs. *Journal of Clinical Investigation* **90:**421–428.
67. Garg UC & Hassid A (1989) Nitric oxide-generating vasodilators and 8-bromo cyclic guanosine monophosphate inhibit mitogenesis and proliferation of cultured rat vascular smooth muscle cells. *Journal of Clinical Investigation* **83:**1774–1777.
68. Samama Ch M, Diaby M, Fellahi JL, Mdhafar A, Eyraud D, Arock M, Guillosson JJ, Coriat P & Rouby JJ (1995) Inhibition of platelet aggregation by inhaled nitric oxide in patients with acute respiratory distress syndrome. *Anesthesiology* **83:**56–65
69. Niu XF, Smith W & Kubes P (1994) Intracellular oxidative stress induced by nitric oxide synthesis inhibition increases endothelial cell adhesion to neutrophils. *Circulation Research* **74:**1133–1140.
70. Kavanach BP, Mouchawar A, Goldsmith J & Pearl RG (1994) Effects of inhaled NO and inhibition of endogenous NO synthesis in oxidant-induced acute lung injury. *Journal of Applied Physiology* **76:**1324–1329.
71. Rimar S & Gillis CN (1992) Pulmonary vasodilation by inhaled nitric oxide after endothelial injury. *Journal of Applied Physiology* **73:**2179–2183.
72. White CW, Nguyen DH & Tuder R (1994) Nitric oxide modulation of hyperoxic injury. *American Journal of Respiratory and Critical Care Medicine* **149(Suppl):**A548 (Abstr).
73. Berisha H, Pakbaz H, Absood A & Said SI (1994) Excess nitric oxide (NO) production in acute lung injury: role of constitutive vs inducible NO synthase. *American Journal of Respiratory and Critical Care Medicine* **149:**A552 (Abstr).
74. Högman M, Frostell CG, Arnberg H & Hedenstierna G (1993) Inhalation of nitric oxide modulates metacholine induced bronchoconstriction in the rabbit. *European Respiratory Journal* **6:**177–180.
75. Puybasset L, Mourgeon E, Segal E, Bodin L, Rouby JJ & Viars P (1993) Effects of inhaled nitric oxide on respiratory resistance in patients with ARDS. *Anesthesiology* **79(Suppl 3A):**A299 (Abstr).
76. Högman M, Frostell CG, Hedenström H & Hedenstierna G (1993) Inhalation of nitric oxide modulates adult bronchial tone. *American Review of Respiratory Disease* **148:**1474–1478.
77. Kilbourn RG, Jubran SS, Griffith OW, Levi R, Adams J & Lodato RF (1990) Reversal of endotoxin mediated shock by N^{G}-methyl-L-arginine, an inhibitor of nitric oxide synthesis. *Biochemical and Biophysical Research Commmunications* **172:** 1132–1138.
78. Kilbourn RG, Gross SS, Jubran SS, Adams J, Griffith OW, Levi R & Lodato RF (1990) N^{G}-Methyl-L-arginine inhibits tumor necrosis factor-induced hypotension: implications for the involvement of nitric oxide. *Proceedings of the National Academy of Sciences USA* **87:**3629–3632.
79. Julou-Schaeffer G, Gray GA, Fleming I, Schott C, Parratt JR & Stoclet JC (1990) Loss of vascular responsiveness induced by endotoxin involves L-arginine pathway. *American Journal of Physiology* **259:**H1038–H1043.
80. Mourgeon E, Roche S, Lu Q, Law-koune JD, Puybasset L, Diaby M, Bodin L, Rouby JJ & Viars P (1994) NO inhalé dans le SDRA: courbes dose–réponse en présence ou en l'absence de choc septique. *Annales Francaises d'Anesthésie et de Réanimation* **13(Suppl):** (Abstr).

81. Gerlach H, Rossaint R, Pappert D & Falke KJ (1993) Time-course and dose–response of nitric oxide inhalation for systemic oxygenation and pulmonary hypertension in patients with adult respiratory distress syndrome. *European Journal of Clinical Investigation* **23:**499–502.
82. Gerlach H, Pappert D, Lewandowski K, Rossaint R & Falke KJ (1993) Long-term inhalation with evaluated low doses of nitric oxide for selective improvement in oxygenation in patients with adult respiratory distress syndrome. *Intensive Care Medicine* **19:**443–449.
83. Journois D, Pouard P, Mauriat P, Malhère T, Vouhé P & Safran D (1994) Inhaled nitric oxide as a therapy for pulmonary hypertension after operations for congenital defects. *Journal of Thoracic and Cardiovascular Surgery* **107:**1129–1135.
84. Sellden H, Winberg P, Gustafsson LE, Lundell BO, Book K & Frostell CG (1993) Inhalation of nitric oxide reduced pulmonary hypertension after cardiac surgery in a 3.2 Kg infant. *Anesthesiology* **78:**577–580.
85. Tiner NN, Etches RC, Kamstra B, Tierney AJ, Peliowski A & Ryan A (1994) Inhaled nitric oxide in infants referred for extracorporeal membrane oxygenation: dose–response. *Journal of Pediatrics* **124:**302–308.

15

Pulmonary Vascular Tone in Ventilated Patients with Chronic Obstructive Pulmonary Disease

Francisco Baigorri
Amato De Monte
Domenec Joseph
Lluis Blanch
Antonio Artigas

INTRODUCTION

Pulmonary vascular tone is a major concern in patients with chronic obstructive pulmonary disease (COPD) because pulmonary arterial hypertension may adversely affect the function of the right ventricle[1] (making it less able to face up to an increase in afterload) and because pulmonary arterial hypertension is associated with poor prognosis,[2,3] probably because it is a reflection of the severity of the disease.[4,5]

Notably, pulmonary artery pressure (PAP) may rise substantially during exacerbations.[6] Moreover, in acute exacerbations of COPD, these critically ill patients may perform intense respiratory efforts, which may lead to a considerable decrease in intrathoracic pressure (ITP). Thus, venous return to the right ventricle increases with pulmonary vascular resistance (PVR). This combination may result in right ventricular failure.[7] Starting mechanical ventilatory support can dramatically affect some of these events.[8] This chapter aims to address the factors that lead to the development of pulmonary arterial hypertension during COPD exacerbations and, specifically, the influence that mechanical ventilation can have on them. Finally, we will discuss the role of selective pulmonary vasodilator therapy by nitric oxide (NO) inhalation in these circumstances.

FACTORS CONTRIBUTING TO THE DEVELOPMENT OF PULMONARY ARTERIAL HYPERTENSION IN COPD

The increase in PAP in patients with COPD probably results from a combination of several factors which passively or actively affect pulmonary hemodynamics. Hypoxia and acidemia act synergistically to produce pulmonary vasoconstriction in patients with COPD.[9] Changes in airway resistance may increase PVR by affecting the alveolar pressure.[10] Polycythemia secondary to chronic hypoxemia can increase blood viscosity. Disruption of the pulmonary vascular bed may also contribute to the pulmonary arterial hypertension which develops during exercise in such patients, so that any increase in cardiac output augments pressure dramatically.

The relative contribution of each of these factors may vary among patients, but hypoxia deserves special consideration as a factor leading to sustained pulmonary hypertension. Acute hypoxia induces pulmonary vasoconstriction, and chronic hypoxia is associated with structural changes that occur in the peripheral arteries. These vessels develop accumulations of vascular smooth muscle cells in their intima.[11]

The mechanism producing hypoxic vasoconstriction and the structural changes which ensue from chronic hypoxia have not been fully elucidated but it seems that the pulmonary endothelial cell has a central role. Endothelial cells release locally active vasodilators and they contribute to the modulation of vasomotor tone through a mechanism that involves NO.[12] There is evidence of loss of pulmonary endothelium-dependent relaxation in rats with chronic hypoxic pulmonary arterial hypertension[13] and there is also evidence of diminished expression of endothelial NO synthase in the lungs of patients with pulmonary arterial hypertension.[14] Moreover, Dinh-Xuan and colleagues[15] showed that endothelium-dependent relaxation *in vitro* is impaired in pulmonary arterial rings from patients with advanced COPD. Notably, in that study, maximal relaxation in rings of COPD patients correlated with the partial pressure of arterial oxygen ($P\text{aO}_2$) and was inversely related to the degree of intimal thickening. Thus, impaired endothelium-dependent relaxation in COPD patients may result from a reduction in NO synthesis as a result of hypoxia. Furthermore, it has been suggested that the reduction in NO synthesis may also influence vascular remodeling.

FACTORS CONTRIBUTING TO THE INCREASE IN PULMONARY ARTERIAL HYPERTENSION IN ACUTE EXACERBATIONS OF COPD

Pulmonary arterial hypertension progresses slowly in patients with COPD, and, even in patients with severe COPD, the increase in PAP is usually rather small.[16] However, during exacerbations it may rise substantially. The mean PAP in patients with stable COPD is 25–35 mmHg[17] but, during exacerbations, it may rise to 45–70 mmHg.[6,18] It is important to note that, when these patients recover from their illness, the PAP falls again. Thus the increase in PAP found during exacerbations cannot be explained solely on the basis of fixed anatomical lesions. Worsening hypoxia, acidosis, and changes in pulmonary mechanics may all contribute to the transitory increase in PAP.

One factor involved in the increase in PAP during exacerbations may be an increment in airway resistance which may augment PVR by affecting the alveolar pressure. As transpulmonary pressure is increased in dogs, at constant blood flow, the relationship between pressure and flow in the pulmonary circulation shifts to the right.[19] The amount by which the curves are shifted is approximately equal to the increase in transpulmonary pressure (Figure 1). This phenomenon has also been shown in subjects with normal hearts and lungs breathing against an increased pressure.[10] The linear relationship between pressure and flow in the pulmonary circulation changes when the alveolar pressure is increased by breathing against an expiratory valve. The slope of the pressure/flow relation becomes steeper, resembling the relation in COPD patients during normal tidal breathing.[10] This effect may be especially notable when ventilation increases as in acute exacerbations of COPD.

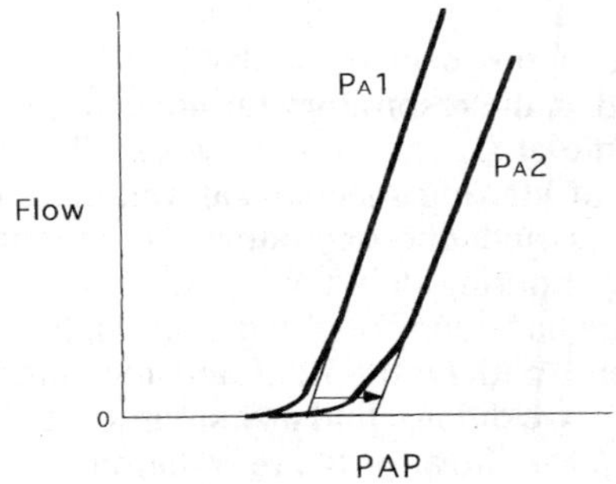

Figure 1. Relationship between mean PAP and flow when alveolar pressure (PA) is increased (PA2 > PA1).

Again hypoxia probably plays a major part in the reversible pulmonary hypertension observed during exacerbations in COPD patients. Abraham and colleagues[6] studied the effects of oxygen on pulmonary hemodynamics and blood gases in COPD patients with acute respiratory failure by serial observations during recovery. The inhalation of 28% oxygen for 30 min resulted in a consistent fall in PAP, often to levels close to those observed after recovery. There was no significant change in cardiac output. These data strongly suggest that the acute pulmonary hypertension seen in these patients may also be related to pulmonary vasoconstriction resulting from hypoxia.[6]

Moreover, because oxygen arterial saturation and content is low, cardiac output increases as a compensating mechanism,[20] contributing to the increase in PAP.

EFFECT OF MECHANICAL VENTILATION ON PULMONARY VASCULAR TONE IN ACUTE RESPIRATORY FAILURE IN COPD

Mechanical ventilation may alter pulmonary vascular tone by changing lung volume and alveolar Po_2. In addition, cardiac output may change. If the application of mechanical ventilation leads to an elimination of the negative inspiratory swings of ITP, venous return will decrease. Right ventricle afterload may also be modified. The balance between changes in ITP and alveolar pressure will determine the magnitude and direction of right ventricle afterload variations with mechanical ventilation.[8]

There are few data in the literature dealing with hemodynamics during acute or chronic respiratory failure requiring mechanical ventilation. We[21] and others[22] recently studied the effect of positive end-expiratory pressure (PEEP) application in patients with COPD during acute ventilatory failure requiring mechanical ventilatory support. The mean PAP values found in these studies were 22–25 mmHg,[21,22] similar to those reported in patients with stable COPD. In these studies[21,22] hypoxemia had been corrected, patients were sedated and paralyzed, and setting of mechanical ventilation were established to minimize air trapping. Thus, most factors capable of increasing PAP had been controlled.

We also performed a prospective study of 10 patients admitted to our intensive care unit with acute respiratory failure caused by acute exacerbation of COPD (A. De Monte et al, unpublished work). The study was performed within the first 24 h of starting mechanical ventilation, and repeated 72 h later. Airway pressures and end-expiratory hemodynamic variables were recorded at baseline and during dobutamine administration. Again, when the study began hypoxemia had been corrected. Although ventilatory support had been stopped in several patients at 72 h and the intrinsic PEEP level had decreased in the others, we did not find any significant change in PAP or PVR (Table 1). Moreover, the flow–pressure relation obtained by increasing cardiac output with dobutamine administration was similar at both steps of the study (Figure 2). Thus, the values of PAP found shortly after starting mechanical ventilatory support were similar to those found during recovery.

Regarding the effect of PEEP application on pulmonary vascular tone in mechanically ventilated COPD patients, Ranieri and colleagues[22] observed that 15 cmH_2O of PEEP caused a significant increase in PVR (from 412 ± 48 to 489 ± 62 dyn s cm^{-5}) (Figure 3A) but, in our study,[21] a total PEEP level about 5 cmH_2O lower than in Rainieri's study did not change PVR (Figure

Table 1. Hemodynamics in COPD patients with acute respiratory failure within the first 24 h of starting mechanical ventilation and 72 h later.

Parameter	First day	72 h later	*P*
CI (liters/min per m^2)	2.5 ± 0.7	3.2 ± 0.6	<0.05
SVI (ml/beat per m^2)	30 ± 10	37 ± 10	< 0.05
RAP (mmHg)	7 ± 5	6 ± 3	NS
PAOP (mmHg)	10 ± 7	11 ± 3	NS
MPAP (mmHg)	21 ± 9	24 ± 5	NS
PVRI (dyn s cm^{-5} m^2)	374 ± 121	320 ± 114	NS

Values are means ± S.D. (n = 10). Abbreviations: CI, cardiac index; SVI, stroke volume index; RAP, right atrial pressure; PAOP, pulmonary artery occlusion pressure; MPAP, mean pulmonary arterial pressure; PVRI, pulmonary vascular resistance index; NS, not significant.

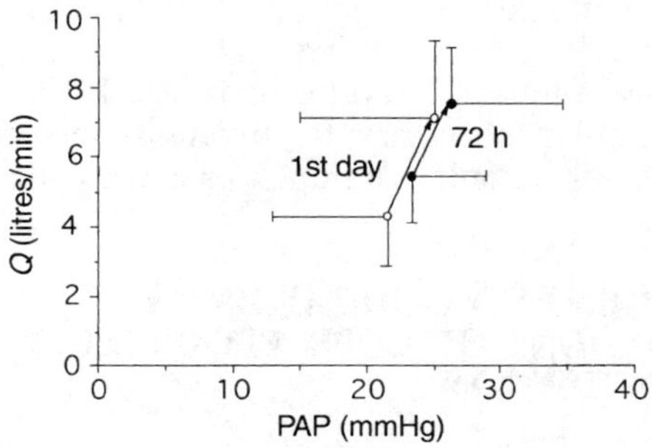

Figure 2. Relationship between mean PAP and flow (Q) obtained by increasing cardiac output by dobutamine administration. Data were recorded within the first 24 h of starting mechanical ventilation (1st day; ○) and 72 h later (72 h, ●).

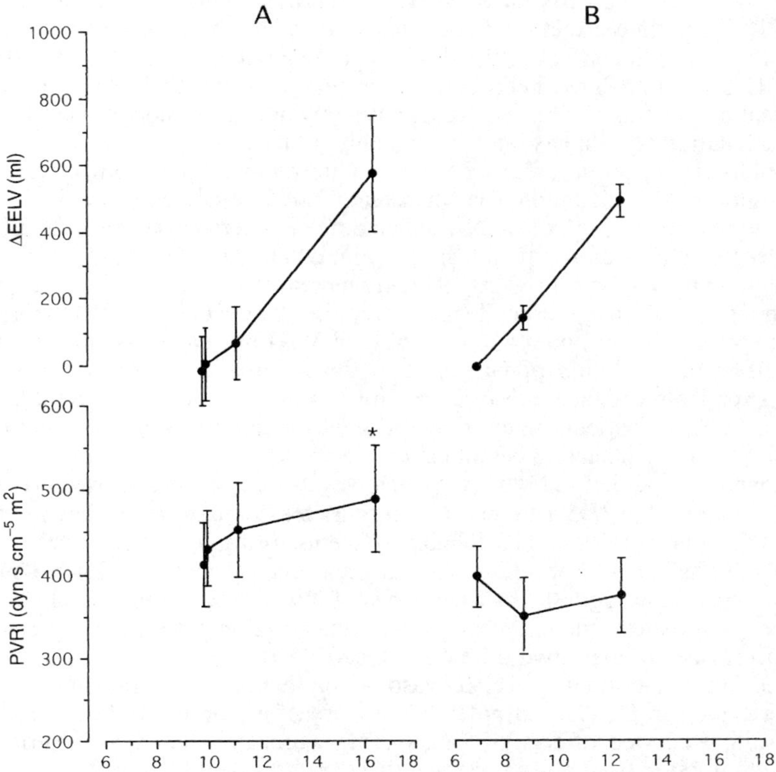

Figure 3. Effect of PEEP application on end-expiratory lung volume (EELV) (top) and PVRI (bottom) in ventilated patients with COPD. A, Data obtained from Ranieri et al.[22] Intrinsic PEEP level 9.8 cmH_2O. B, Data obtained from Baigorri et al.[21] Intrinsic PEEP level 6.6 cmH_2O. *$P < 0.05$, compared with 10 cmH_2O.

3B). Nevertheless, both studies[21,22] showed that PEEP application to levels close to the level of intrinsic PEEP does not significantly modify PAP and cardiac output. Thus, a matched level of extrinsic PEEP used to reduce the respiratory muscle effort necessary to initiate spontaneous inspiration or trigger an assisted breath should not impair cardiovascular function.

SELECTIVE PULMONARY VASODILATION IN ACUTE EXACERBATIONS OF COPD REQUIRING MECHANICAL VENTILATION

In a nonhomogeneous system with uneven local ventilation, the hypoxic vasoconstriction could be a means of improving gas exchange. Drugs that inhibit hypoxic vasoconstriction may worsen the hypoxemia because of an increased perfusion to lung units with a lower than normal V_A/Q ratio. This is a well-known effect of the vasodilator therapy of pulmonary arterial hypertension in COPD.[23] The final effect of vasodilator therapy on arterial oxygenation will also depend on the effect of the drug on cardiac output. Recently, the effects of NO inhalation have been studied in patients with COPD under stable clinical conditions.[24–26] Inhaled NO is a directly acting pulmonary vasodilator. NO inhalation vasodilates lung vessels only in the ventilated lung areas without inducing systemic effects because of its rapid affinity with circulating hemoglobin. NO inhalation was consistently found to decrease PAP in COPD patients[24–26] but the effect of NO inhalation on arterial oxygenation differs between studies. Adnot and colleagues[24] found that inhalation of a gas mixture containing up to 40 ppm NO significantly increased $Pa\text{O}_2$ (from 57 ± 3 to 60 ± 3 mmHg) but Barberá and colleagues[26] reported a reduction in $Pa\text{O}_2$ (from 56 ± 7 to 53 ± 7 mmHg) due to a worsening of V_A/Q mismatch. We also studied the effect of inhalation of NO on hemodynamics and gas exchange in 10 COPD patients with acute respiratory failure requiring mechanical ventilatory support and 11 patients with adult (or acute) respiratory distress syndrome (ARDS).[27] NO inhalation significantly decreased PAP, and cardiac output remained unmodified in both groups. However, $Pa\text{O}_2$ increased by more than 20% in 73% of ARDS patients, but only increased in 20% of patients with COPD (Figure 4). Since NO inhalation seems to improve gas exchange by inducing vasodilation of ventilated areas and decreased blood flow to shunt areas, our results suggest that when areas of low V_A/Q and pure shunt coexist in the same patient, the net result of NO inhalation on gas exchange depends on the balance of these two different effects.

The other important aspect of vasodilator therapy of pulmonary arterial hypertension in COPD is a potential salutary effect on the right ventricular function. Reported effects of vasodilating agents on the right ventricular ejection fraction (RVEF) suggest that these drugs do not sufficiently decrease pulmonary vascular tone to improve right ventricular function.[23] Even oxygen does not change RVEF in patients with stable and decompensated cor pulmonale.[28] However, two recent studies have shown that NO inhalation is able to increase RVEF in patients with ARDS.[29,30] We tested the effect of inhalation of a gas mixture containing 20 ppm NO on right ventricular

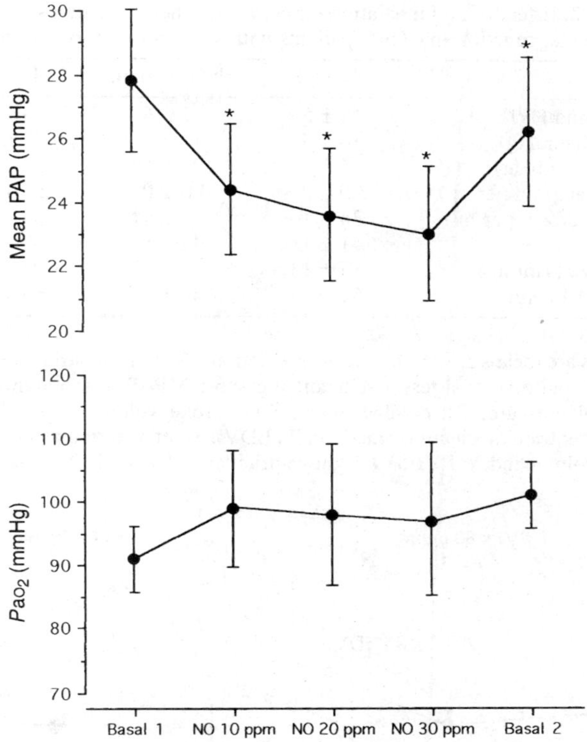

Figure 4. Effect of NO inhalation (10–20–30 ppm) on PAP and PaO_2 in ventilated patients with COPD. NO inhalation significantly reduced PAP but did not significantly change PaO_2. $*P < 0.05$, compared with basal.

function by the thermodilution method in eight COPD patients with acute respiratory failure on requiring mechanical ventilatory support (F. Baigorri et al, unpublished work). Again, NO inhalation was followed by a significant reduction in PAP without change in either cardiac output or oxygenation. RVEF and right ventricular volumes did not significantly change either (Table 2). However, the observed effect of NO inhalation and PAP reduction on RVEF was different when patients with right heart dysfunction (stroke volume < 30 ml/m^2) were compared with those without right heart dysfunction (stroke volume ≥ 30 ml/m^2). The RVEF increased from 29 to 34% in patients with low stroke volume but remained unmodified in those with normal stroke volume (from 48 to 47%). The reduction in RVEF observed in patients with right ventricular dysfunction was related to a larger reduction of right ventricular end-systolic volume (Figure 5). This suggests that NO inhalation does not significantly modify the right ventricular function in COPD patients requiring mechanical ventilation, but NO inhalation may be useful in reducing the loading conditions of the right ventricle in those patients with right ventricular dysfunction.

Table 2. Effect of NO inhalation on pulmonary hemodynamics and right ventricular function in COPD patients with acute respiratory failure.

	Base 1	NO 20 ppm	Base 2
RAP (mmHg)	8 ± 5	7 ± 6	8 ± 6
PAOP (mmHg)	10 ± 4	11 ± 4	11 ± 4
MPAP (mmHg)	27 ± 7	23 ± 6*	25 ± 7
CI (liters/min per m²)	3.0 ± 0.8	3.0 ± 0.8	2.9 ± 0.9
SVI (ml/beat per m²)	34 ± 10	35 ± 9†	32 ± 11
RVEF (%)	41 ± 11	42 ± 8	36 ± 13
RVEDVI (ml/m²)	85 ± 13	83 ± 13	97 ± 32
RVESVI (ml/m²)	51 ± 13	49 ± 9	65 ± 35

*$P < 0.05$ vs base 1; † $P < 0.05$ vs base 2.
Values are means ± S.D. ($n = 8$). Abbreviations: RAP, right atrial pressure; PAOP, pulmonary artery occlusion pressure; MPAP, mean pulmonary arterial pressure; CI, cardiac index; SVI, stroke volume index; RVEF, right ventricular ejection fraction; RVEDVI, right ventricular end-diastolic volume index; RVESVI, right ventricular end-systolic volume index.

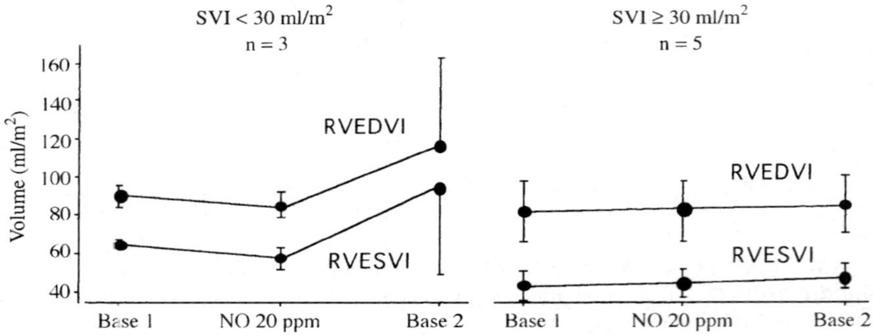

Figure 5. Effect of NO inhalation (20 ppm) on right ventricular volumes in ventilated COPD patients with right ventricular dysfunction (stroke volume index (SVI) < 30 ml/m²) (n = 3) and without right ventricular dysfunction (stroke volume index ≥ 30 ml/m²) (n = 5). RVEDVI, right ventricular end-diastolic volume index, RVESVI, right ventricular end-systolic volume index.

SUMMARY

Data presented in this chapter show that, although PAP may rise substantially during exacerbations of COPD, PAP values observed in COPD patients requiring mechanical ventilation are very similar to those reported in patients with stable COPD. Mechanical ventilation may contribute to the control of pulmonary arterial hypertension during COPD exacerbations allowing the improvement of alveolar Po_2 and restoring functional residual capacity. In these conditions, PEEP application to levels approaching the level of intrinsic PEEP does not result in a further clinically significant increment in PAP.

Regarding the role of selective pulmonary vasodilation with NO inhalation in COPD patients with acute respiratory failure, the benefit of this intervention should be considered on an individual basis according to the level of shunt and/or right ventricular dysfunction existing in each case. However, NO inhalation does not seem to be useful in either improving $Pa\mathrm{O}_2$ in most patients, or significantly improving RVEF and right ventricular output.

ACKNOWLEDGEMENTS

This work was supported in part by grants 92/1076 and 95/1390 from Fondo de Investigaciones Sanitarias de la Seguridad Social.

REFERENCES

1. Marangoni S, Scalvini S, Schena M, Vitacca M, Quadri A & Levi G (1992) Right ventricular diastolic function in chronic obstructive lung disease. *European Respiratory Journal* **5:**438–443.
2. Burrows B, Kettel LJ, Niden AH, Rabinowitz M & Diener CF (1972) Patterns of cardiovascular dysfunction in chronic obstructive lung disease. *New England Journal of Medicine* **286:**912–918.
3. Weitzenblum E, Hirth C, Ducolone A, Mirhom R, Rasaholinjanahary J & Ehrhart M (1981) Prognostic value of pulmonary artery pressure in chronic obstructive pulmonary disease. *Thorax* **36:**752–758.
4. France AJ, Prescott RJ, Biernacki W, Muir AL & MacNee W (1988) Does right ventricular function predict survival in patients with chronic obstructive pulmonary disease? *Thorax* **43:**621–626.
5. MacNee W (1994) Pathophysiology of cor pulmonale in chronic obstructive pulmonary disease. *American Journal of Respiratory Critical Care Medicine* **150:**833–852.
6. Abraham AS, Cole RB, Green ID, Hedworth-Whitty RB, Clarke SW & Bishop JM (1969) Factors contributing to the reversible pulmonary hypertension of patients with acute respiratory failure studied by serial observations during recovery. *Circulation Research* **24:**51–60.
7. Pinsky MR & Kramer D (1992) Cardiopulmonary interactions. In Tinker J & Zapol WM (eds) *Care of the Critically Ill Patient*, pp 41–58. New York: Springer Verlag.
8. Armaganidis A, Kotanidou A & Roussos C (1995) Mechanical ventilation in circulatory failure. In Vincent JL (ed) *Yearbook of Intensive Care and Emergency Medicine*, pp 185–208. Berlin: Springer Verlag.
9. Enson Y, Guintini C, Lewis ML, Morris TQ, Ferrer MI & Harvey RM (1964) The influence of hydrogen ion concentration and hypoxia on the pulmonary circulation. *Journal of Clinical Investigation* **43:**1146–1162.
10. Harris P, Segel N, Green J & Housley E (1968) The influence of the airways resistance and alveolar pressure on the pulmonary vascular resistance in chronic bronquitis. *Cardiovascular Research* **2:**84–94.
11. Magee F, Wright JL, Wiggs BR, Paré PD & Hogg JC (1988) Pulmonary vascular structure and function in chronic obstructive pulmonary disease. *Thorax* **43:**183–189.
12. Din-Xuan AT (1992) Endothelial modulation of pulmonary vascular tone. *European Respiratory Journal* **5:**757–762.
13. Adnot S, Raffestin B, Eddahibi S, Braquet P & Chabrier PE (1991) Loss of endothelium-dependent relaxant activity in the pulmonary circulation of rats exposed to chronic hypoxia. *Journal of Clinical Investigation* **87:**155–162.

14. Giaid A & Saleh D (1995) Reduced expression of endothelial nitric oxide synthase in the lungs of patients with pulmonary hypertension. *New England Journal of Medicine* **333:**214–221.
15. Dinh-Xuan AT, Higenbottam TW, Clelland CA, Pepke-Zaba J, Cremona G, Butt AY, Large SR, Wells FC & Wallbork J (1991) Impairment of endothelium-dependent pulmonary artery relaxation in chronic obstructive pulmonary disease. *New England Journal of Medicine* **324:**1539–1547.
16. Weitzenblum E, Loiseau A, Hirth C, Mirhom R & Rasaholinjanahary J (1979) Course of pulmonary haemodynamics in patients with chronic obstructive pulmonary disease. *Chest* **75:**656–662.
17. Biernacki W, Flenley DC, Muir AL & MacNee W (1988) Pulmonary hypertension and right ventricular function in patients with COPD. *Chest* **94:**1169–1175.
18. Herles F, Jezek V & Daum S (1968) Site of pulmonary resistance in cor pulmonale in chronic bronchitis. *British Heart Journal* **30:**654–660.
19. Graham R, Skoog C, Oppenheimer L et al (1982) Critical closure in the canine pulmonary vasculature. *Circulation Research* **50:**1277–1283.
20. Aubier M, Murciano D, Milic-Emili J et al (1980) Effects of the administration of O_2 on ventilation and blood gases, in patients with chronic obstructive pulmonary disease during acute respiratory failure. *American Review of Respiratory Disease* **122:**747–754.
21. Baigorri F, De Monte A, Blanch L, Fernández R, Vallés J, Mestre J, Saura P & Artigas A (1994) Hemodynamic responses to external counterbalancing of auto-positive end-expiratory pressure in mechanically ventilated patients with chronic obstructive pulmonary disease. *Critical Care Medicine* **22:**1782–1791.
22. Ranieri VM, Giuliani R, Cinnella G, Pesce C, Brienza N, Ippolito EL, Pomo V, Fiore T, Gottfried SB & Brienza A (1993) Physiologic effects of positive end-expiratory pressure in patients with chronic obstructive pulmonary disease during acute ventilatory failure and controlled mechanical ventilation. *American Review of Respiratory Disease* **147:**5–13.
23. Naeije R (1992) Should pulmonary hypertension be treated in chronic obstructive pulmonary disease. In Weir EK, Archer SL & Reeves JT (eds) *The Diagnosis and Treatment of Pulmonary Hypertension* pp 209–239. Mount Kisco, NY: Futura Publishing Inc.
24. Adnot S, Kouyoumdjian C, Defouilloy C, Andrivet P, Sediame S, Herigault R & Fratacci MD (1993) Hemodynamic and gas exchange response to infusion of acetylcholine and inhalation of nitric oxide in patients with chronic obstructive lung disease and pulmonary hypertension. *American Review of Respiratory Disease* **148:**310–316.
25. Moinard J, Manier G, Pillet O & Castaing Y (1994) Effect of inhaled nitric oxide on hemodynamics and V/Q inequalities in patients with chronic obstructive pulmonary disease. *American Journal of Respiratory and Critical Care Medicine* **149:**1482–1487.
26. Barberá JA, Roger N, Roca J, Rovira I, Diaz O, Masclans JR & Rodriguez-Roisin R (1995) Inhaled nitric oxide may worsen gas exchange in chronic obstructive pulmonary disease. *American Journal of Respiratory and Critical Care Medicine* **151:**A727.
27. Blanch L, Joseph D, Fernández R, Jubert P, Mas A, Martínez M, Vallés J & Artigas A (1995) Hemodynamic and gas exchange responses to inhalation of nitric oxide in severe hypoxemic ARDS and COPD patients. *Intensive Care Medicine* **21:**S45.
28. Macnee W, Wathen CG, Flenley DC & Muir AD (1988) The effects of controlled oxygen therapy on ventricular function in patients with stable and decompensated cor pulmonale. *American Review of Respiratory Disease* **137:**1289–1295.

29. Rossaint R, Slama K, Steudel W, Gerlach H, Pappert D, Veit S & Falke K (1995) Effects of inhaled nitric oxide on right ventricular function in severe acute respiratory distress syndrome. *Intensive Care Medicine* **21:**197–203.
30. Fierobe L, Brunet F, Dhainaut JF, Monchi M, Belghith M, Mira JP, Dall'ava-Santucci J & Dinh-Xuan AT (1995) Effect of inhaled nitric oxide on right ventricular function in adult respiratory distress syndrome. *American Journal of Respiratory and Critical Care Medicine* **151:**1414–1419.

Part IV

The Alveolar Interface: Doorway to the Circulation

16

Consequences of Leukocyte Migration in the Lungs: a Reappraisal

Thomas R. Martin

INTRODUCTION

We depend on leukocyte migration for our survival. Leukocyte migration through the microvasculature and into the extravascular spaces is one of the important features of acute inflammatory responses. Patients with congenital abnormalities of leukocyte adhesion[1] and oxidative metabolism develop severe recurrent infections of skin, lungs and other tissues, and often die at an early age.[2,3] Neutrophils (PMNs) are required for the clearance of Gram-negative organisms from the lungs of animals,[4] and patients with acquired neutropenia are at high risk for pyogenic and fungal infections. Thus, mechanisms have evolved that permit leukocytes to migrate through vessel walls and into surrounding tissues in order to defend the host against microbial invasion. At what price to the host does this occur? Neutrophils contain potent effector systems, including reactive oxygen species and proteases, that are designed to contact, ingest and eliminate potential pathogens.[3] When these products are formed and released in a protected intracellular environment such as the phagolysosome, they destroy ingested bacteria. However, when these products are released into the extracellular milieu they have the potential to damage nearby normal structures. The balance between 'appropriate' and 'inappropriate' release of PMN products has received a great deal of attention from investigators interested in the pathogenesis of acute lung injury.[5,6] This chapter summarizes some of the recent developments that clarify the role of PMN migration in lung defense and lung injury.

Leukocyte recruitment into the airspaces is one of the classical features of the inflammatory response that accompanies acute lung injury. Normally, more than 90% of the leukocytes in the airspaces of the lungs are alveolar macrophages (AMs), and only 1–2% are PMNs.[7] In patients with acute lung injury (acute (or adult) respiratory distress syndrome (ARDS)), up to 90% of the airspace leukocytes are PMNs,[8,9] and products of activated PMNs are present in bronchoalveolar lavage fluid.[10–12] ARDS is characterized by a severe injury to both the endothelial and epithelial barriers of the lungs, with the accumulation of protein and fibrin-rich exudates in the airspaces.[13,14] This results in severe ventilation/perfusion abnormalities, and clinical manifestations that include diffuse bilateral infiltrates and critical hypoxemia.

The presence of PMNs and their products in the airspaces of patients with ARDS led to the 'PMN hypothesis',[6] which proposes that the migration of PMNs from the vascular space into the airspaces causes the changes in microvascular and epithelial permeability that are characteristic of ARDS. In the last two decades, many investigators have studied this hypothesis. Although initial studies supported the relationship between PMN migration and lung injury, recent studies in animals and humans have provided a more balanced perspective on the role of PMN migration through the pulmonary microvasculature and the pathogenesis of acute lung injury.

ANATOMY AND FUNCTION OF THE ALVEOLAR BARRIER IN THE LUNGS

One of the unique anatomic features of the lung is the juxtaposition of microvascular endothelial cells and alveolar epithelial cells on opposite sides of a thin basement membrane. Each of these structures provides a barrier to the movement of fluid and proteins into the airspaces, and the consequences of leukocyte movement across these two barriers differ (Table 1). The understanding of the contribution of PMNs to lung injury must take into account the effects of PMN migration on each of these barriers, and the relative contributions of endothelial injury and epithelial injury to changes that occur in experimental systems. For example, changes in endothelial permeability can occur rapidly in response to intravascular stimuli, resulting in increased lung lymph flow, extravascular water, and weight gain.[15] On the other hand, the epithelium forms a relatively tight barrier to fluid and solute,[16,17] and does not readily change permeability.[18] Injury to the epithelium by inflammatory products or other means results in alveolar flooding with proteinaceous

Table 1. Consequences of endothelial and epithelial injury in the lungs.

Endothelial injury
- plasma moves into the interstitium
- increased intravascular lung water
- increased lung lymph flow
- altered V_A/Q relationships, with hypoxemia
- relatively rapidly reversible, with transient decrease in lung function

Epithelial injury
- alteration in the tight epithelial barrier
- plasma movement into airspaces results in alveolar flooding
- altered V_A/Q relationships with sustained hypoxemia
- slowly reversible with sustained loss of function

exudates, surfactant abnormalities, alveolar collapse, and prolonged pulmonary dysfunction.

The alveolar epithelium consists of Type I pneumocytes, which make up most of the alveolar surface, and Type II pneumocytes, which produce surfactant and surfactant-associated proteins and give rise to Type I pneumocytes during pulmonary repair processes. Recent observations indicate that the alveolar epithelium is not a passive barrier to fluid movement, but rather is a dynamic cellular layer that expends energy to reabsorb proteins, solutes, and water from the alveolar spaces. Studies by Matthay et al[19–21] have established that alveolar protein clearance is relatively slow, occurring at a rate of about 1–2%/h in several animal species. The normal epithelium has sieving properties, as small molecules like cyanocobalamin (1.4 kDa) pass through the epithelium relatively rapidly, whereas molecules equal to or greater than the size of albumin (>67 kDa) pass much more slowly.[22] Larger molecules such as immunoglobulin (Ig)G (150 000 kDa) are present in the airspaces, but large molecules such as IgM and α_2-macroglobulin (900 000 kDa) are relatively excluded.[23] The protein-sieving function of the alveolar membrane is lost in patients with acute lung injury,[24] and large concentrations of IgM and α_2-macroglobulin are present in bronchoalveolar lavage fluid.

Solutes are cleared from the alveolar spaces through active transport mechanisms. Active sodium transport has been demonstrated in the lungs of animals[25] isolated lung preparations,[26] and Type II pneumocytes *in vitro*.[27–30] Oxidant injury impairs sodium transport in Type II pneumocytes,[31] raising the possibility that injury to solute transport mechanisms in acute lung injury may have important effects on normal homeostatic mechanisms that keep the airspaces dry.

In addition to solute clearance, recent evidence indicates that the alveolar epithelium reabsorbs water through regulated water channel proteins. The CHIP28 protein is a mercury-sensitive water channel that is present in the kidney, erythrocytes, and other cell membranes.[32] The CHIP28 protein has been identified by immunocytochemistry on the surface of normal Type I pneumocytes.[32] This finding has led to the suggestion that a major function of the Type I pneumocytes may be to remove water from the airspaces of the lungs. This function may be critical in normal homeostasis, promoting the removal of water that moves into otherwise normal airspaces. Damage to the epithelial barrier should impair water transport out of the airspaces, providing an additional mechanism for failure of net fluid clearance out of the airspaces in patients with lung injury.

A growing amount of information indicates that epithelial function is as important as endothelial injury in the resolution of pulmonary edema and lung injury in humans and animals.[33,34] Matthay et al[33] discovered that alveolar edema fluid can be sampled by aspirating gently through a catheter wedged deeply into a basal bronchus of the lungs of intubated patients. This led to the important observation that the alveolar protein concentration rises during the early hours following the onset of pulmonary edema in patients who subsequently improve.[33] In contrast, protein concentration remains unchanged or actually falls over the first 12–24 h in patients who fail to resolve their lung injury. This observation suggested that the change in protein concentration in the edema fluid reflects the balance between net water reabsorption, which is relatively rapid across normal alveolar epithelium, and net protein clearance, which is slower than water reabsorption[33]. This hypothesis is supported by experimental data in animals, and may explain the extremely high protein concentrations in bronchoalveolar lavage fluid of patients with high altitude pulmonary edema who recovered rapidly with treatment at altitude.[23]

EVIDENCE LINKING PMNs WITH ACUTE LUNG INJURY (Table 2)

The pathology of the lungs of patients who die with ARDS consistently shows disruption of the alveolar epithelial and endothelial barriers, and infiltration of the airspaces with PMNs.[13,14] PMNs and their products are consistently found in the bronchoalveolar lavage fluids of patients with ARDS. At the onset of ARDS in humans following sepsis, trauma, or other risks, PMNs represent up to 90% of airspace leukocytes,[9] and PMN-derived oxidants and proteases are present in airspace fluids.[10–12] The key question that has received a great deal of attention is whether migrating PMNs cause the injury in ARDS, or whether the presence of airspace PMNs reflects other mechanistic events that mediate lung injury.

Evidence supporting a role for PMNs in lung injury derives from *in vitro* studies using cell culture systems, and from experimental studies in animal preparations.[5,35] Oxidants from PMNs attack target cells *in vitro*, inducing damage to cell membranes and nuclear DNA.[36] Activated PMNs alter the permeability of endothelial monolayers to albumin *in vitro*.[37] PMN-derived oxidants[37] and arachidonic acid[38] have been implicated. PMNs also induce detachment of Type II pneumocytes from adherent monolayers by a protease-dependent mechanism.[39] While these studies are important in establishing the concept that PMNs can injure endothelial and epithelial cells *in vitro*, the relationship between the relatively simple tissue-culture conditions in which such experiments are conducted and the complex environments *in vivo* in which PMNs function is not clear. Hence, the extent to which these studies actually reflect *in vivo* events is difficult to ascertain.

Table 2. Evidence linking PMN and lung injury.

In vitro
- PMN oxidants and proteases injure endothelial monolayers *in vitro*

In vivo
- activated PMNs cause weight gain and albumin leak in isolated rabbit lungs, and PMN depletion blocks this effect

In ARDS
- circulating PMNs are activated in some patients with ARDS
- PMNs accumulate in large numbers in the lungs of patients with ARDS
- PMN products (oxidants, proteases, granular enzymes) are present in bronchoalveolar lavage fluid of patients with ARDS

Animal studies also have provided experimental links between PMNs and acute lung injury. For example, Shasby et al[40] reported that human PMNs activated with phorbol myristate acetate (PMA) caused weight gain and increased movement of albumin into the airspaces of isolated buffer-perfused rabbit lungs.[40] The observation that PMNs from a patient with chronic granulomatous disease, which do not produce oxidants normally, did not affect the lungs suggested that PMN-derived oxidants were mechanistically involved. Antioxidants blocked the effects of intravascular PMNs, providing further support for the role of PMN-derived oxidants in altering lung permeability in this model. The activating agent used in these and other studies was phorbol myristate acetate PMA, which is a potent and irreversible trigger of the respiratory burst in leukocytes.[41] PMA activates protein kinase C-dependent cellular mechanisms, including activation of the membrane oxidase that produces superoxide anion, upregulation of major adhesion molecules on the leukocyte surface, and degranulation of primary granules that contain myeloperoxidase and leukocyte proteases.[4,42] PMA also has leukocyte-independent vascular effects that confound the interpretation of experiments using PMA. For example, PMA caused lung weight gain independently of leukocytes when infused directly into buffer-perfused lung preparations.[43] Thus, although PMA is a useful tool for studying leukocyte activation in experimental systems, the results must be interpreted with caution, as it produces sustained and unregulated leukocyte activation that simulates the extreme of leukocyte activation. In addition, direct effects on other cells in the experimental preparations may confound the interpretation of the results.

Studies using PMN depletion provide an alternative approach to studying the role of PMNs in lung injury and have provided further support for a causal link between PMN activation in the lung microvasculature and lung injury.[40,44–46] In general, antimetabolites such as nitrogen mustard or vinblastine have been used to deplete PMNs *in vivo* by blocking marrow production. Neutrophil depletion with nitrogen mustard prevented the lung weight gain induced by PMA in intact rabbits.[40] Induction of neutropenia with hydroxyurea prevented increased lymph flow (which reflects altered endothelial permeability) induced by endotoxin[44] and thrombin[47] in sheep. Similarly, PMN depletion blocked hyperoxic lung injury in rabbits.[45] Not all investigators have found that PMN depletion blocks lung injury, however, as PMN depletion did not block the increased protein flux that occurred with lung injury in sheep.[48]

One of the key advances in this area was the recognition that the mechanisms that control PMN emigration through the microcirculation of the lungs are different from those that control emigration in the systemic circulation.[49] In the skin and the peritoneum, PMN migration is dependent on the initial adhesion of PMNs to the vascular endothelium via integrins (CD18) on PMNs and intercellular adhesion molecules (ICAM-1) on vascular endothelial cells. Blockade of CD18 prevents vascular injury in the systemic circulation in a variety of injury models.[50] In the lungs, however, PMN emigration is not necessarily dependent on CD18 or ICAM-1, and both CD18-dependent and -independent pathways exist. For example, PMN migration into the airspaces in response to *S. pneumoniae* is CD18-independent, whereas PMN migration in response to *E. coli* is CD18-independent.[49]

The molecules that mediate the CD18-independent pathways in the lungs have not been identified.

STUDIES OF PMNs IN PATIENTS WITH ARDS

As noted previously, pathologic studies showed that PMNs are present in the airspaces of patients who die with ARDS,[13,51] and clinical studies using bronchoalveolar lavage established that PMNs are present in the airspaces at the onset of ARDS, and persist during the course of ARDS.[8–10] Studies with ^{111}In-labeled PMNs showed that PMN recruitment is an active process in patients with ARDS.[52] Interleukin (IL)-8, an important cytokine that recruits PMNs, is present in the airspaces of patients with ARDS,[53,54] and correlates with PMN recruitment.[55] Circulating PMNs in patients with ARDS produce increased amounts of oxidants[56] in response to the chemotactic peptide *N*-formylmethionyl-leucyl-phenylalanine (FMLP), a membrane stimulus, suggesting that circulating PMNs are activated within the intravascular spaces. However, the responses of circulating PMNs to the protein kinase C activator, PMA, were similar in patients with ARDS and normal volunteers.[57] Airspace PMNs produced less superoxide anion and hydrogen peroxide than central venous blood PMNs from the same individuals, suggesting that the PMNs had been activated either in transit through the lungs or in the airspaces.[57] These observations support the concepts that circulating mediators activate PMNs in the vascular compartment of patients with ARDS, but that the activity of airspace PMNs is downregulated, most likely by stimuli that cause rapid degranulation of migrating PMNs.[57]

Neutrophils are not required for the development of ARDS, however, as ARDS develops in neutropenic patients who have been treated with radiation and cytotoxic drugs.[58,59] This emphasizes the concept that the lung endothelial and epithelial barriers are sensitive to a variety of injuries that occur in the presence, as well as the absence, of circulating PMNs. Not all acute lung injuries are associated with PMN recruitment. Patients who develop acute high-altitude pulmonary edema (HAPE) have extremely high protein concentrations in the airspaces, higher than many patients with ARDS, yet patients with HAPE have only small increases in airspace leukocytes, including PMNs.[23] This presumably results from a primary injury to the alveolar barrier mediated by extremely high intravascular pressures, with movement of protein and fluid from the intravascular to the alveolar compartment. Reabsorption of water more rapidly than protein by normal epithelial pneumocytes may further increase the airspace protein concentration.[23]

EVIDENCE THAT PMN MIGRATION DOES NOT NECESSARILY INJURE THE LUNGS

Despite the evidence suggesting an association between PMNs and acute lung injury in humans and animals, recent evidence indicates that PMN movement through the pulmonary microvasculature does not necessarily cause 'injury', as reflected by increased protein leakage. When PMNs migrate into the lungs of normal humans in response to the low molecular mass lipid chemoattractant, leukotriene B_4 (LTB_4), only a minor increase in protein occurs in the airspace. High molecular mass proteins such as IgM do not appear in the airspace, indicating that the sieving properties of the epithelium are intact.[60] Morphometric measurement on the PMNs recovered from the lungs indicated that the airspace PMNs had lost the smaller specific granules, but contained normal amounts of the larger primary granules that contain myeloperoxidase and proteolytic enzymes.[60] These changes are also typical of PMNs that migrate into skin.[61] The airspace PMNs migrated normally in response to the bacterial chemotactic peptide signal, FMLP, indicating that PMNs that had recently migrated into the airspaces could recognize and move toward secondary bacterial signals. Airspace PMNs also produced normal amounts of superoxide anion in response to PMA, so that they had arrived in the airspaces with intact oxidative mechanisms. Chest radiographs were normal in all of the subjects, although this is an insensitive measure of alveolar edema. This study was the first demonstration that PMNs can migrate into the lungs of normal human volunteers without causing significant injury.

This concept, that PMN migration can occur without substantial injury to the lungs, has also been demonstrated by Wiener-Kronish et al[62] in studies of the effects of bacterial lipopolysaccharide (LPS) and *Pseudomonas aeruginosa* instilled into the lungs of sheep. The airspace and intravascular compartments were labeled with ^{125}I-albumin or ^{131}I-albumin, respectively, so that albumin flux in each direction across the alveolar membrane could be measured. Either LPS or *P. aeruginosa* was added to the alveolar instillate, containing radiolabeled albumin. In these studies, PMN migration into the lungs was not associated with a significant increase in epithelial permeability, even when endothelial permeability increased substantially.[62] Instillation of bacterial endotoxin caused a large increase in airspace PMNs, but no increase in the movement of albumin in either direction across the epithelium. Because LPS is a potent inducer of proinflammatory cytokines from alveolar macrophages, e.g. tumor necrosis factor α (TNF-α), IL-1β, IL-8 and others, this study provides indirect evidence that these proinflammatory cytokines in the airspaces do not induce major changes in epithelial permeability in this animal model. Intravascular LPS increased albumin movement across the endothelium and into lymph, but not across the epithelium. In contrast with the effects of LPS, the instillation of *P. aeruginosa* directly into the airspaces caused a large increase in epithelial permeability with significant movement of the alveolar tracer into the bloodstream.[62] This study suggests that bacterial products in the airspaces may be more important in regulating epithelial permeability than either migrating PMNs or the host cytokines that regulate the inflammatory response. Interestingly, instillation of *P. aeruginosa* into the vasculature caused an increase in endothelial permeability, as expected, but did not cause a consistent change in epithelial permeability.[63] This established that the lung epithelium is relatively resistant to attack by bacteria and their products in the vascular space.

Subsequent studies using mutant derivatives of *P. aeruginosa* have shown that lung injury is lost in a mutant strain that lacks the regulatory gene for an important pseudomonas exoenzyme, identified as ExoS.[64] ExoS appears to be more important in causing injury than pseudomonas elastase, as strains that lack elastase still induce epithelial injury in this system.

In recent experiments, we have found that when increasing doses of *E. coli* are instilled into the airspaces of rabbits via a catheter placed in the right mainstem bronchus, there was a dose-dependent increase in airspace leukocytes within 4 h of the instillation of bacteria.[65] In contrast, the alveolar protein concentration did not increase as a linear function with the increase in leukocytes. Instead, protein concentration increased with dose at the lower doses of instilled bacteria, but was lower in the animals treated with the highest dose of instilled *E. coli* (1×10^{10} colony-forming units/ml). Thus, at high concentrations of instilled bacteria there was a definite dissociation between PMN migration and protein permeability. The protein concentrations mirrored the concentration of TNF-α in the lung lavage fluid, suggesting that TNF-α contributes in some way to the increase in protein permeability in this model. This is consistent with recent observations in rats[66] that link TNF-α with the pathogenesis of lung injury following the instillation of bacteria into the airspaces. Some evidence indicates that TNF-α does not cause direct injury to the lung microvasculature, but initiates events that require the participation of other factors to induce injury.[67,68]

SUMMARY

In summary, a substantial amount of information links PMNs in the lungs with lung injury, but recent information in human and whole animal systems suggests that PMN migration alone, whether in response to endogenous or exogenous stimuli, accounts for only a minor portion of the increase in permeability that occurs with acute lung injury in humans. PMN migration may have a major influence on the permeability of the endothelium, promoting exudation of plasma proteins into the lymphatic spaces, but PMN migration by itself does not appear to have a major effect on lung epithelial permeability. Other stimuli in conjunction with PMNs appear to be necessary to substantially alter the permeability of the epithelial barrier in the lungs.

ACKNOWLEDGEMENTS

This work was supported in part by the Medical Research Service of the Department of Veterans' Affairs, and by grants HL30542, AI29103 and GM37696 from the National Institutes of Health.

REFERENCES

1. Beatty PG, Harlan JM, Rosen JM et al (1984) Absence of monoclonal antibody defined protein complex in a boy with abnormal leukocyte function. *Lancet* **i**:535–537.
2. Gallin JI, Buescher ES, Seligmann BE, Nath J, Gaither T & Katz P (1983) NIH

conference: recent advances in chronic granulomatous disease. *Annals of Internal Medicine* **99:**657–674.
3. Borregaard N (1988) The human neutrophil. Function and dysfunction. *European Journal of Haematology* **41:**401–413.
4. Rehm S.R, Gross GN & Pierce AK (1980) Early bacterial clearance from murine lungs. Species-dependent phagocyte response. *Journal of Clinical Investigation* **66:**194–199.
5. Boxer LA, Axtell R & Suchard S (1990) The role of the neutrophil in inflammatory diseases of the lung. *Blood Cells* **16:**25–42.
6. Repine J.E & Beehler C.J (1991) Neutrophils and the adult respiratory distress syndrome: two interlocking perspectives. *American Review of Respiratory Disease* **144:**251–252.
7. Cherniak RM, Banks DE, Bell DY, Davis GS, Hugh JM & King TE Jr (1990) The Bronchoalveolar Lavage Cooperative Study Group. Bronchoalveolar lavage constituents in healthy individuals, idiopathic pulmonary fibrosis and selected comparison groups. *American Review of Respiratory Disease* **141:**S169–S202.
8. Weiland J.E, Davis WB, Holter JF, Mohammed JR, Dorinsky PM & Gadek JE (1986) Lung neutrophils in the adult respiratory distress syndrome. Clinical and pathophysiologic significance. *American Review of Respiratory Disease* **133:**218–225.
9. Steinberg KP, Milberg JA, Martin TR, Maunder RJ, Cockrill BA & Hudson LD (1994) Evolution of bronchoalveolar cell populations in the adult respiratory distress syndrome. *American Journal of Respiratory and Critical Care Medicine* **150:**113–122.
10. Cochrane CG, Spragg RG, Revak SD, Cohen AB & McGuire WW (1983) The presence of neutrophil elastase and evidence of oxidation activity in bronchoalveolar lavage fluid of patients with adult respiratory distress syndrome. *American Review of Respiratory Disease* **127:**S25–S27.
11. McGuire WW, Spragg RG, Cohen AM & Cochrane CG (1982) Studies on the pathogenesis of the adult respiratory distress syndrome. *Journal of Clinical Investigation* **69:**543–553.
12. Lee CT, Fein AM & Lippman M (1981) Elastolytic activity in pulmonary lavage fluid from patients with the adult respiratory distress syndrome. *New England Journal of Medicine* **304:**192–196.
13. Bachofen M & Weibel ER (1982) Structural alterations of lung parenchyma in the adult respiratory distress syndrome. *Clinical Chest Medicine* **3:**35–56.
14. Tomashefski JF Jr (1990) Pulmonary pathology of the adult respiratory distress syndrome. *Clinical Chest Medicine* **11:**593–619.
15. Winn R, Harlan J, Nadir B, Harker L & Hildebrandt J (1983) Thromboxane A2 mediates lung vasoconstriction but not permeability after endotoxin. *Journal of Clinical Investigation* **72:**911–918.
16. Taylor AE, Guyton AC & Bishop VS (1965) Permeability of the alveolar membrane to solutes. *Circulation Research* **16:**353–362.
17. Gorin AB & Stewart PA (1979) Differential permeability of endothelial and epithelial barriers to albumin. *Journal of Applied Physiology* **47:**1315–1324.
18. Johnson MC II, Goodman RB, Kajikawa O, Wong VA, Mongovin SM & Martin TR (1994) Cloning of two rabbit GRO homologues and their expression in rabbit alveolar macrophages. *Gene* **151:**337–338.
19. Matthay MA, Berthiaume Y & Staub NC (1985) Long-term clearance of liquid and protein from the lungs of unanesthetized sheep. *Journal of Applied Physiology* **59:**928–934.
20. Berthiaume Y, Broaddus VC, Gropper MA, Tanita T & Matthay MA (1988) Alveolar liquid and protein clearance from normal dog lungs. *Journal of Applied Physiology* **65:**585–593.

21. Berthiaume Y, Albertine KH, Grady M, Fick G & Matthay MA (1989) Protein clearance from the airspaces and lungs of unanesthetized sheep over 144 h. *Journal of Applied Physiology* **67:**1887–1897.
22. Hastings RH, Grady M, Sakuma T & Matthay MA (1992) Clearance of different-sized proteins from the alveolar space in humans and rabbits. *Journal of Applied Physiology* **73:**1310–1316.
23. Schoene RB, Swenson ER, Pizzo CJ et al (1988) The lung at high altitude: bronchoalveolar lavage in acute mountain sickness and pulmonary edema. *Journal of Applied Physiology* **64:**2605–2613.
24. Holter JF, Weiland JE, Pacht ER, Gadek GE & Davis WB (1986) Protein permeability in the adult respiratory distress syndrome. Loss of size selectivity of the alveolar epithelium. *Journal of Clinical Investigation* **78:**1513–1522.
25. Matthay MA, Landolt CC & Staub NC (1982) Differential liquid and protein clearance from the alveoli of anesthetized sheep. *Journal of Applied Physiology* **53:**96–104.
26. Bassset G, Crone C & Saumon G (1987) Significance of active ion transport in transalveolar water absorption: a study on isolated rat lung. *Journal of Physiology (London)* **384:**311–324.
27. Mason RJ, Williams MC, Widdicombe JH, Sanders MJ, Misfeldt DS & Berry LC (1982) Transepithelial transport by pulmonary alveolar type II cells in primary culture. *Proceedings of the National Academy of Sciences USA* **79:**6033–6037.
28. Cheek JM, Kim KJ & Crandall ED (1989) Tight monolayers of rat alveolar epithelial cells: bidirectional properties and active sodium transport. *American Journal of Physiology* **256:**C688.
29. Effros RM, Mason GR, Sietsema K, Hukkaen J & Silverman P (1988) Pulmonary epithelial sieving of small solutes in rat lungs. *Journal of Applied Physiology* **65:**640–648.
30. Matalon S (1991) Mechanisms and regulation of ion transport in adult mammalian alveolar type II pneumocytes. *American Journal of Physiology* **261:**C727–C738.
31. Matalon S, Beckman JS, Duffey ME & Freeman BA (1989) Oxidant inhibition of epithelial active sodium transport. *Free Radical Biology and Medicine* **6:**557–564.
32. Folkesson HG, Matthay MA, Hasegawa H, Kheradmand F & Verkman AS (1994) Transcellular water transport in lung alveolar epithelium through mercury-sensitive water channels. *Proceedings of the National Academy of Sciences USA* **91:**4970–4974.
33. Matthay MA & Wiener-Kronish JP (1990) Intact epithelial barrier function is critical for the resolution of alveolar edema in humans. *American Review of Respiratory Disease* **142:**1250–1257.
34. Matthay MA, Folkesson HG, Campagna A & Kheradmand F (1993) Alveolar epithelial barrier and acute lung injury. *New Horizons* **1:**613–622.
35. Weiss SJ (1989) Tissue distruction by neutrophils. *New England Journal of Medicine* **320:**365–376.
36. Schraufstatter IU, Browne K, Harris A et al (1990) Mechanisms of hypochlorite injury of target cells. *Journal of Clinical Investigation* **85:**554–562.
37. Shasby DM, Shasby SS & Peach MJ (1983) Granulocytes and phorbol myristate acetate increase permeability to albumin of cultured endothelial monolayers and isolated perfused lungs. *American Review of Respiratory Disease* **127:**72–76.
38. Shasby DM, Shasby SS & Peach MJ (1985) Polymorphonuclear leukocyte: arachidonate edema. *Journal of Applied Physiology* **59:**47–55.
39. Ayars G.H, Altman LC, Rosen H & Doyle T (1984) The injurious effect of neutrophils on pneumocytes *in vitro*. *American Review of Respiratory Disease* **129:**964–973.

40. Shasby DM, Vanbenthuysen KM, Tate RM, Shasby SS, McMurtry I & Repine JE (1982) Granulocytes mediate acute edematous lung injury in rabbits and in isolated rabbit lungs perfused with phorbol myristate acetate: role of oxygen radicals. *American Review of Respiratory Disease* **125:**443-447.
41. Gerard C, McPhail LC, Marfat A, Stimler-Gerard NP, Bass DA & McCall CE (1986) Role of protein kinases in stimulation of human polymorphonuclear leukocyte oxidative metabolism by various agonists: differential effects of a novel protein kinase inhibitor. *Journal of Clinical Investigation* **77:**61–65.
42. Nishizuka Y (1986) Studies and perspectives of protein kinase C. *Science* **233:**305.
43. Johnson A (1988) PMA-induced pulmonary edema: mechanisms of the vasoactive response. *Journal of Applied Physiology* **65:**2302–2312.
44. Heflin AC Jr & Brigham KL (1981) Prevention by granulocyte depletion of increased vascular permeability of sheep lung following endotoxemia. *Journal of Clinical Investigation* **68:**1253–1260.
45. Shasby DM, Fox RB, Harada RN & Repine JE (1982) Reduction of the edema of acute hyperoxic lung injury by granulocyte depletion. *Journal of Applied Physiology* **52:**1237–1244.
46. Perkett EA, Brigham KL & Meyrick B (1990) Granulocyte depletion attenuates sustained pulmonary hypertension and increased pulmonary vasoreactivity caused by continuous air embolization in sheep. *American Review of Respiratory Disease* **141:**456–465.
47. Garcia-Szabo RR, Johnson A & Malik AB (1986) Leukocytes are required for the trypsin-induced increase in lung vascular permeability. *American Journal of Pathology* **124:**377–383.
48. Glauser FL, Bechard DE, Fisher BJ, Davis D & Fowler III AA (1988) Bronchoalveolar lavage in an animal model of acute lung injury. Relationship between enhanced membrane permeability and transvascular neutrophil flux. *American Journal of Pathology* **131:**404–410.
49. Doerschuk CM, Winn RK, Coxson HO & Harlan JM (1990) CD18-dependent and -independent mechanisms of neutrophil emigration in the pulmonary and systemic microcirculation of rabbits. *Journal of Immunology* **144:**2327–2333.
50. Talbott GA, Sharar SR, Harlan JM & Winn RK (1994) Leukocyte–endothelial interactions and organ injury: the role of adhesion molecules. *New Horizons* **2:**545–554.
51. Tomashefski JF Jr, Davies P, Boggis L et al (1983) The pulmonary vascular lesions of the adult respiratory distress syndrome. *American Journal of Pathology* **112:**112–126.
52. Warshawski RJ, Sibbald WJ, Driedger AA & Cheung H (1986) Abnormal neutrophil-pulmonary interaction in the adult respiratory distress syndrome. Qualitative and quantitative assessment of pulmonary neutrophil kinetics in humans with in vivo ^{111}indium neutrophil scintigraphy. *American Review of Respiratory Disease* **122:**797–804.
53. Miller EJ, Nagao S, Griffith D et al (1992) Elevated levels of NAP-1/interleukin-8 are present in the airspaces of patients with the adult respiratory distress syndrome and are associated with increased mortality. *American Review of Respiratory Disease* **146:**427-432.
54. Donnelly S.C, Strieter RM, Kunkel S et al (1993) Interleukin-8 and development of adult respiratory distress syndrome in at-risk groups. *Lancet* **341:**643–647.
55. Goodman RB, Strieter RM, Steinberg KP et al (1996) Inflammatory cytokines in patients with persistence of the acute respiratory distress syndrome. *American Journal of Respiratory and Critical Care Medicine* In press:
56. Zimmerman GA, Renzetti AD & Hill HR (1983) Functional and metabolic activity of granulocytes from patients with adult respiratory distress syndrome. *American Review of Respiratory Disease* **127:**290–300.

57. Martin TR, Pistorese BP, Hudson LD & Maunder RJ (1991) Function of lung and blood neutrophils in patients with the adult respiratory distress syndrome. Implications for the pathogenesis of lung infections. *American Review of Respiratory Disease* **144:**254–262.
58. Maunder RJ, Hackman RC, Riff E, Albert RK & Springmeyer SC (1986) Occurrence of the adult respiratory distress syndrome in neutropenic patients. *American Review of Respiratory Disease* **133:**313-316.
59. Ognibene FP, Martin SE, Parker MM et al (1986) Adult respiratory distress syndrome in patients with severe neutropenia. *New England Journal of Medicine* **315:**547-551.
60. Martin TR, Pistorese BP, Chi EY, Goodman RB & Matthay MA (1989) Effects of leukotriene B4 in the human lung. Recruitment of neutrophils into the alveolar spaces without a change in protein permeability. *Journal of Clinical Investigation* **84:**1609–1619.
61. Wright DG & Gallin JI (1979) Secretory responses of human neutrophils: exocytosis of specific (secondary) granules by human neutrophils during adherence in vitro and during exudation in vivo. *Journal of Immunology* **123:**285–294.
62. Wiener-Kronish JP, Albertine KH & Matthay MA (1991) Differential responses of the endotheilal and epithelial barriers of the lung in sheep to *Escherichia coli* endotoxin. *Journal of Clinical Investigation* **88:**864–875.
63. Pittet JF, Wiener-Kronish JP, Serikov V & Matthay MA (1995) Resistance of the alveolar epithelium to injury from septic shock in sheep. *American Journal of Respiratory and Critical Care Medicine* **151:**1093–1100.
64. Kudoh I, Wiener-Kronish JP, Hashimoto W, Pittet JF & Frank D (1994) Exoproduct secretions of *Pseudomonas aeruginosa* strains influence severity of alveolar epithelial injury. *American Journal of Physiology (Lung Cell. Mol. Physiol.)* **267:**L551–L556.
65. Fox-Dewhurst R, Alberts M, Kajikawa O et al (1995) Dissociation between lung cytokines and bacterial burden in rabbits with gram negative pneumonia. *American Journal of Respiratory and Critical Care Medicine* **151:**A452.
66. Li XY, Donaldson K, Brown D & MacNee W (1995) The role of tumor necrosis factor in increased airspace epithelial permeability in acute lung inflammation. *American Journal of Respiratory and Critical Care Medicine* **13:**185–195.
67. Lo SK, Everitt J, Gu J & Malik AB (1992) Tumor necrosis factor mediates experimental pulmonary edema by ICAM-1 and CD18-dependent mechanisms. *Journal of Clinical Investigation* **89:**981–988.
68. Bonsignora MR, Valenti A & Spatofora M (1992) Tumor necrosis factor-alpha does not cause lung edema in rabbits. *Journal of Applied Physiology* **73:**173-178.

17

Pulmonary Edema and Alveolar Overdistension

Didier Dreyfuss
Georges Saumon

INTRODUCTION

Mechanical ventilation is a technique which, although frequently life-saving, carries nevertheless the potential risk of severe complications.[1] Among these adverse effects, some are the direct consequence of pulmonary pressure and/or volume changes induced by mechanical insufflation of diseased lungs. Barotrauma is the usual term for such complications, and refers to the presence of extra-alveolar air (manifesting as interstitial emphysema, pneumomediastinum or pneumoperitoneum, pneumothorax, etc.). In addition to these 'macroscopic' alterations, it has been experimentally demonstrated that lung distension during mechanical ventilation may induce alterations in lung fluid balance, increases in endothelial and epithelial permeability, and severe ultrastructural damage. These abnormalities may culminate in the production of a pulmonary permeability-type edema accompanied by a diffuse alveolar damage.

PULMONARY EDEMA DURING HIGH-PRESSURE/HIGH-VOLUME VENTILATION

Webb and Tierney[2] have shown that rats mechanically ventilated with intermittent positive pressure ventilation with a peak airway pressure of 30 cmH_2O developed pulmonary edema very rapidly. Hence, after only 1 h of such ventilation, there was an increase in the extravascular lung water content, as assessed by post-mortem weighing. When the lungs of these animals were examined by light microscopy, only interstitial edema was present. In contrast with these mild alterations induced by moderate increases in airway pressure, ventilating the animals with 45 cmH_2O peak pressure resulted even more rapidly (in less than 40 min) in a very severe pulmonary edema, responsible for massive tracheal flooding and hypoxemia leading to the death of most animals. Extravascular lung water was considerably increased (nearly 3-fold normal values). Histologic examination confirmed this severity, by disclosing widespread alveolar edema.

Closely related observations have been made by Kolobow et al[3] on a sheep model of acute respiratory failure. They ventilated the animals with intermittent positive pressure ventilation and a peak inspiratory pressure of 50 cmH_2O for 2 days. This resulted in large alterations in lung compliance and gas exchange, leading to the death of some animals. At gross examination, the lungs appeared severely damaged. The same team has also confirmed, on larger animals, the observations by Webb and Tierney that peak inspiratory pressure of moderate range, but applied for longer periods, could also be deleterious to the lungs.[4] Indeed, sheep ventilated with a peak inspiratory pressure of only 30 cmH_2O for 48 h showed a progressive deterioration in total static lung compliance, functional residual capacity, and arterial blood gases. Post-mortem examination disclosed severe pulmonary atelectasis, increased wet lung weight, and an increase in the surface tension of saline lung lavage fluid (reflecting altered surfactant function).

Several studies aimed at assessing the nature (hydrostatic or permeability origin) of ventilation-induced edema. An increased microvascular permeability has been demonstrated in isolated lung lobes after ventilation with high peak airway pressure.[5] Alveolar epithelial permeability may increase as the result of lung distension, and may even allow free diffusion of albumin when high levels of distension are reached.[6] These permeability alterations at the endothelial and epithelial levels might reflect a 'stretched pore' phenomenon, resulting from high tension in cell connection.

In order to assess whether pulmonary edema is of the hydrostatic or permeability type, we conducted experiments on intact rats ventilated for various lengths of time (5, 10, and 20 min) with intermittent positive pressure ventilation with a peak inspiratory pressure of 45 cmH_2O.[7] In addition to measuring indices of pulmonary edema such as extravascular lung water content and the distribution space of ^{22}Na in lungs, we also estimated microvascular permeability by measuring the post-mortem extravascular dry lung weight (an increase in which reflects the amount of extravasated proteins) and the uptake by lungs of intravenously injected radiolabeled albumin. Permeability edema was present within 5 min of challenge, as attested by significant increases in all the edema and permeability indices. The severity of these alterations worsened with the duration of the experiment. Hence, after 20 min of such ventilation, a significant increase in edema was observed. The animals had copious amounts of tracheal fluid, with an albumin concentration close to that of plasma. Electron microscopic examination of lungs of rats that had received 20 min of intermittent positive pressure ventilation with 45 cmH_2O peak airway pressure disclosed a pattern of diffuse alveolar damage, with Type I cell destructions and hyaline membranes.

Other authors using different approaches have confirmed the presence of altered microvascular permeability during mechanical ventilation-induced pulmonary edema.[8,9] In addition to permeability alterations, hydrostatic force changes may also contribute to edema formation. Parker et al[8] have shown in open-chest dogs that ventilation with very high (64 cmH_2O) peak inspiratory pressure resulted in a combination of the two effects (i.e. hydrostatic and permeability changes) on lung microcirculation. Indeed, they observed, first, an increase in estimated mean microvascular pressure of 12.5 cmH_2O (derived from Swan–Ganz measurements), and second an increase in microvascular permeability. Increases in vascular pressure of the same magnitude have been reported by others during ventilation with high peak airway pressure in closed-chest lambs.[9] This mild to moderate increase in vascular pressure seems unable to produce a permeability-type edema, especially of the severity observed after high-volume ventilation, but can enhance the extravasation of fluid and proteins through an altered microvasculature.

RESPECTIVE ROLES OF HIGH AIRWAY PRESSURE AND HIGH LUNG VOLUME

High peak airway pressure, such as that used in our study, results in lungs with a normal compliance in a high tidal volume. It seemed therefore important to determine the respective roles of pressure and volume in the genesis of high permeability edema. We addressed this point in experiments where airway pressure and lung volume were made to vary independently.[10] We compared the effects of high-pressure/high-volume ventilation as previously described with those of high airway pressure alone (ventilating the animals with intermittent positive pressure ventilation with 45 cmH_2O peak pressure, but with a normal tidal volume obtained by thoracoabdominal strapping), and with those of high-volume ventilation with low (negative) airway pressure (ventilating the animals by means of an iron lung).

Permeability edema occurred in both groups submitted to high-volume ventilation, whether airway pressure was high or low. At the ultrastructural level, dramatic alterations in the alveolar–capillary barrier were present. In contrast, after high-pressure/low tidal volume ventilation, both extravascular lung water and indices of microvascular permeability remained within normal range, and no ultrastructural damage was observed. The observation that volume changes are responsible for both edema and permeability changes and that high airway pressure has no deleterious effect *per se* was confirmed in larger animals by other teams.[9,11]

EFFECTS OF THE DIFFERENT COMPONENTS OF LUNG VOLUME

The effects of positive end-expiratory pressure (PEEP) during acute lung injury are controversial. Indeed, during mechanical ventilation-induced pulmonary edema, for the same teleinspiratory pressure, less edema was present in animals ventilated with PEEP than in those ventilated with zero end-expiratory pressure (ZEEP).[2,10] Does it mean that PEEP would have some 'protective' effect against volutrauma (in contrast with the absence of reduction or even the increase in edema observed with PEEP during most types of experimental edema), or is it simply the result of hemodynamic alterations due to the higher mean intrathoracic pressure during ventilation with PEEP? This question pertains to the problem of the respective responsibility of large pressure/volume excursions and of the absolute level of lung distension in the genesis of ventilator-induced lung injury. To assess this point, rats were ventilated with increasing tidal volumes starting from different levels of PEEP.[12] Pulmonary edema with permeability alterations occurred regardless of the level of PEEP, provided that the increase in tidal volume was large enough. Similarly, edema occurred even during normal tidal volume ventilation provided that the increase in PEEP was large enough. It is worth noting that moderate increases in tidal volume or PEEP that were innocuous when applied alone, produced edema when combined. Similar observations were made in animals ventilated with negative inspiratory pressure indicating that the effect of PEEP was not the consequence of raised airway pressure but of the increase in functional residual capacity. Thus, it appears that end-inspiratory volume is probably the main determinant of ventilation-induced edema, rather than level of functional residual capacity or tidal volume. However, although permeability alterations were similar, edema was less marked in animals ventilated with PEEP than in those ventilated with ZEEP with the same end-inspiratory pressure. This 'beneficial' effect of PEEP was probably the consequence of hemodynamic alterations. Indeed, infusion of dopamine to correct the drop in systemic arterial pressure that occurred during PEEP ventilation resulted in a significant increase in pulmonary edema.

EFFECTS OF MECHANICAL VENTILATION ON PREVIOUSLY INJURED LUNGS

Most previously mentioned studies were conducted on animals with healthy lungs. It is conceivable that diseased lungs are more susceptible than healthy ones to the deleterious effects of mechanical ventilation. Bowton and Kong[13] studied the effects of varying tidal volume during mechanical ventilation of oleic acid-injured isolated perfused rabbit lungs. Lungs ventilated with a high tidal volume of 18 ml/kg had a significantly greater weight gain than those ventilated with a small tidal volume of 6 ml/kg. Hernandez and colleagues[14] studied the effects of oleic acid alone, mechanical ventilation alone and a combination of both interventions on the capillary filtration coefficient of isolated perfused young rabbits lungs. Low doses of oleic acid or mild overinflation during mechanical ventilation did not significantly affect the filtration coefficient when studied separately. In contrast, when oleic acid administration was followed by mechanical ventilation, a significant increase in this coefficient was observed. These studies were conducted on isolated lungs and did not address the problem of the nature of the interaction between previous lung injury and lung overinflation. Indeed, this interaction may be only additive (i.e. the resulting effect is the net sum of each separate injury) or synergistic (i.e. the resulting effect is larger than the sum of each separate injury). A synergistic interaction was recently demonstrated in intact rats:[15] animals received mechanical ventilation with three different tidal volumes resulting in lung overinflation of various degrees. Some animals were only ventilated whereas others were ventilated after having their lungs mildly injured with a small dose of α-naphthylthiourea. Additivity of the two types of injury was observed for the lower tidal volumes. At very high tidal volume, there was an obvious synergy between the two injuries with a very much more severe edema than would be expected from the simple addition of both effects.

MECHANISMS OF PULMONARY EDEMA DURING HIGH-PRESSURE/HIGH-VOLUME VENTILATION

As explained above, changes in hydrostatic forces are involved to a minor degree (on a quantitative basis) in the genesis of this edema. Two mechanisms can lead to increased vascular pressure during lung distension. First, surfactant abnormalities, which have been demonstrated after high-volume ventilation,[16,17] can promote an increase in alveolar surface tension. This leads in turn to a decrease in the pressure surrounding alveolar microvessels and therefore to an increased transmural pressure of these vessels. Second, lung distension results in augmentation of the transmural pressure of extra-alveolar vessels,[18] which in turn enhances fluid filtration at this level.

A possible explanation for the large permeability alterations observed during mechanical ventilation-induced edema may be the occurrence of mechanical failure of both alveolar epithelium and microvascular endothelium due to the very high alveolar distending pressures. Indeed, the similarities in the ultrastructural aspect of the lungs observed during mechanical ventilation-induced lung injury and during the capillary stress failure that occurs after very large increases in capillary transmural pressure (40 mmHg or more)[19] are quite remarkable and may indicate that both are manifestations of the same spectrum of mechanical lung failure. Thus, pulmonary edema after high-pressure/high-volume ventilation is likely to be the result of the synergistic effects of a very substantial alteration in microvascular permeability and increased filtration pressure. This would explain the fulminating course of such edema which may be produced by very short periods of overinflation in small animals.[20]

In conclusion, cyclic lung overinflation results in pulmonary edema. This edema is of the permeability type and associated with diffuse alveolar damage. It is worth noting that such injury is not the consequence of 'barotrauma' but rather of 'volutrauma'. These observations might be clinically relevant. Indeed, it has been shown that, during acute (or adult) respiratory distress syndrome, the distribution of lung lesion is inhomogeneous.[21] Therefore, owing to uneven distribution of pulmonary compliance, some overdistension of the less damaged zones may occur during mechanical ventilation of such patients, especially when high peak airway pressures are required. The possibility that protracted regional overinflation may worsen preexisting lesions is worthy of consideration.

REFERENCES

1. Pingleton SK (1988) Complications of acute respiratory failure. *American Review of Respiratory Disease* **137:**1463–1493.
2. Webb HH & Tierney DF (1974) Experimental pulmonary edema due to intermittent positive pressure ventilation. Protection by positive end-expiratory pressure. *American Review of Respiratory Disease* **110:**556–565.
3. Kolobow T, Moretti MP, Fumagalli R, Mascheroni D, Prato P, Chen V & Joris M (1987) Severe impairment in lung function induced by high peak airway pressure during mechanical ventilation. An experimental study. *American Review of Respiratory Disease* **135:**312–315.
4. Tsuno K, Prato P & Kolobow T (1990) Acute lung injury from mechanical ventilation at moderately high airway pressures. *Journal of Applied Physiology* **69:**956–961.
5. Parker JC, Townsley MI, Rippe B, Taylor AE & Thigpen J (1984) Increased microvascular permeability in dog lungs due to high peak airway pressures. *Journal of Applied Physiology* **57:**1809–1816.
6. Egan EA, Nelson RM & Olver RE (1976) Lung inflation and alveolar permeability to non-electrolytes in the adult sheep *in vivo*. *Journal of Physiology (London)* **260:**409–424.
7. Dreyfuss D, Basset G, Soler P & Saumon G (1985) Intermittent positive-pressure hyperventilation with high inflation pressures produces pulmonary microvascular injury in rats. *American Review of Respiratory Disease* **132:**880–884.
8. Parker JC, Hernandez LA, Longenecker GL, Peevy K & Johnson W (1990) Lung edema caused by high peak inspiratory pressures in dogs. Role of increased microvascular filtration pressure and permeability. *American Review of Respiratory Disease* **142:**321–328.
9. Carlton DP, Cummings JJ, Scheerer RG, Poulain FR & Bland RD (1990) Lung overexpansion increases pulmonary microvascular protein permeability in young lambs. *Journal of Applied Physiology* **69:**577–583.
10. Dreyfuss D, Soler P, Basset G & Saumon G (1988) High inflation pressure pulmonary edema. Respective effects of high airway pressure, high tidal volume, and positive end-expiratory pressure. *American Review of Respiratory Disease* **137:**1159–1164.
11. Hernandez LA, Peevy KJ, Moise AA & Parker JC (1989) Chest wall restriction limits high airway pressure-induced lung injury in young rabbits. *Journal of Applied Physiology* **66:**2364–2368.
12. Dreyfuss D & Saumon G (1993) Role of tidal volume, FRC, and end-inspiratory volume in the development of pulmonary edema following mechanical ventilation. *American Review of Respiratory Disease* **148:**1194–1203.
13. Bowton DL & Kong DL (1989) High tidal volume ventilation produces increased lung water in oleic acid-injured rabbit lungs. *Critical Care Medicine* **17:**908–911.
14. Hernandez LA, Coker PJ, May S, Thompson AL & Parker JC (1990) Mechanical ventilation increases microvascular permeability in oleic-acid injured lungs. *Journal of Applied Physiology* **69:**2057–2061.
15. Dreyfuss D, Soler P & Saumon G (1995) Mechanical ventilation-induced pulmonary edema: interaction with previous lung alterations. *American Journal of Respiratory and Critical Care Medicine* **151:**1568–1575.
16. Forrest JB (1972) The effect of hyperventilation on pulmonary surface activity. *British Journal of Anaesthesiology* **44:**313–319.

17. Wyszogrodski I, Kyei Aboagye K, Taeusch HW Jr & Avery ME (1975) Surfactant inactivation by hyperventilation: conservation by end-expiratory pressure. *Journal of Applied Physiology* **38:**461–466.
18. Permutt S (1979) Mechanical influences on water accumulation in the lungs. In Fishman AP & Renkin EM (eds) *Pulmonary Edema*. Clinical Physiology Series, pp 175–193. Bethesda: The American Physiological Society.
19. West JB, Tsukimoto K, Mathieu-Costello O & Prediletto R (1991) Stress failure in pulmonary capillaries. *Journal of Applied Physiology* **70:**1731–1742.
20. Dreyfuss D, Soler P & Saumon G (1992) Spontaneous resolution of the pulmonary edema caused by short periods of cyclic overinflation. *Journal of Applied Physiology* **72:**2081–2089.
21. Maunder RJ, Shuman WP, Mc Hugh JW, Marglin SI & Butler J (1986) Preservation of normal lung regions in the adult respiratory distress syndrome. Analysis by computed tomography. *Journal of the American Medical Association* **255:**2463–2465.

18

Role of Arachidonic Acid Metabolites in Vascular and Airway Tone During States of Systemic Inflammation

Gordon R. Bernard

INTRODUCTION

Studies of animal models of sepsis have repeatedly demonstrated that treatment with inhibitors of the cyclooxygenase enzyme improves survival, although the biochemical and physiological mechanisms responsible for this beneficial effect have not been well understood until recently.[1–8] Along with the substantial improvements in analytical techniques as well as increasingly specific metabolic blockers, interpretations of the physiologic effects of cyclooxygenase inhibition have been placed on a more secure biochemical basis.[4,5] There are now substantial data available that link abnormalities of prostaglandin metabolism with airway mechanics abnormalities, pulmonary hypertension and the associated hypoxemia, cardiovascular collapse, and multiple organ failure.[5,8–14]

It is now established that there is continual release of constrictor products of arachidonic acid, especially thromboxane A_2 (TXA_2), into the lung in human sepsis resulting in increased airflow resistance, decreased dynamic compliance, hypoxemia, and increased work of breathing. In addition, potent dilator prostaglandins, especially prostacyclin (PGI_2), are released into the circulation by vascular endothelium and act systemically to produce persistent systemic vasodilation and shock, thus contributing to progressive ischemic damage in the lung and other organs. Both constrictor and dilator effects can coexist in the same organism because of the extremely short half-lives of these compounds, requiring activity proximal to the site of production, and because of differential effects (perhaps by differences in receptor concentrations) across systemic and pulmonary vascular beds.[1,12] This feature of prostaglandin metabolism makes whole animal investigations relating to mechanism difficult. In spite of this, we and others have accumulated a body of laboratory evidence which demonstrates the bronchodilator and pulmonary vasodilator effects of thromboxane inhibition resulting from use of either cyclooxygenase inhibitors or the more specific thromboxane receptor antagonists in sheep.[1,14] In models where systemic vasodilation is the more prominent response to endotoxin, such as the primate and septic dog, cyclooxygenase inhibition with ibuprofen or other cyclooxygenase inhibitors causes (or allows) systemic vasoconstriction and results in restoration of blood pressure and improved survival.[13] Finally, that TXA_2 and PGI_2 can be produced in different amounts and in varying proportions from cells of different origins has been shown in studies comparing macrophages from different species and different sites (e.g. pulmonary resident macrophage versus peritoneal resident macrophage) and may have different effects depending on the nature of the target cell.[15–17]

This discussion will focus on the lung and on the role of ibuprofen because we have had significant experience with this agent in our animal and human studies of acute lung injury. It is likely that substitution of another cyclooxygenase inhibitor for ibuprofen would achieve the same results.

STUDIES IN ANIMALS

The following summary refers to animal studies extensively discussed for two reasons. First of all, appropriate animal models of human disease offer a controlled situation in which to study pulmonary pathophysiology. Second, extensive study has only been conducted in the animal model, and clinical studies at this point are very limited in number and scope. It is important to note that while most of these studies involve 'pretreatment' with ibuprofen, we and others have been able to confirm similar effects when ibuprofen is administered as a 'post-treatment' after the initiation of sepsis syndrome and in a time frame consistent with the realities of clinical medicine and clinical research. Studies described below in which ibuprofen was given after endotoxin or other insults are cited as such.

Pulmonary hypertension

Alterations in pulmonary hemodynamics are a major component of the whole animal response to the administration of a number of agents including endotoxin, glass beads, air emboli, and others, although not oleic acid.[1] The sheep model of endotoxin-induced adult (or acute) respiratory distress syndrome (ARDS) has been particularly useful in studying and elucidating the mechanisms responsible for these changes. Infusion of *Escherichia coli* endotoxin produces a consistent major increase in pulmonary artery pressure (PAP) and pulmonary vascular resistance (PVR) beginning approximately 30–45 min after infusion and persisting for at least 4–5 h. Tumor necrosis factor (TNF) produces a strikingly similar effect except that the response is nearly immediate, a finding compatible with the scenario that endotoxin activates macrophages to produce TNF, therefore suggesting that the endotoxin induced changes in the pulmonary vasculature are TNF mediated. Regardless of the model of acute pulmonary hypertension, cyclooxygenase inhibitors have been capable of causing major attenuation and even total blockade of this response whether delivered prior to or following endotoxin administration.[1,18] Furthermore, studies have suggested that the majority of TXA_2 produced after endotoxin originates in the lung and, possibly because of the short half-life of this compound, it does not cause significant systemic vasoconstriction.[1]

Airway mechanics

Changes in dynamic compliance and airflow resistance are also well-documented responses to administration of endotoxin in the sheep model of ARDS. These changes are severe: a halving of dynamic compliance and a 5–10-fold increase in airflow resistance occurs within 30–45 min of endotoxin infusion and persists for at least 4–5 h.[8,18] These changes can be reversed by nitroprusside, a nonspecific smooth muscle dilator, suggesting that some of these changes are due to bronchospasm rather than to pulmonary edema, airway secretions, or atelectasis.[19] The remainder of the effects may indeed be due to the pulmonary edema component.[20]

Lung microvascular permeability (leak)

Although studies in the sheep endotoxin model show that pretreatment with ibuprofen and other cyclooxygenase inhibitors reduces pulmonary lymph flow, this effect appears to be hydrostatic in nature, i.e. secondary to major reductions in pulmonary microvascular pressure, rather than due to prevention of endothelial cell damage. Beneficial effects of ibuprofen therapy on permeability have been shown in the rat endotoxin alveolitis model[21] as well as the smoke-induced pulmonary edema model.[22]

Gas exchange

Studies in various models of experimentally induced hypoxemia have shown that cyclooxygenase blockade improves oxygenation. In the ethchlorvynol-induced unilateral acute lung injury model in dogs, ibuprofen was shown to both prevent the development of hypoxemia if given as pretreatment and restore oxygenation to control levels if given 60 min after injury.[23] In the canine lobar atelectasis model of hypoxemia, indomethacin restored pulmonary shunt to normal levels compared with controls.[24] In the sheep endotoxin model, pretreatment with ibuprofen prevents the development of hypoxemia after endotoxin.[8]

Multiple organ failure

Although it is difficult to determine cause and effect relationships in complex models of multisystem failure, there is evidence of a more systemic involvement of arachidonic acid metabolites from a variety of models. Studies in rats given infusions of live *E. coli* had significantly improved 24 h survival rates over control animals.[25] Studies in the newborn rat given Group B streptococci (a model of neonatal sepsis) show significantly improved survival if the rats are given ibuprofen at the time of bacterial injection, and a trend toward improved survival if the rats are treated as late as 4 h after bacterial injection. Investigations using the peritonitis and endotoxin models have shown that ibuprofen, whether given as pretreatment or several hours to 1 day after development of sepsis syndrome, is capable of improving systemic blood pressure, decreasing lactic acidosis, and restoring systemic vascular resistance.[12,13] There is even the suggestion that the massive resuscitation given patients in shock can activate the arachidonic acid cascade. Sheep (and humans) given very rapid infusions of concentrated albumin develop pulmonary hypertension, and increased PAWP which are blocked by pretreatment with ibuprofen. There is also evidence that some of the myocardial dysfunction occurring in sepsis is prostaglandin related and may be reversible.[14]

STUDIES IN HUMANS

The cyclooxygenase system

Man has not been well studied with regard to the participation of prostaglandins in the pulmonary, cardiovascular, and other organ dysfunction of sepsis syndrome. Available data suggest that levels of both TXB_2 (a stable metabolite of TXA_2) and 6-keto-prostaglandin $F_{1\alpha}$ (6-keto-$PGF_{1\alpha}$) (a stable metabolite of prostacyclin) are elevated in sepsis in man and that there is a positive correlation between plasma levels and mortality.[25] These studies were conducted in small numbers of patients and relied on plasma values which can be contaminated by prostaglandin products generated *ex vivo* during sampling, especially thromboxane.[26] Only very recently have reliable techniques become readily available to study prostaglandin metabolism in man. The ability to measure metabolites indicative of *in vivo* prostaglandin production but which are not produced *ex vivo* in blood samples, and measurements of metabolites in urine, a fluid generally free of cells that can cause *ex vivo* production, constitute a major advance in this area.[26]

Airway mechanics

Abnormal lung mechanics are an important feature of ARDS, a clinical syndrome of diverse etiology. Studies of gas exchange abnormalities in ARDS have focused on parenchymal alterations resulting from atelectasis, edema, and cellular infiltration. The contribution of active airway dysfunction (bronchospasm) to ARDS has only recently been studied.[27] We performed a second set of studies in order to characterize the airway mechanics abnormalities of ARDS patients receiving mechanical ventilation both inclusive and exclusive of the effects of the endotracheal tube.[27] Others have looked at effects of endotracheal tubes in non-ARDS patients, but no such studies are available in ARDS patients. We found that, even excluding the endotracheal tube resistance, patients with ARDS have airflow resistances more than five times those in other intubated patients, and that dynamic compliance (also grossly abnormal) correlates with $Pa\text{O}_2/P\text{A}\text{O}_2$. Not surprising, but useful clinically, was the fact that peak airway pressure correlates with airflow resistance. In a prospective randomized cross-over design study, we recently examined the effects of aerosolized metaproterenol in patients with established ARDS.[28] Our studies indicated that airflow resistance was approximately 5–6-fold greater in ARDS than in otherwise normal patients intubated for reasons other than lung disease. A 15 min aerosol of 1 mg of metaproterenol reduced airflow resistance by approximately 50%, although values did not reach normal. These data indicate that bronchoconstriction is present in ARDS. Presumably, inhibition of constrictor prostaglandins also allows better ventilation–perfusion matching through dilation of the airways. In addition to potential benefits secondary to improved gas exchange, bronchodilation may lower peak and mean airway pressure, reduce the associated risk of barotrauma, prevent further parenchymal injury, and reduce the work of breathing.[28]

Hypoxemia

Studies in man with regard to the role of prostaglandins in the modulation of ventilation–perfusion matching and hence hypoxemia in sepsis or ARDS have not been forthcoming. However, studies in patients with respiratory failure secondary to pneumonia have revealed significant benefits to gas exchange through the use of cyclooxygenase inhibitors. Hanley et al[29] studied 10 such patients requiring mechanical ventilation and found an increase in $Pa\text{O}_2/F_i\text{O}_2$ from 128±51 to 155±53 mmHg (mean±SD) when patients were given indomethacin 1 mg/kg either orally or rectally, $P < 0.005$. This effect on oxygenation persisted for at least 2 h (no data were collected after this time).

Pulmonary hypertension and edema

There have been no studies in man attempting to establish the role of cyclooxygenase inhibitors in the development of or the persistence of pulmonary edema. If, as the animal studies would suggest, at least some of the pulmonary edema seen is a result of pulmonary hypertension secondary to venoconstriction, then it is possible that reduction in pulmonary microvascular pressure may benefit these patients. Further, if afterload on the right ventricle is reduced by lowering pulmonary vascular resistance from often extremely high levels, then there would be the potential for improving cardiac output and oxygen delivery.[30]

Shock and multiple organ failure

There have been no studies of the effect of cyclooxygenase inhibitors on human shock. However, studies in normal human volunteers given endotoxin clearly show that endotoxin causes release of tumor necrosis factor into the systemic circulation. The timing of this release correlates with increased temperature (2 °F), an increase in heart rate of more than 20 beats per minute, and a doubling of plasma adrenocorticotropin (ACTH) and epinephrine levels. Although shock did not develop at these doses of endotoxin, pretreatment with orally administered ibuprofen blocked all symptoms, attenuated the fever, tachycardia, ACTH peak and epinephrine peak even though the TNF peak was not blocked. These findings led the authors to conclude that the effects of endotoxin administration to humans is mediated through the elaboration of TNF which in turn produces physiologic responses through activation of the cyclooxygenase pathway.[32]

CURRENT CLINICAL STUDIES

We conducted a study relevant to this discussion in patients with established ARDS, the majority of whom were either septic at entry or developed sepsis during the study. Entry and exclusion criteria were as follows: (1) a chest radiograph revealing bilateral diffuse infiltrates consistent with pulmonary edema; (2) a $Pa\text{O}_2 \leq 70$ mmHg with the patient breathing ≥ 40% oxygen or a $Pa\text{O}_2/PA\text{O}_2$ of ≤ 0.3; (3) a pulmonary artery wedge pressure ≤ 18 mmHg; (4) a clinical setting known to be associated with ARDS.

Because corticosteroids are often used in the therapy of ARDS in humans and because some studies have suggested that at least part of the mechanism of these drugs is related to inhibition of prostaglandin production, we thought it would be appropriate to examine the effect of methylprednisolone in our patients. We conducted a multicenter double-blind trial of methylprednisolone (30 mg/kg for four doses versus placebo) in patients with established ARDS as defined above.[32] We found that neither survival nor reversal of ARDS was affected by such therapy. In addition, we examined the data to see if any component of ARDS was ameliorated by therapy. A comparison of the placebo-treated and methylprednisolone-treated patients with regard to measurements of static compliance, oxygenation, and chest radiograph score show no trends toward a treatment effect from methylprednisolone. There was no statistical difference between the groups during the 5 days immediately after therapy.[32]

Finally we conducted pilot studies of the effect of ibuprofen on patients with sepsis syndrome.[33] These studies were intended to provide clinical evidence that cyclooxygenase inhibition in humans (1) is possible, (2) results in clinically measurable positive results, and (3) is reasonably safe in the patient population under consideration here. We found that urinary concentrations of the major metabolites of prostacyclin and thromboxane were markedly increased over normal and that ibuprofen-treated patients experienced a marked decline in these levels. Abnormal physiology such as tachycardia, increased minute ventilation, high peak airway pressure, and oxygenation, and hypotension tended to improve with therapy. No adverse effects of therapy were noted with regard to either bleeding abnormalities or impairment of renal function.

Furthermore, as presented at the American Thoracic Society meeting in May 1996, ibuprofen had no effect on mortality or development/duration of ARDS or shock. It did effectively treat clinical manifestations of the hypermetabolic state of sepsis including the hyperpyrexia, tachycardia, tachypnea and lactic acidosis. Patients who entered the trial hypothermic (temperature < 96°F) did experience a statistically significant reduction in mortality.

In summary, extensive basic scientific and animal research has been conducted into the question of whether or not, as well as how, cyclooxygenase inhibition might work to reduce lung injury in sepsis syndrome. Clinical data in this area are scant but are beginning to accumulate, and the results of our own pilot work suggest that ibuprofen may prove very beneficial in the intensive care setting with regard to blood pressure stabilization, reduction in airway resistance, tachycardia, minute ventilation and fever. Although the preliminary data look promising, the more global effects of cyclooxygenase inhibition on the ultimate survival of the critically ill patient must be examined before routine use of such agents can be recommended.

REFERENCES

1. Brigham KL & Meyrick B (1986) State of the art: endotoxin and lung injury. *American Review of Respiratory Disease* **133:**913–927.
2. Fletcher JR & Ramwell PW (1977) Modification, by aspirin and indomethacin, of the hemodynamic and prostaglandin releasing effects of *E. coli* endotoxin in the dog. *British Journal of Pharmacology* **61:**175–181.
3. Parratt JR & Sturgess RM (1975) *E. coli* endotoxin shock in the cat; treatment with indomethacin. *British Journal of Pharmacology* **53:**485–488.
4. Harris RH, Zmudka M, Maddox Y, Ramwell PW & Fletcher JR (1980) Relationships of TXB_2 and 6-Keto PGF_{1a} to the hemodynamic changes during baboon endotoxic shock. *Advances in Prostaglandin, Thromboxane and Leukotriene Research* **7:**843–849.
5. Bowers RE, Ellis EF, Brigham KL & Oates JA (1979) Effects of prostaglandin cyclic endoperoxides on the lung circulation of sheep. *Journal of Clinical Investigation* **63:**131–137.
6. Northover BJ & Subramanian G (1962) Analgesic-antipyretic drugs as antagonists of endotoxin shock in dogs. *Journal of Pathology and Bacteriology* **83:**463–468.
7. Hinshaw LB, Solomon LA, Erdos EG, Reins DA & Gunter BJ (1967) Effects of acetylsalicylic acid on the canine response to endotoxin. *Journal of Pharmacology and Experimental Therapy* **157:**665–671.
8. Snapper JR, Hutchison AA, Ogletree ML & Brigham KL (1983) Effects of cyclooxygenase inhibitors on the alterations in lung mechanics caused by endotoxemia in the unanesthetized sheep. *Journal of Clinical Investigation* **72:**63–76.
9. Mizus I, Michael J, Summer W & Gurtner G (1983) Acid aspiration induced pulmonary artery pressure rise is attenuated by hypoxia or ibuprofen. *Critical Care Medicine* **11:**241.
10. Perkowski SZ, Havill AM, Flynn JT & Gee MH (1983) Role of intrapulmonary release of eicosanoids and superoxide anion as mediators of pulmonary dysfunction and endothelial injury in sheep with intermittent complement activation. *Circulation Research* **53:**574–583.
11. Perlman MB, Johnson A & Malik AB (1987) Ibuprofen prevents thrombin-induced lung vascular injury: mechanism of effect. *American Journal of Physiology* **252:**H605–H614.

12. Kopolovic R, Thrailkill KM, Martin DT, Ambrose T, Vento M, Carey LC & Cloutier CT (1984) Effects of ibuprofen on a porcine model of acute respiratory failure. *Journal of Surgical Research* **36:**300–305.
13. Jacobs ER, Soulsby ME, Bone RC, Wilson FJ Jr & Hiller FC (1987) Ibuprofen in canine endotoxin shock. *Journal of Clinical Investigation* **70:**536–541.
14. Soulsby ME, Jacobs ER, Perlmutter BH & Bone RC (1984) Protection of myocardial function during endotoxin shock by ibuprofen. *Prostaglandins and Leukotrienes in Medicine* **13:**295–305.
15. Rouzer CA, Scott WA, Hamill AL & Cohn ZA (1982) Synthesis of leukotriene C and other arachidonic acid metabolites by mouse pulmonary macrophages. *Journal of Experimental Medicine* **155:**720–733.
16. Brown KA & Collins AJ (1977) Action of nonsteroidal, anti-inflammatory drugs on human and rat peripheral leucocyte migration *in vitro*. *Annals of Rheumatic Diseases* **36:**239–243.
17. Kaplan HB, Edelson HS, Korchak HM, Given WP, Abramson S & Weissmann G (1984) Effects of non-steroidal anti-inflammatory agents on human neutrophil functions *in vitro* and *in vivo*. *Biochemical Pharmacology* **33:**371–378.
18. Wright PW & Bernard GR (1988) Effects of metaproterenol, atropine and ibuprofen on lung function during the late phase of endotoxemia in sheep. *American Review of Respiratory Disease* **137:**179.
19. Wright P, Ishihara Y & Bernard GR (1988) Effects of nitroprusside on lung mechanics and hemodynamics after endotoxemia in awake sheep. *Journal of Applied Physiology* **64:**2026–2032.
20. Bernard, GR, Pou AN, Coggeshall, JW, Carroll, FE & Snapper JR (1995) Comparison of the pulmonary dysfunction caused by cardiogenic and noncardiogenic pulmonary edema. *Chest* **108:**798–803.
21. Rinaldo JE & Pennock B (1986) Effects of ibuprofen on endotoxin-induced alveolitis. *American Journal of Medical Sciences* **291:**29–38.
22. Shinozawa Y, Hales C, Jung W & Burke J (1986) Ibuprofen prevents synthetic smoke-induced pulmonary edema. *American Review of Respiratory Disease* **134:**1145–1148.
23. Sprague RS, Stephenson AH, Dahms TE, Asner NG & Lonigro AJ (1987) Effects of ibuprofen on the hypoxemia of established ethchlorvynol-induced unilateral acute lung injury in anesthetized dogs. *Chest* **92:**1088–1093.
24. Garrett RC & Thomas HMIII (1983) Meclofenamate uniformly decreases shunt fraction in dogs with lobar atelectasis. *Journal of Applied Physiology* **540:**284–289.
25. Cook JA, Wise WC, Butler RR, Reines HD, Rambo W & Halushka PV (1984) The potential role of thromboxane and PGI_2 in endotoxic and septic shock. *American Journal of Emergency Medicine* **2:**28–37.
26. FitzGerald GA, Pedersen AK & Patrono C (1983) Analysis of prostacyclin and thromboxane biosynthesis in cardiovascular disease. *Circulation* **67:**1174–1177.
27. Wright PW, Marini JJ & Bernard GR (1988) Increased airway resistance contributes to impaired lung mechanics in the ARDS. *American Review of Respiratory Disease* **137:**137.
28. Wright PE, Carmichael LC & Bernard GR (1994) Effect of bronchodilators on lung mechanics in the acute respiratory distress syndrome (ARDS). *Chest* **106:**1517–1523.
29. Hanly PJ, Roberts D, Dobson K & Light RB (1987) Effect of indomethacin on arterial oxygenation in critically ill patients with severe bacterial pneumonia. *Lancet* 351–354.
30. Hasselstrom LJ, Eliasen K, Mogensen T & Andersen JB (1985) Lowering pulmonary artery pressure in a patient with severe acute respiratory failure. *Intensive Care Medicine* **11:**48–50.

31. Michie HR, Manogue KR, Spriggs DR, Revhaug A, O'Dwyer S, Dinarello CA, Cerami A, Wolff SM & Wilmore DW (1988) Detection of circulating tumor necrosis factor after endotoxin administration. *New England Journal of Medicine* **318:**1481–1486.
32. Bernard GR, Luce JM, Sprung CL, Rinaldo JE, Tate RM, Sibbald WJ, Kariman K, Higgins S, Bradley R, Metz CA, Harris TR & Brigham KL (1987) High-dose corticosteroids in patients with the adult respiratory distress syndrome. *New England Journal of Medicine* **317:**1565–1570.
33. Bernard GR, Reines HD, Halushka PV, Higgins SB, Metz CA, Swindell BB, Wright PE, Watts FL, & Vrbanac JJ (1991) Prostacyclin and thromboxane A_2 formation in human sepsis syndrome: Effects of cyclooxygenase inhibition. *American Review of Respiratory Disease* **144:**1095–1101.

19

Pulmonary Edema Reabsorption: New Therapeutic Strategies

Luis Oppenheimer
A. Smit
A. Palomar

INTRODUCTION

We have developed diagnostic and therapeutic strategies based on the application of well-known physiologic principles of transvascular fluid and macromolecular exchange. These are passive principles which do not specifically include more recent knowledge regarding the participation of transcellular ionic and water exchange.

EXPERIMENTAL BASIS FOR OUR CLINICAL APPROACH

The concepts to be presented in this work were developed from information obtained from isolated canine lobe preparations, which are commonly used to estimate transvascular fluid exchange. Excised pulmonary lobes are suspended from force transducers for continuous weight estimates (Figure 1). They are perfused with blood, and pulmonary capillary pressure (P_c) is changed by adjustments in the venous reservoir. In this preparation, we have interposed a spectrophotometric device capable of obtaining very accurate determinations of on-line hematocrit.[1] This device continuously measures the proportion of 815 nm light emitted by a 100 mW CW laser diode, which is transmitted across the column of perfusate. We have demonstrated a very good correlation between the logarithm of the signal proportional to light transmission and hematocrit.[1] We have also shown that changes in hematocrit

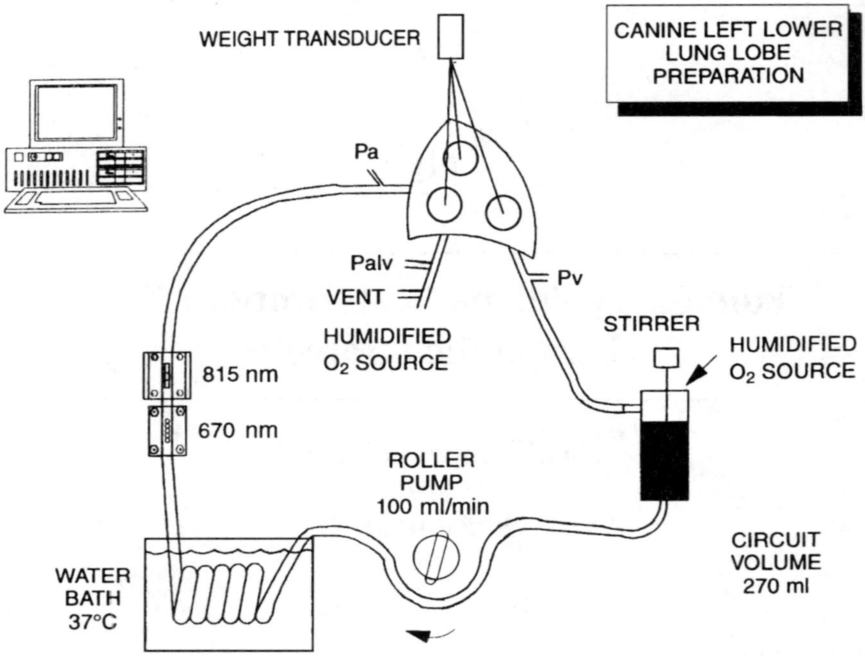

Figure 1. Isolated lobe preparation with two spectrophotometric devices.

(Hct) correspond very well to the volume of fluid exchanged with the lobe (V_E) according to the following equation:

$$V_E = C_V(1 - \text{Hct}_i/\text{Hct}_{(t)}) \tag{1}$$

where C_V represents the initial circuit volume, and Hct_i and $\text{Hct}_{(t)}$ represent initial and on-line changes in Hct at any given time (t). A representative experiment is summarized in Figure 2. At any given time, the rate of edema formation (Q_F) can be obtained as follows:

$$Q_F = \Delta V_E/\Delta t \tag{2}$$

Note that Q_F is proportional to P_c and that for each P_c, Q_F (the slope of the curve) is relatively constant, suggesting stable conditions.

As described in the Starling equation (eqn. 3),

$$Q_F = K_F\,(\Delta P - \sigma\Delta\pi) \tag{3}$$

Q_F is not only related to the transvascular hydrostatic gradient (ΔP), but is also influenced by the transmural colloid osmotic gradient ($\Delta\pi$), which is the result of protein concentration differences across the vessel wall, and must be related to the membrane permeability to protein by the reflection coefficient (σ). The filtration coefficient (K_F) takes into account membrane permeability and surface area.

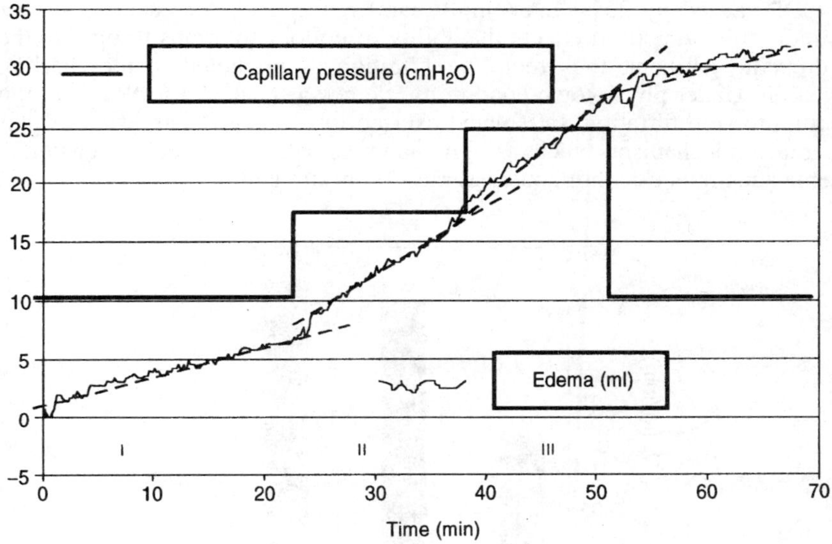

Figure 2. Filtration time courses after three step increases in P_c.

The role of transvascular colloid osmotic pressure (COP) in transvascular fluid exchange remains controversial, particularly in the clinical literature. We have previously reported decreases in Q_F for comparable capillary hydrostatic pressures (P_c) when 25% human serum albumin (25%HSA) was added to the perfusate.[2] However, these were not direct estimates of Q_F. We have repeated these experiments using the spectrophotometric technique described above. The addition of 25%HSA (30 ml) doubled COP from an average of 16±2 mmHg to 31±2 mmHg (Figure 3).

As shown in Figure 4, when compared with control (solid bars) the increase

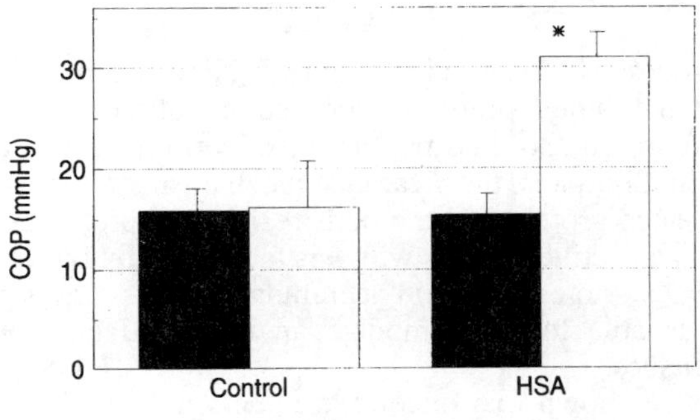

Figure 3. Addition of 25% HSA significantly increased COP. ■, Baseline; □, after intervention. *Significantly different from control and baseline.

in COP caused by 25%HSA (empty bars) reduced Q_F for each P_c. In our opinion, this reduction reflects the ability of colloid solutions to oppose the hydrostatic gradient, thus retarding filtration as predicted in the Starling equation. Under physiologic conditions, we never reached a COP level high enough to stop filtration. In isolated excised lobe preparations, where water clearance mechanisms such as lymphatic vessels have been interrupted, edema accumulates continuously at rates proportional to P_c.

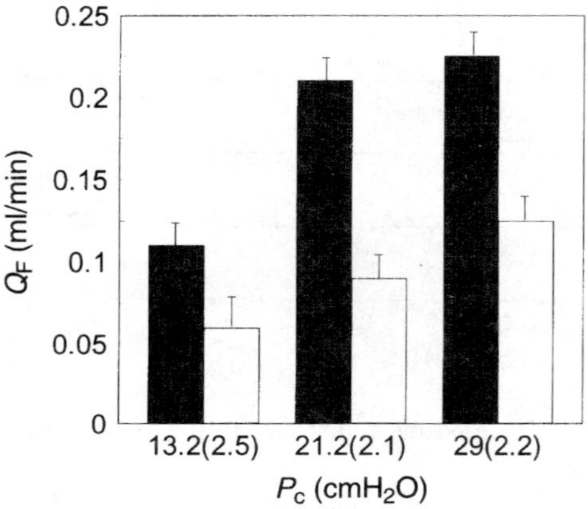

Figure 4. Rates of edema formation before and after the addition of 25% HSA for each P_c. ■, Control; □, 25% HSA. Values in parentheses are standard deviations.

Tissue hydration, oncotic gradients and fluid clearance

Even though oncotic gradients partially off-set hydrostatic forces, as explained above, there is always net filtration into the tissues. To maintain the tissues at optimal hydration, fluid-clearance mechanisms (Q_{Cl}) have been developed. The best understood (but likely not the only one) is the lymphatic system. At any time, hydration (Q_H) is the net result of filtration and clearance:

$$Q_H = Q_F - Q_{Cl} \qquad (4)$$

This general process is illustrated in Figure 5. Note two important features: (1) except for the blood–brain barrier, the membrane is not completely impermeable to protein, so, in time, the oncotic gradient would be gradually dissipated; (2) in all organs, the clearance mechanisms return the excess fluid and the extravasated protein to the bloodstream. As represented by a pump in the figure, this is an active process which is facilitated by lymphatic pumping. So long as $Q_F = Q_{Cl}$, no edema fluid accumulates. If a point is reached where Q_{Cl} no longer is able to accommodate an increased Q_F, net edema fluid accumulation ensues.

So far, we have shown that oncotic gradients induced by plasma protein reduce Q_F for each P_c in normal lungs. We have also explored the possibility of reducing Q_F when permeability is increased.

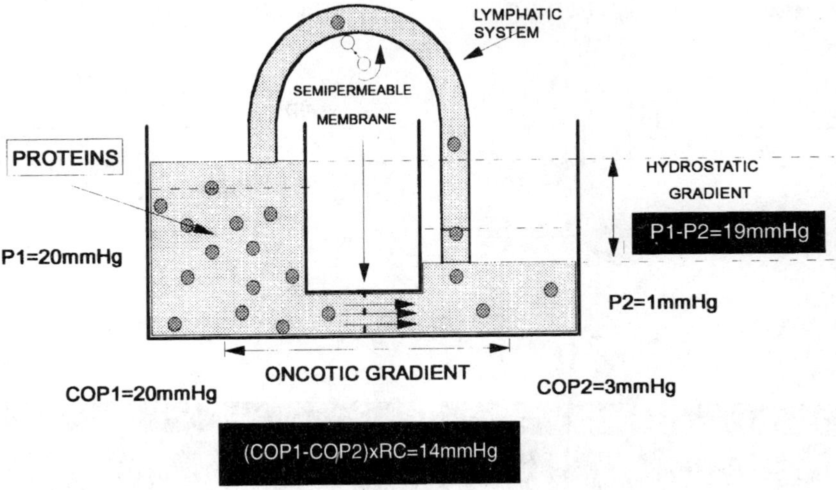

Figure 5. Idealized model of fluid exchange between intra- and extravascular compartments. RC denotes reflection coefficient and could be substituted by σ.

ONCOTIC MANIPULATIONS IN ACUTE LUNG INJURY (ALI)

Early ALI is characterized by increased alveolocapillary permeability and a corresponding decrease in the transvascular oncotic gradient. The resulting increase in transvascular filtration is such that clearance mechanisms are overwhelmed and pulmonary edema ensues. Theoretically, and depending on the severity of the ALI, it may be possible to reduce filtration by manipulation of transvascular forces. Filtration would be decreased with reductions in pulmonary capillary hydrostatic pressure (P_c) or increases in effective colloid oncotic pressure.

In very severe ALI induced with intravenous oleic acid (OA), Prewitt et al[3] successfully treated lung edema with significant reductions in P_c. This treatment approach has been used in patients with some degree of success.[4] In Prewitt's study, the addition of human serum albumin to increase COP failed to reduce edema, presumably because in this lesion the increase in microvascular permeability precluded the development of an effective oncotic gradient with the addition of such a small macromolecule.

We have been successful in re-establishing oncotic gradients in conditions of increased permeability to protein in dogs. This was accomplished with the use of 6% Hetastarch, a commercially available polydisperse solution. As shown in Figure 6, by presenting the injured membrane with a wide range of fractions, we expected some to leak, but hoped the larger ones would be retained. Conceivably, the retained fractions would be able to re-establish an oncotic gradient sufficient to allow Q_{Cl} to bring the affected organ back to normal hydration. Since the oncotic effect (a molar property) is inversely related to molecular weight (MW), how much colloid is needed to normalize the oncotic gradient in conditions of increased permeability is contingent on

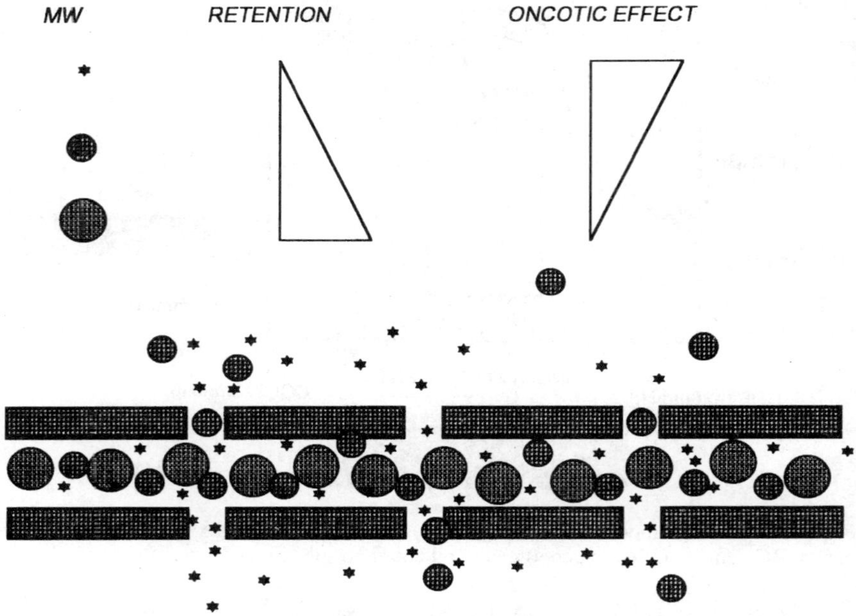

Figure 6. Idealized representation of transvascular macromolecular exchange. Small particles leak, whereas larger fractions may be retained. The oncotic effect decreases as size increases.

the MW of the retained fractions. Polysaccharide macromolecular solutions are widely used as plasma substitutes. As opposed to plasma proteins, which represent a mixture of discrete molecular weights), the above mentioned solutions are polydisperse, i.e. they include a wide range of molecular sizes. We hypothesized that, when such a solution is added to the circulation in the presence of severe ALI, the injured membrane may be able to retain large macromolecules, while smaller species would cross the microvascular membrane. If so, it may be possible to develop an effective transvascular oncotic gradient based on the retained macromolecules, if appropriate amounts of the polydisperse solution are infused. To test this hypothesis, after severe ALI was induced with intravenous OA as described by Prewitt et al,[3] we infused 6% Hetastarch (6%HS), which includes hydroxyethyl starch molecules ranging in MW from 10 000 to 2 000 000. The infusion was maintained until COP had increased by about 25 mmHg. This arbitrary goal was selected assuming a net macromolecular retention of the order of 50%, and consequently, an effective transvascular oncotic gradient about half the increase in COP (about 12.5 mmHg). Such an increase in the transvascular oncotic gradient was expected to counteract or even exceed the transvascular hydrostatic gradient and reduce edema accumulation. Because of the large volumes of 6%HS required to achieve this goal, circulating blood volume (CBV) was maintained constant with the use of continuous hemofiltration (CH). In this way, increases in transvascular hydrostatic pressure or decreases in plasma protein concentration were prevented. Since CH has been used as a method of eliminating circulating mediators[5,6] in a treatment control group, we infused and ultrafiltered comparable volumes of normal saline.

One hour after the infusion of OA, a severe ALI developed characterized by hypoxemia. On average, the $P\text{aO}_2$ decreased by about 70%, whereas no significant hemodynamic or gas-exchange abnormalities developed in the control group. Sieve chromatographic analysis of dextran 40 000 (D40) and dextran 500 000 (D500) fractions suggested preferential loss of the D40 fraction, which decreased significantly ($P<0.05$) from 51.3±6.4 to 39.7±7.3% in the ALI group, while no significant changes occurred in the control experiments (Figure 7). The preferential loss of small fractions suggested that oncotic gradients may be developed through the large fractions.

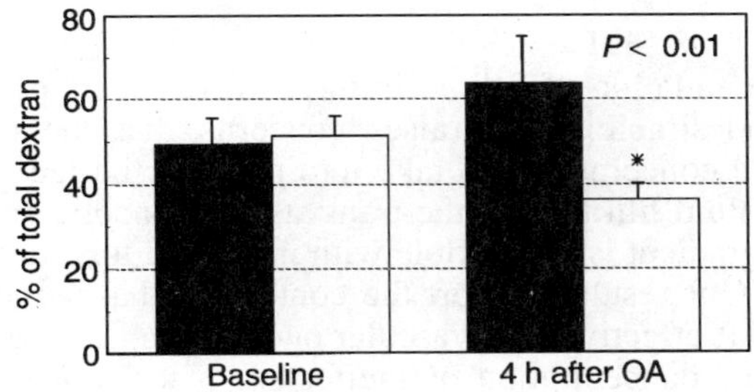

Figure 7. Preferential loss of D40 after OA infusion. ■, D500; □, D40.

This was confirmed in the gravimetric analysis of the lungs at the end of the experiments (Figure 8), where the wet weight to body weight ratio (WW/BW) of 6%HS-treated animals (24.9±5.8 g/kg) was about 30% lower ($P<0.05$) than that of controls (34.3±11.8 g/kg). Note that the dry weight to body weight ratio (DW/BW) of the 6%HS-treated group (2.81±0.29 g/kg) was significantly increased over the controls (2.33±0.3 g/kg), presumably reflecting significant extravasation of colloid into the extravascular space (Figure 9).

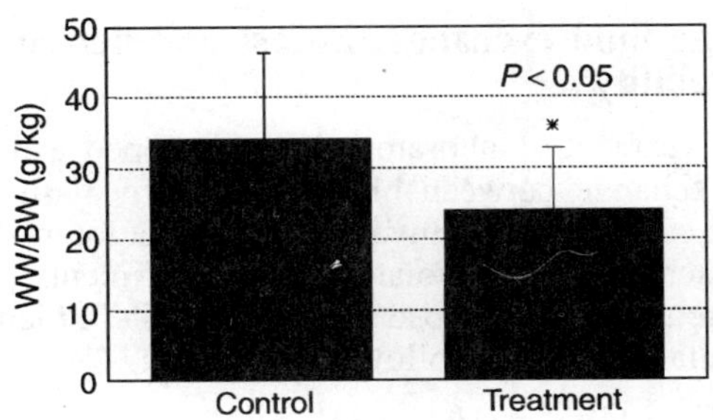

Figure 8. Effect of 6%HS treatment on lung edema in dogs.

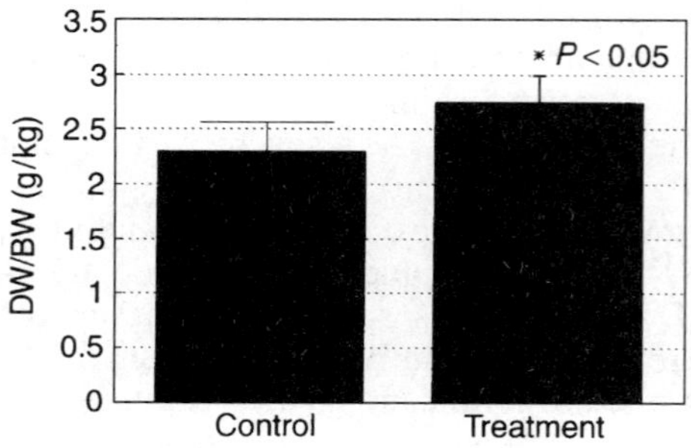

Figure 9. Effect of 6%HS treatment on dry weight/body weight ratio in dogs. Significant extravasation of macromolecules occurred.

Potential accumulation of colloid in the extravascular space is commonly regarded as undesirable, as it raises concerns that the disease may be worsened. These concerns fail to take into account the fact that the driving force opposing fluid filtration is the transvascular oncotic gradient, and that increasing this gradient is compatible with increased final lung tissue colloid concentrations. Our results support the contention that reductions in edema can be achieved if effective transvascular oncotic gradients are reestablished, even if the tissue concentration of ineffective macromolecular fractions is increased.

CLINICAL STUDY

Successful mobilization of edema increases the CBV and filling pressures (P_c), and dilutes the oncotic agent. In other words, when successful, this process is self-limiting because it will result in increases in P_c and decreases in COP, both of which favor filtration. Consequently, the approach needs to include a way to remove the mobilized edema fluid in order to prevent auto-dilution of the oncotic agent, and also to prevent increases in CBV. To address all the above mentioned issues we have developed a monitoring approach.

Monitoring of the fluid exchange process and determination of capillary permeability

Over the last 10 years, this laboratory has developed a device capable of following fluid exchange between blood and bodily tissues. This methodology is based on continuous noninvasive determination of Hct and is based on the device described in the isolated lobe experiments. It is included in extracorporeal circuits such as those used in dialysis. Fractional changes in CBV can be calculated with the following equation:

$$CBV = (Hct_{final} - Hct_{initial})/Hct_{initial} \quad (5)$$

We have taken advantage of continuous renal replacement modalities, such as continuous arteriovenous (CAVH) or venovenous (CVVH) hemofiltration. Because there was a question as to whether the establishment of extracorporeal circuits (an invasive procedure which requires heparinization) could be justified in this patient population, initially we used periodic determinations of microhematocrit to guide our treatment, and relied on diuresis to eliminate excess reabsorbed fluid. This approach proved very labor intensive and impractical. We also found that oncotic manipulations influence diuresis and we could not rely on normal kidneys to effectively eliminate the mobilized edema fluid, particularly at rates required to prevent increases in CBV. We therefore now feel justified in establishing ultrafiltration circuits in all patients about to undergo oncotic manipulations, but allow an initial trial with diuresis. In our experience, the CVVH modality is the most reliable. We interpose our hematocrit monitor in all circuits, not only to monitor the fluid-exchange process, but also to assist in determinations of capillary permeability, the choice of oncotic agent, and the dose of colloid to be administered.

General protocol presently in use

Over time, and as the number of treated patients for many of the various conditions listed above increased, our general approach has become better defined with the experience gained. Patients must not be actively bleeding. We have now developed the general protocol shown in Figure 10 in patients with clinical criteria for ALI.

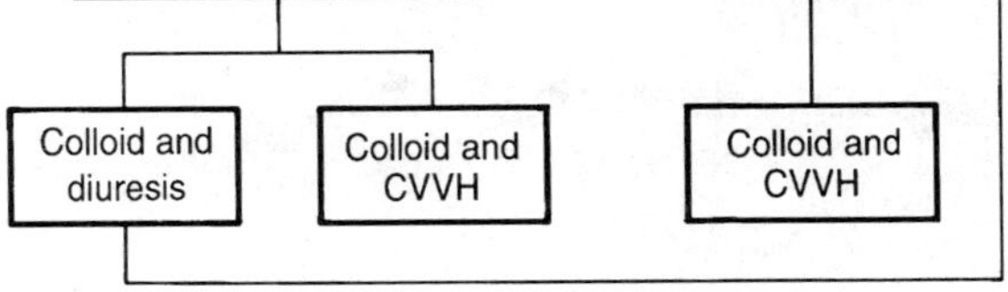

Figure 10. Treatment algorithm for patients with clinical criteria for acute lung injury.

Patients with $Pa\text{O}_2/F_i\text{O}_2$ ratio less than 100

At the time of recruitment, these patients were already on maximal therapy. Our approach was as follows.

Loading phase

After insertion of a hemodialysis catheter, patients were placed on a CVVH circuit. Pentastarch was infused at a rate of 1 liter/h, which was matched by the rate of ultrafiltration. Consequently, patients should remain euvolemic and CBV should not change. As the COP increases (Figure 11A; ◇) a point is reached where CBV increases progressively towards 20% greater than control (Figure 11A; ■). In conditions where the rate of infusion was matched by the rate of ultrafiltration, we accepted this increase in CBV as proof that the colloid infusion had achieved its goal of fluid mobilization, stopped the infusion and proceeded to the mobilization phase. The pentastarch infusion was also stopped if there was significant improvement in the $Pa\text{O}_2/F_i\text{O}_2$ ratio, or if 2 liters were infused without change in CBV. This would be consistent with a massive macromolecular leak, which would preclude the success of this approach. Unless there was a specific contraindication, heparin was used to prevent clotting of the extracorporeal circuit.

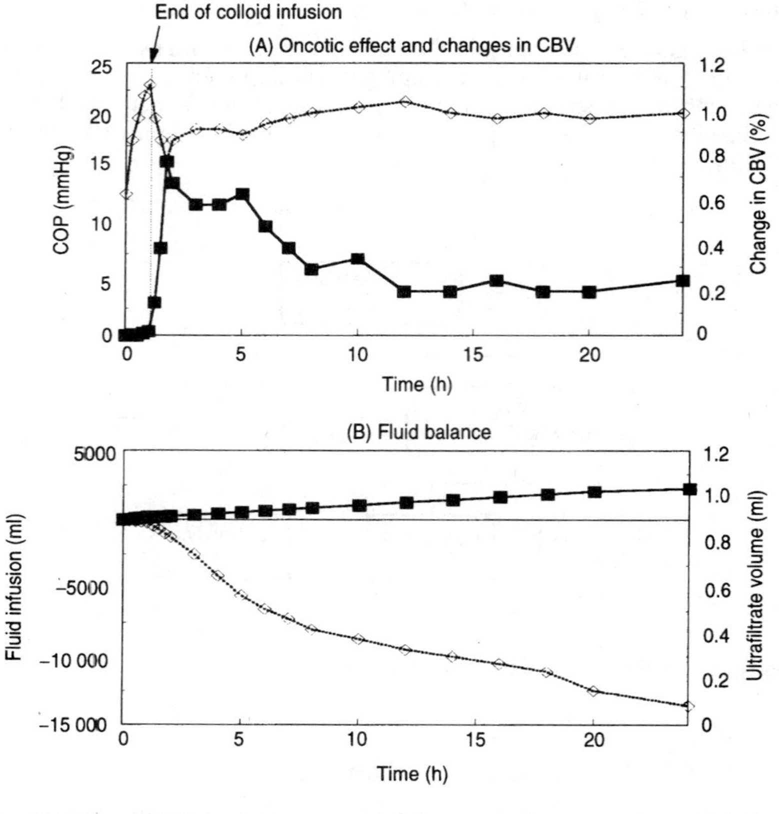

Figure 11. Effect of infusion of Pentastarch on COP and CBV (A) and fluid balance (B). In (A) ■, change in CBV; ◇, COP. In (B) ■, infusion; ◇, removal.

Mobilization phase

Once the infusion of pentastarch was stopped, ultrafiltration was continued to achieve fluid mobilization, until CBV returned towards normal (Figure 11A). Note how the COP remains constant for a long period of time. The procedure was repeated, if necessary, until the $Pa{O_2}/F_i{O_2}$ ratio improved, or it became evident that the approach would not be successful. Typically, significant negative fluid balances were required to improve the condition (Figure 11B). These negative balances were achieved without negative hemodynamic consequences. This was due to the fact that our approach ensures that CBV is never below baseline. On the contrary, it has become our experience that, as CBV increases with successful fluid resuscitation, hemodynamics improve and the need for inotropes and vasopressors is reduced. Presumably, many of these patients are kept relatively hypovolemic.

Other patients with the clinical diagnosis of ALI

All other patients were randomized into diuresis and CVVH groups. The principles outlined above were followed, except that diuresis was used for fluid mobilization. If diuresis became difficult to achieve, or the condition continued to deteriorate, patients were placed on CVVH.

Summary of clinical results

A summary of our clinical results to date is shown in Table 1. Overall, this approach was particularly successful in patients with exclusive pulmonary lesions, where both the lung improvement and survival figures were excellent. In patients with multiorgan disease, we were able to achieve pulmonary improvements in about 80%. However, almost 40% did die ultimately from other causes. So far, these figures do not seem to represent a significant improvement over accepted outcomes, except for the fact that most patients in this category were treated when all other measures had failed. In this context, our approach may offer better results if started earlier. Of particular interest to us was the fact that, invariably, our adjustments of CBV allowed us to reduce the need for inotropes and vasopressors. If this exercise is started earlier, perhaps it will decrease the incidence of multiorgan failure.

The most common side effect of oncotic manipulations was oliguria and a

Table 1. Summary of clinical results.

Problem	No. of patients	Mode (D/CVVH)	Negative balance (liters)	No. improved	No. survived
Burns	3	1/2	12.8(2.3)	3	2
Lung rejection	3	1/2	4.5(1.6)	3	3
Lung contusion	2	2/0	6.7(2.2)	2	2
Aspiration	3	2/1	5.6(1.8)	3	3
Sepsis	11	5/6	9.6(3.6)	9	7
Total	22	10/12		20	17

D, diuresis.

biochemical picture consistent with prerenal failure. This phenomenon likely reflects colloid-induced reduction in glomerular filtration. It was always present when COP was increased above 30 mmHg. However, in all cases, baseline renal function was recovered as the COP returned to baseline levels.

This is still a preliminary study. However, the results are encouraging and warrant further study, perhaps on a multicenter basis.

REFERENCES

1. Oppenheimer L & Huebert D (1993) Near-infrared spectrophotometric device to measure fluid exchange in blood-perfused organs. *Journal of Applied Physiology* **74:**2205–2213.
2. Hancock BJ Hoppensack M & Oppenheimer L (1989) Do transvascular forces in isolated lobe preparations equilibrate? *Journal of Applied Physiology* **67:**628–635.
3. Prewitt RM, McCarthy J & Wood LD (1981) Treatment of acute low pressure pulmonary edema in dogs. *Journal of Clinical Investigation* **67:**409–418.
4. Sznajder JI & Wood LD (1991) Beneficial effects of reducing pulmonary edema in patients with acute hypoxemic respiratory failure (editorial; comment). *Chest* **100:**890–892.
5. Gotloib L, Barzilay E, Shustak A & Lev A (1984) Sequential hemofiltration in nonoliguric high capillary permeability pulmonary edema of severe sepsis: preliminary report. *Critical Care Medicine* **12(11):**997–1000.
6. Gotloib L, Barzilay E, Shustak A, Jaichenko J & Lev A (1986) Hemofiltration in septic ARDS. The artificial kidney as an artificial endocrine lung. *Resuscitation* **13(2):**123–132.

Index

Numbers in italics refer to tables or illustrations; numbers in bold refer to main discussion

A23187, calcium ionophore, 132
acetylcholine, 18, *19*, 26, 35, 87, 111, 128, 140
  fetal lamb response, 28
  reduced effect in hypoxia, 132
acetylsalicylic acid, *181*, 182
acidemia in COPD, 230
acute lung injury, 4, 6–7, 33, 37, **77**, **81–2**
  alterations of vasomotor control, 35, 37
  alveolar membrane, loss of protein-sieving function, 243
  ANP levels, 47
  associated conditions and factors, *78*
  endothelial lesions, 215
  hypoxic pulmonary vasoconstriction (HPV), 86
  increased respiratory resistance, 216–17
  NO inhalation, 41, 42
    co-administration with almitrine, 194, 195–6, *197*
  oncotic manipulations, 275–8
    treatment protocol, *279*
  pathogenesis, 82–4
  pathophysiology, 85–6
  role of PMNs, 241, 244–5
acute (or adult) respiratory distress syndrome (ARDS), 3, 5, 148, 189
  airway mechanics, 264–5
  almitrine, 190–2, 193, 194
  associated conditions and factors, *78*
  CD11/CD18 expression on granulocytes, 84
  cyclooxygenase inhibitors
    animal models, 262–3
    clinical studies, 266–7
  diagnostic criteria, *85*
  high pressure/high volume ventilation, 257–8
  hypoxic pulmonary vasoconstriction (HPV), 86
  inhaled NO, 139, 141, 203, 208, 209, 234
    co-administration of almitrine, 190, **194–8**
    dose-response curves, 218–22
    effect on right ventricular function, 148–9
    increased respiratory resistance, 217
    neonates 115
    pulmonary thromboemboli prevention, 215
    trial, 41
  intravenous PGE_1, 45
  intravenous PGI_2, 44
  neutrophils (PMNs), 6–7, 241, 242, 244, **246**
  pulmonary hypertension, 175–6
    experimental, 178–9
    mechanisms of, 179–81
  pulmonary vascular tone
    and gas exchange, 181–3
    role of endothelium, 77–97
  role of ET-1, 67, 70
  sepsis, 77, 81, 82
  TXA_2 and leukotrienes, 95
  ventricular coupling, 183–5
acute renal failure, 69
adenylate cyclase, 45

adhesion molecules (CAM)
  adhesion cascade, 82, 84
alkalosis-induced mechanical hyperventilation, 116
almitrine, 5–6, **182–3**, **191–4**
  co-administration with NO, 189, 190, **194–8**
alveolar
  barrier, anatomy and function, 242–4
  dead space, decrease in, NO inhalation, 213, *214*
  distension and pulmonary edema, 253–8
  edema, 206
  hypoxia, 126, 130, 144, **190**, **191**
  interface, 6–7
  macrophages, 241, 247
  pressure increase, relationship with mean PAP, *231*
  recruitment, 6
    PEEP-induced, 212
aminoguanidine, 91
amyl nitrite, 18
angina pectoris, 18
antiplatelet effects
  NO, 41, 215
  PGE_1, 45
  PGI_2, 43
aortic
  pulse pressure, 183
  smooth muscle cells, ET-1, 61
apparent outflow pressure, 178
arachidonic acid metabolites
  eicosanoids, 63, 70, 95
    fetal and transitional circulation, 109
    in HPV, 96
  role in vascular tone
    ARDS, 95–6
    systemic inflammation, 261–7
  see also cyclooxygenase (COX); leukotrienes; prostaglandins; thromboxane
arginine *see* L-arginine
arterial
  oxygenation, effect NO inhalation, 195
  PO_2, NO inhalation, 142
  pressure, systemic, inhibition of L-arginine pathway, 23
arterial to venous ET-1 ratio, **65–6**, 70
arterioles, systemic, NO production, 26
aspirin, *181*, 182
asthma
  aerosolized PGI_2, 44
  cNOS levels, 4
  exhaled NO, **11**, 129, 140
  inhaled NO, 141, 206, 217
  role of ET-1, 67, 70
ATP, 18, 132, **192**
  mesenteric ischemia-reperfusion, 37
atrial natriuretic peptide (ANP), 35
  as therapeutic vasodilator, **46–7**, 107
auto-inhalation NO, endotracheal intubation, 2, 12
autoregulation, fetal pulmonary circulation, 107–8

β-adrenergic signal transduction, hypoxia, 37
balloon occlusion angiography, 180
barotrauma, 7, 253
  see also volutrauma
BE-18257A, cyclic pentapeptide, 68
BE-18257B, cyclic pentapeptide, 68
big ET-1, 57, 58, 60, 112
  fetal hemodynamic response, 113
birth
  onset of ventilation, 108
  PGI_2 synthesis, 109–10
  pulmonary vascular resistance (PVR), 108, 109, 111
  spike release of ET-1, 114
bleeding time, NO inhalation, 215, *216*
BM 13505, TXA_2 receptor antagonist, 64
BN52021, PAF receptor antagonist, 64
bosentan, 69
BQ-123, ET_A receptor antagonist, 62, 67, **68**, 69, 92
  hemodynamic effects, fetal lung, 113–14
BQ-788, ET_B-specific antagonist, 68
bradykinin (BK), 18, **64–5**
8-bromo-cGMP, 107
bronchiolar smooth muscle, ET-1, 70
bronchoalveolar lavage fluid
  IgM and α_2-macroglobulin, 243
  inflammatory cells, NO inhalation, 206
  neutrophils (PMNs), 242, 246
  protein concentration HAPE, 244
bronchoconstriction, metacholine-induced, 216

calcium
  activation of NOS,, 38
  elevation of cytosolic 65
  and endothelial shear, 25–7
calmodulin, 20, 38

cAMP *see* cyclic adenosine monophosphate (cAMP)
capillary permeability, determination of, 278–9
cardiac
  catheterization
    hemodynamic study, oxygen therapy devices, 160, 164, *165*
    NO inhalation, preoperative, 150, 152
  index, NO inhalation in ARDS, 149
  output
    co-administration almitrine and NO, 195, 196
    COPD exacerbations, 231
    NO inhalation, 209
  see also heart
catecholamines, 222
CD11 molecules, 84
CD18 molecules, 84
  blockade, 245
cGMP *see* cyclic guanosine monophosphate (cGMP)
CGS 27830, ET receptor blocker, 114
characteristic impedance Z_c, 183–4
chemiluminescence, 21, *22*, 204
  continuous recordings, NO concentrations, *205*
  exhaled NO, 10
  intratracheal NO_2 concentrations, 206, *207*
CHIP28 protein, 243
chronic lung lymph model, NO inhalation, 42
chronic obstructive pulmonary disease (COPD), 33, 182
  hypoxia, 37
    chronic hypoxic pulmonary hypertension, 126
  nasal prongs versus oxygen-saving devices study, 157–68
  PGE_1 administration, 45
  pulmonary vascular tone, ventilated patients, 229–37
    selective vasodilation, acute exacerbations, 234–6
  role of NO, 139–44
    inhaled, 4, 6, **141–4**, 189, 203
    reduced synthesis, 139–41
  structural changes, pulmonary artery intima, 132
circulating blood volume (CBV), oncotic manipulations, 276, 278, 279, 280, 281
  calculating changes in, 278
citrulline, 2, 20, *21*, 110
closing pressure, vascular, 5, **177**, **178**
cNOS *see* constitutive NOS (cNOS)
collagen
  production, 65
  vascular disease, systemic, 45
colloid osmotic pressure (COP), 7, 278, 282
  Hetastarch (6% HS) infusion, 276
  human serum albumin (25% HSA) infusion, **273–4**, 275
  Pentastarch infusion, *280*
conduit arteries, 192
congenital diaphragmatic hernia (CDH)
  inhaled NO, 115
  surfactant therapy, 116
congenital heart disease, inhaled NO effect on right ventricular function, 150–1
constitutive NOS (cNOS), 2, 3, 4, 9, 12, 38, 84, 87, 110, 128
  airway-exhaled, 4
  characteristics, *88*
  sepsis, 90
continuous hemofiltration, 276–7
  arteriovenous (CAVH), 279, 280, 281
  venovenous (CVVH), 279
cor pulmonale, 167, 168, 234
coronary arteries, constriction with L-NMMA, 23, *24*
cremaster artery, vessel diameter and intracellular Ca^{2+}, 26
critical closing pressure *see* closing pressure, vascular
cryptographic fibrosing alveolitis (CFA), ET-1 expression, 66
CV-6209, PAF receptor antagonist, 63
cyanocobalamin, 243
cyclic adenosine monophosphate (cAMP)
  acute lung injury, 35, 37
  vasodilation, 34–5
cyclic guanosine monophosphate (cGMP), 38, 39, 87, **110–11**
  breakdown catalysed by PDE_5, 28
  cGMP PDE
    activity, 114
    inhibition, 112
  vasodilation, 18, *19*, 20, 34, **35**, 37
cyclic pentapeptide ET antagonists 68
cycloheximide, 92
cyclooxygenase (COX), 65, 84, **95**
  inhibitors, 7, 63, 96, 110, 182, 261
    systemic inflammation, 262–4, 265–7

cyclooxygenase (COX) (*cont.*)
  products in sepsis, 96
  system, humans, 264
cytokines, 82, 84, 96, 246, 247

diltiazem, 180, 181
dipyridamole, 112, 116
diuresis and oncotic manipulations, 279, 281
dobutamine administration, COPD patients, 232, *233*
dose-response curves, inhaled NO, 217–22
double-lumen endotubes, split lung VCO_2 measurement, 172
ductus arteriosus, 107, 114
  compression, 26, *27*
  patency, PGE_1, 110

E. coli, animal models
  cyclooxygenase inhibitors, 262–3, 264
  PMN migration, 245, 248
E-selectin, 84
echocardiography, home oxygen therapy study, 159, 164, 167
edema formation (Q_F), rate of, 272, 273, 274
eicosanoids, 63, 70, 95
  fetal and transitional circulation, 109
  in HPV, 96
  see also leukotrienes; prostaglandins
ejection fraction (EF)
  home oxygen therapy study, 159, 161, 164, 167
    mean values, *161*
  right ventricular, 147, 148, 149, 185, 234, 235
electrochemical monitoring, NO toxicity, 204
emphysema-like lesions, 206
end-tidal carbon dioxide tension ($PetCO_2$), NO inhalation, 213, *214*
endopeptidase, 46
endothelial cells, 57, 242
  ET release, 70, **94**
    inhibition, endogenous BK, 65
  ET_{B1} receptor activation, 62
  fetal circulation, 108
    role in regulating vascular tone, 108–14
  hypoxia, 34, 127, 230
  injury, ultrastructural changes, 82, 127
  metabolism of L-arginine to NO, *22*
  NO release, 132, 203, **215**
  PMN injury, 244
  preproET-1 mRNA expression, 66
  shear stress, **25–7**, 131
endothelial NOS (eNOS), 28, 114
endothelial–leukocyte adhesion molecule-1 (E-selectin), 84
endothelin receptors, 4, **61–3**, 66, **92**, 95, 112
  distribution and function, *62*
  fetal and newborn lung, 112, 113–14
endothelin-converting enzyme (ECE), 58, 60, 92, 112
endothelins (ETs), 3, 4, **47–8**, **57**, 84, **91–5**, 125, 127, 208
  amino acid sequence, *59*
  antagonists and inhibitors, **68–9**, 70–1
  ET-1, 47, 48, **57**, 62, 63, 64, 92, *93*
    hemodynamic response in fetus, 112, 113, 114, 115
    in HPV, 94, 95
    as mediator of pulmonary pathology, 65–7
    regulation of vascular tone, *58*
    secondary mediators of actions, 63–5
    in sepsis, 94
    synthesis and clearance, 58–61
  fetal circulation, 112–14
  in HPV, 94–5
  in sepsis, 93–4
endothelium, 125, 127
  dysfunction and pulmonary vasoreactivity, 132–3
  local and global function, 2–3
  permeability, 242, 247
  role of in ARDS, 77–97
    modulation of vascular tone, 3–5, **87–91**
endothelium-derived contracting factor (EDCF), 125
endothelium-derived relaxing factor (EDRF), 9, 87, 125
  NO as, **17–30**, 34
  see also nitric oxide (NO)
endotoxemia
  ANP levels, *47*
  NOS activity, 4, **89–90**
  sepsis patients with ARDS, 82
endotoxin, 42, 82
  animal models
    cyclooxygenase inhibitors, 262–3, 264
    PMN migration, 245, 247, 248

effect on exhaled NO, 12
ET release, 93–4
TNF release, 266
endotracheal intubation, 264–5
auto-inhalation of NO, 2, 12
double-lumen endotubes, split-lung VCO_2 measurments, 172
epithelium, 6, 247
alveolar permeability, lung distension, 254
injury in lungs, 242, 243, 244
epoprostenol *see* prostaglandins: PGI_2
ethanol intake, exhaled NO, 11
ethchlorvynol-induced lung injury model, ibuprofen therapy, 263
exercise
COPD patients, 230
exhaled NO, 11
home oxygen therapy study, 158–9, 162, 163, 166
pulmonary blood flow regulation, 2, 126
exhaled air
endogenously produced NO, **10–11**, **12**, 129, 140–1
factors influencing NO concentration, 11–12
ExoS, pseudomonas exoenzyme, 248
extracorporeal membrane oxygenation (ECMO), 115, 176
dose-response curves, 218, 220, 222

fetal and perinatal circulation, **107–14**, 133
fetus, lamb
changes in NOS content of endothelium, 28, *29*
effects of L-NA, 24, *25*
vascular shear stress response, 26, *27*
fibrosis, role of ET-1, 65, 66
filtration coefficient (K_F), 272
fluid
clearance, isolated lobe experiments, 274
exchange, monitoring, 278–9
flurbiprofen, 96
formylmethionyl–leucyl–phenylalanine (FMLP), 246, 247
FR 139317, ET_A antagonist, 64, **68**
fraction inspired O^2 (F_iO_2)
NO inhalation, 195
co-administration with almitrine, 196, 198
PaO_2/FiO_2 ratio, 148, *219*

oncotic manipulations, 279–81
unilung venous admixture measurement, 173

gas exchange
ARDS, **181–3**, 264
cyclooxygenase blockade, 263
NO inhalation
ARDS, 181–3
COPD, 141–4
predictive factors of effects, 210–14
gestation, NO production, 28–9, 111
granulocyte-associated membrane protein (P-selectin), 84
granulocytes, CD11/CD18 expression in ARDS, 84
group B streptococcal models
ibuprofen therapy, 264
NO inhalation, 42
thromboxane, 110
guanylate cyclase, 65, 87, 110, 208
ANP stimulation, 46
NO stimulation, 18, 35
gut, NO formation, 11, 12

half-life
^{125}I-ET-1, 93
almitrine, 191
nitric oxide, 38
prostaglandin I_2, 43, 44, 45
heart
ET-1 clearance and metabolizing capacity, *61*
failure, 33, 69, 175
left ventricular, 152, 210
right ventricular, 147, 150, 151, 152, 175, 229
severe congestive, NO inhalation, 41
surgery
adults, NO inhalation, 151, 203, 208
CHD, postoperative NO inhalation, 150
infant, PGE_1 administration, 45
transplantation, 41, 45
inhaled NO, 151–3
see also cardiac
heart-lung transplantation, 41, **44**, **139–40**, 152
hematocrit determinations, spectrophotometric device, 271, 272, 278
ultrafiltration circuits, 279

hemoglobin
NO affinity, 20, 21
relaxation blocked by, *19*, 20
scavenged endogenous NO, 10–11
Hetastarch 6%, acute lung injury, 275, 276, 277, *278*
high altitude pulmonary edema, 244, **246**
high-frequency oscillatory ventilation (HFOV), 115
persistent pulmonary hypertension of newborn, 116
histamine, 64
home oxygen therapy, cardiopulmonary response, 157–68
HS 142–1, selective ANP inhibitor, 47
human serum albumin administration, **273–4**, 275
hyaline membrane disease, NO inhalation, 115
hydrostatic
capillary pulmonary pressure, 215
pulmonary edema, alveolar distension, 254, 255, 257
hypertension, systemic
effect of L-NAME, 23, 24
see also pulmonary hypertension
hypertrophy, vascular, 3, 210
hyperventilation
alkalosis-induced mechanical, 116
PGI_2 release, 43
hypoxemic respiratory failure
cyclooxygenase inhibitors, 265
neonatal
inhaled NO trial, 115
total or partial liquid ventilation, 116
hypoxia, **37**, **133**, 191, 192, 193
ANP, 46
chronic, 130, *131*, 132
COPD, 230, 231
effects on pulmonary circulation, 126–7
inadvertant airway disconnection, 182
NO
exhaled, 11, 12
impaired release, 132
influence on vasculature, 2, **9–10**
pulmonary endothelial-smooth muscle interface, 3–5
vasoconstriction, 34, 35
hypoxic pulmonary vasoconstriction (HPV), 34, 35, **86–7**, **126**
in acute lung injury, 86
almitrine, 192, 193, 198
COPD, 230
eicosanoids, 96
endothelins, 94–5
NO, 91, **125–33**, **190–1**
inhaled, 44, 143, 144, 210

ibuprofen, 262
animal studies, 262–4
human studies, endotoxin administration, 266
immunoglobulins, 243, 247
indomethacin, 63, 64, 65, 96, 110, 129, 182
inducible NOS (iNOS), 2, 9, 12, 38, 87, 128, 206
asthma and bronchiectasis, 140
bacterial stimulation, 12, **89–90**
characteristics, *88*
selective blockade, 91
sepsis, 39, 84
inhaled
aerosolized metaproterenol, 265
aerosolized prostaglandin I_2, 44
NO, 4, 40, **41–3**, 68, 70
acute respiratory failure, factors predicting response, 203–22
combined with pulmonary vasconstriction enhancement, 189–98
COPD, 234, 235, **236**
fetal and transitional circulation, 111
persistent pulmonary hypertension of the newborn (PFC), **115**, 116–17
pulmonary hemodynamics and gas exchange, **141–4**, 181–2, **210–14**
respiratory system resistance, 141, *142*
right ventricular function, 4, **147–53**
severe congestive heart failure, 41
toxicity, 40–1, **205–8**
unilateral lung injury, 5–6
iNOS *see* inducible NOS (iNOS)
integrins, 84, 245
intercellular adhesion molecules (ICAM-1 and -2), 84
intermittent positive pressure ventilation, pulmonary edema, 253, 254, 255
interstitial
lung fibrosis, ET-1 expression, 66
pulmonary edema, 180
intragastric formation NO, 11
intrapulmonary shunt, 148, **181–2**, 208, 210, 211
as determinant of hypoxemia, 144
sepsis, 39, 42

IRL-1620, ET_B-selective antagonist, 69
isolated lung experiments
  NOS inhibitors, 129, 130, 190, 191
  pulmonary edema, 271–4
isoproterenol, 132, 180, 181

Kartagener's syndrome, 11
ketanserin, 180
6-keto-prostaglandin $F_{1\alpha}$ (6-keto-$PGF_{1\alpha}$), 264
kidney, ET-1 clearance and metabolizing capacity, *61*

L-arginine, 2, 4, 9, 10, 20, 38, 87, 110, 190, 191
  conversion to citrulline, 20, *21*, 28
  NO-induced vasodilation, 21, *22*, 23–5
L-arginine analogs, **10**, **23–5**, 26, 87, 90, 129
  L-NA (*N*-nitro-L-arginine), 24, *25*, 65, 90, 111, 182
  L-NAME (N^{ω}-nitro-L-arginine methyl ester, 10, 23, 64, 87, 90, 129
  L-NMMA (*N*-monomethyl-L-arginine), 23, *24*, *39*, 64, 90, 91, 92, 94, 129, 140, 182
L-selectin, 84
left ventricular failure, 152, 210
leukocyte
  migration in lungs, 7, 82, 84, 215, **241–8**
  trafficking, 45
leukotrienes, 95, 217
  fetal pulmonary circulation, 109
  LTB_4, 96, 247
  LTD_4, 64
lipopolysaccharide (LPS), 84
  challenge
    iNOS mRNA expression, 90
    PMN migration, 247
  sepsis, 82
liver, ET-1 clearance and metabolizing capacity, *61*
long-term
  home oxygen therapy study, 157–68
  NO therapy, risks, 206
lung
  ET-1 clearance and metabolizing capacity, *61*
  function, interaction between vasodilators and, 33–48
  high resting tone, fetal, 107
  injury, *81*
    pathogenesis, 82–4
    see also acute lung injury
  microvascular permeability, cyclooxygenase inhibitors, 263
  transplantation, 45
    pulmonary blood flow, 171–4
  weight gain
    6% HS treatment edema, 277, *278*
    PMA-induced, 245

macrophages, alveolar, 241, 247
mean arterial pressure
  NO inhalation
    ARDS, 149
    heart transplant patients, 152
mean pulmonary artery pressure (MPAP)
  inhaled NO, 208–9, 210
    dose-response curves, *218*
meclofenamate, 110, 182
meconium aspiration syndrome (MAS), 115, 116
mesenteric ischemia-reperfusion model, 35, 37
metabolic alkalosis, 181
metacholine, 132
  -induced bronchoconstriction, inhaled NO inhibition, 216
metaproterenol, aerosolized in ARDS, 265
methemoglobin, 39, **41**, 206
methylene blue, 18, 20, 65, 129
methylprednisolone, 266
microemboli
  platelet, 37
  pulmonary hypertension model, spectrum of PVZ, 84
mitochondria, respiratory assemblies, 192
molecular weight and oncotic effect, 275–6
multiple organ failure (MOF), **77**, 86
  arachidonic acid metabolites, animal models, 263–4
  cyclooxygenase inhibitors, 265–6
  sepsis-induced endothelium-mediated circulatory failure, 81
mutagenic potential, NO, 206
myocardium, iNOS in sepsis, 90

N-monomethyl–L-arginine (L-NMMA), 23, *24*, *39*, 64, 90, 91, 92, 94, 129, 140, 182
N-nitro–L-arginine (L-NA), 24, *25*, 65, 90, 111, 182

NADH–cytochrome Q reductase complex, 192
nasal prongs versus oxygen-saving devices study, 157–68
  discussion, 165–8
  materials and methods, 158
  protocol, 158–60
  results, 160–5
nasopharyngeal excretion, NO 11, 12
neonates
  ET-1 infusion, 112, 113
  inhaled, NO
    ARDS, 115
    long-term, patient registration, 206
    methemoglobin reductase deficiency, 41
    pulmonary hypertension, 41, 220
    suprasystemic pulmonary hypertension, 150
  NO nasal concentrations, 12
  persistent pulmonary hypertension of the newborn (PFC), 109, 110, 111, **114–17**, 139
neutropenia, 82, 241, 245, 246
neutrophils (PMNs), migration, 7, 82, 84, **241–8**
  inhaled NO inhibition, 215
  not causing injury, 246–8
nitric oxide (NO), 1, 2, 57, *58*, **87–90**, 180
  antiplatelet effects, 41, 215
  endogenous production, 9–12
  endothelial-smooth muscle interactions, 3
  hypoxic pulmonary vasoconstriction, 91, **125–33**
  perinatal circulation, 110–12
  and pressure-flow relations, acute respiratory failure, 175–85
  as principal endothelium-derived relaxing factor (EDRF), **17–30**, 34
    formation and characteristics, 20–1
    historical perspective, 17–20
  in sepsis, 89–90
  as therapeutic pulmonary vasodilator, 38–43
  see also inhaled: NO
nitric oxide synthase (NOS) inhibitors, 87, **129**, 130, 190, 191
  L-arginine analogs *see* L-arginine analogs
  paraquat lung injury, prevention of, 215–16
  sepsis, 90–1
nitric oxide synthase (NOS) species
  characteristics, *88*
  see also constitutive NOS (cNOS); endothelial NOS (eNOS); inducible NOS (iNOS)
nitrogen mustard, PMN depletion, 245
nitrogen oxide toxicity, 40
nitroglycerin, 18, 35, 148
  effect on exhaled NO, 11–12
nitroprusside, 35, 132, 140, 152, 181
  effect on exhaled NO, 11–12
nocturnal oxygen flow requirements, home oxygen therapy study, *160*, 161
nonadrenergic noncholinergic (NANC) receptors, 2
N^{ω}-nitro–L-arginine methyl ester (L-NAME), 10, 23, 64, 87, 90, 129

oleic acid acute lung injury models
  acetylsalicylic acid, *181*, 182
  almitrine, 182, 193
  PGE_1 and nitroprusside, 181
  plasma ET-1 levels, 67
  pulmonary edema, 178
    6% Hetastarch infusion, 275, 276
  pulmonary hypertension, 178–*9*
    NO inhalation, 42
  sieve chromatographic analysis, dextran, 277
  ventilated tidal volume variation, 256
oncotic gradients, isolated lobe experiments, 274
oncotic manipulations, acute lung injury, 7, **275–8**
  clinical study, 278–82
    summary of results, 281–2
oxidative phosphorylation, almitrine effects, 192, 194
oxygen
  delivery (DO_2), ARDS and sepsis, 85–6
  flow determination, home oxygen therapy study, 158–9
  tension, NO release, 34, 133
  therapy, long-term, home oxygen therapy study, 4, **157–68**
  see also fraction inspired oxygen (F_iO_2); partial pressure of oxygen (PaO_2)
oxygenation index (OI), response to inhaled NO, 115
oxymetric thermodilution pulmonary artery catheter, 195

P-selectin, 84
paraquat-induced lung injury, 216
partial pressure of oxygen (PaO_2)
  almitrine effects, 192, 193, 194, 196, 198
  intrapulmonary shunt, 148
  NO inhalation, 210–11, 212
    acute lung injury, 196, 198
    acute respiratory failure, 208
    ARDS, 190, 234
    congenital heart disease, 150
    COPD, **142**, 234, *235*
    dose-response curves, *218*
  PaO_2/F_iO_2 ratio, 148, *219*
    oncotic manipulations, 279–81
  transtracheal catheter, 162, 166
PD 142893, peptide antagonist, 68–9
PD 145065, peptide antagonist, 68–9
Pentastarch infusion, 280
perinatal pulmonary circulation, pathophysiology, 107–17
peripheral oxygen uptake (VO_2), ARDS and sepsis, 85–6
permeability edema and alveolar distension, 254, 255, 256
  roles of high airway pressure and high lung volume, 255, 257
peroxynitrite, 41, 206
persistent pulmonary hypertension of the newborn (PFC), 111, **114–17**, 139
  high ET-1 levels, 114, 115
  leukotrienes, 109
  management strategies, 116
  thromboxane, 110
phenylephrine, 90
phorbal myristate acetate (PMA) activation of PMNs, 245, 246
phosphatase, 114–15
phosphodiesterase (PDE_5), 28–9
  cGMP PDE
    activity, 114
    inhibition, 112
phospholipase C activation, 92
phosphoramidon, 58, 60, 92
platelet microemboli, 37
platelet-activating factor (PAF), **63**, **64**, 127, 208
  receptor antagonists, 63, 64
platelet–endothelial cell adhesion molecule (PECAM-1), 84
plexogenic pulmonary arteriopathy, 66, 140
pneumocytes, Type I and II, 243, 244
pneumonia, 189
  aerosolized PGI_2, 44
  almitrine plus NO inhalation, 194
  NO_2 inhalation in mice, 206, 208
  surfactant therapy, 116
pneumonitis, acute interstitial, 40
polycythemia, 230
polymorphonuclear activation *see* neutrophils (PMNs)
polysaccharide macromolecular solutions, 276
positive end-expiratory pressure (PEEP), 5, 189, 195, 196, 236
  and alveolar recruitment, NO inhalation, 211, 212, *213*, *214*
  effect of increased on PAP/Q plots, 178, *179*
  effect on pulmonary vascular tone, COPD patients, 232, *233*, 234
  ventilation-induced pulmonary edema, 255, 256
preproET-1, 112
  mRNA expression, 66, 67, 68
pressure-flow relations and NO, acute respiratory failure, 175–85
prostacyclin *see* prostaglandins: PGI_2
prostaglandins, **109–10**, 261, 264
  6-keto-$PGF_{1\alpha}$, 264
  PGE_1, **45–6**, 152, 180, 181
    fetal lung, 110
  PGE_2, 46
  PGI_2, 18, 26, 35, 62, 63, 92, 127, 261–2
    fetal lung, 109–10
    as therapeutic pulmonary vasodilator, **43–5**, 95, **148–9**, 152, 153, 181, 182
protein clearance, alveolar, 243
  pulmonary edema, 243–4
Pseudomonas aeruginosa sepsis
  ANP effects, 46–7
  PMN migration, 247
pulmonary arterial pulse pressure, 183
pulmonary arteries, 86, 210
  effects of almitrine, 192–3
  electrical field stimulation-induced contractile response, L-NMMA, 129
  endothelium-dependent relaxation of isolated, 127–9
    different animal species, *128*
  ET-1-induced vasoconstriction, 62
  reduced expression NO synthase, pulmonary hypertension, 140
  structural changes, hypoxia, **126–7**, 132, 230

pulmonary artery pressure (PAP), 5
  ARDS
    instantaneous measurement, 183
    PAP/Q relationship, 175, 176, 178
  co-administration NO and almitrine, 196
  COPD
    exacerbations, 229, **230–1**
    respiratory failure, effects of PEEP on, 232, 234
  hypoxemia, 175
  infusions of vasodilators, 147–8
  long-term oxygen therapy, 164, 167
  NO inhalation effect on, 151
    ARDS, 148–9
    congenital heart disease, 150
    COPD, 142, 143, 144, 234, *235*
    mean PAP (MPAP), 208–9, 210, *218*
  PAP–PAOP/Q plots, 176–7, 181
  shear stress measurements, 26, *27*
pulmonary circulation, 1–7
  blood flow, 5–6
  effects of hypoxia, 126–7
  effects of NO
    predictive factors, 208–10
    remodeling limitation, 215
  fetal and perinatal, **107–14**, 133
  hypoxic pulmonary vascular bed, 130–2
  mechanisms of vasomotor control, 34–5
  physiological roles of NO, 127–9
  see also pulmonary arteries
pulmonary edema, 37
  alveolar overdistendion, 253–8
  cyclooxygenase inhibitors, 265
  epithelial function, 243–4
  high altitude (HAPE), 244, 246
  NO inhalation, 206, 210, 215
  reabsorption, new therapeutic strategies, 271–82
    clinical study, 278–82
    experimental basis for clinical approach, 271–4
  smoke inhalation, models, 41, *43*, 262
pulmonary function tests (PFTs), home oxygen therapy study, 158, 162, *163*, 166
pulmonary hypertension, 3, 39, 128, 130
  acute canine microembolic model, spectrum of PVZ, 184
  acute lung injury, 33
  ANP effects, 46–7
  ARDS, 85, 148, **175–6**
    experimental, 178–9
  children, plasma ET-1 levels, 66
  chronic hypoxic, **126–7**, 130, *131*, 132, 133
  congenital heart disease, 150
  COPD, 139, 229
    acute exacerbations, 230–1
    development of, 230
    vasodilator therapy, 234
  cyclooxygenase inhibitors, 265
    animal models, 262–3
  ET-1, role of, 47, **65–7**, 70
    animal models, 66–7
  inhaled NO, **41**, 68, 151, 203
    congenital heart disease, 150, 151
    dose-response curves, 221
    postoperative heart transplantation, 152
  NO synthase, reduced expression, 9, **140**
  persistent pulmonary hypertension of the newborn (PFC), 109, 110, 111, **114–17**, 139
  PGI_2, 44, 45
  RVEF in sudden, 147
pulmonary vascular impedance (PVZ), 183, *184*
pulmonary vascular resistance (PVR)
  almitrine effects on, 193
  ARDS, 85, **175–6**, 180–1, 215
  at birth, **108**, 109, 111, 117
    COX inhibition, 110
  baseline, 208, 209, 211
  COPD, 231
    PEEP application, 232, *233*
  elevated in transplant candidates, 152
  in fetus, 114
  flow relationships, 176–7
    PAP–PAOP/Q plots, 177
  inhaled NO, 209, 210, *219*
    dose-response curves, *218*, 221–2
    PEEP-induced alveolar recruitment, 212
  long-term oxygen therapy, 164
  TXA_2-mediated increases, 96
pulmonary vascular tone, 3–5
  arachidonic metabolites in systemic inflammation, 261–7
  ARDS
    gas exchange, 181–3
    role of endothelium, 77–97
  COPD, ventilated patients, 229–37
  inhibition of NO activity, 129, 130
  see also vasoconstriction; vasodilation
pulse oximetry, 166

RES-701-1, ET_B receptor antagonist, 62
respiratory failure
  COPD, 231
    effect of ventilation on pulmonary vascular tone, 231–4
  cyclooxygenase inhibitors, 265
  inhaled NO, factors predicting response to, 203–22
    monitoring methods, 204–5
    toxicity, 205–8
  intravenous almitrine, 193
  neonatal hypoxemic
    inhaled NO trial, 115
    total or partial liquid ventilation, 116
  pressure-flow relations and NO, 175–85
  sheep model, IPPV-induced lung injury, 254
respiratory resistance
  acute lung injury, 216–17
  effect of inhaled NO, 141, *142*
  see also pulmonary vascular resistance (PVR)
restenosis, 69
resting tone, fetal lung, 107
reverse transcription polymerase chain reaction (Rt–PCR), iNOS mRNA expression, 90
right ventricle free wall stress (RVFWS) index, 159, 164
right ventricular ejection fraction (RVEF)
  NO inhalation
    COPD, 234, 235
    severe ARDS, 148, 149, 185
  sudden pulmonary hypertension, 147
right ventricular failure, 147, 150, 175, 229
  elevated PVR, transplant candidates, 152
  reversal, assist device with NO inhalation, 151
right ventricular (RV) function
  congenital heart disease, 150–1
  inhaled NO, 4, **147–53**
    in COPD, 234, 235, *236*
Ro 46–2005, nonpeptide ET receptor antagonist, 69

S. pneumoniae, PMN migration, 245
Sarafotoxin S6c, hemodynamic effects, fetal lung, 113–14
SB 209670, nonpeptide antagonist, 69
SB 217242, nonpeptide antagonist, 69
selectins, 84
sensory peripheral neuropathy, almitrine, 191–2
sepsis, 77, 81, 82, 314
  cardiovascular physiology of, *79*
  definitions, clinical syndromes, *80*
  endothelins, 93–4
  group B streptococcal models
    ibuprofen therapy, 264, 266
    NO inhalation, 42
    thromboxane, 110
  iNOS, 39, 84
  inter-relationship between associated syndromes, *79*
  intrapulmonary shunt, 39, 42
  NO, 89–90
    inhaled in neonates, 115
    NOS inhibitors, 90–1
  pathogenesis of lung injury, 82–4
    interaction pathway for mediators, *83*
  Pseudomonas aeruginosa, ANP effects, 46–7
  role of arachidonic acid metabolites, 261–7
sepsis syndrome, 7, *80*, **262–4**
  ibuprofen therapy, 264, 266
septic shock, *80*, 81, 89
  ARDS associated with, dose-response curves inhaled NO, 221–2
shear stress, stimulus for NO production, **25–7**, 35
silo filler's disease, 40
single-breath analysis, NO concentration, 10
skin, PMN migration, 245, 246
smoke inhalation injury models, pulmonary edema
  ibuprofen therapy, 262
  inhaled NO, 41, *43*
smokers
  cNOS reduction, 4
  exhaled NO, 11, 140
sodium transport, Type II pneumocytes, 243
spectrophotometric device, on-line hematocrit determinations, 271, 272
split-lung VOC_2 measurements, 172, *173*
staurosporine, 92
structural changes, pulmonary vessels, **126–7**, 132, 230
superoxide anion, 206, 246, 247
suprasystemic pulmonary hypertension, CHD, 150
surfactant, 243, 257
  therapy, 116

systemic collagen vascular disease, PGE_1 administration, 45
systemic inflammatory response syndrome (SIRS), 77, *80*, 81
systolic pressure increase, 183

tachyphylaxis, pulmonary vasodilator responses to ET-1 and ET-2, 63
technetium perfusion scans, 172
thiorphan, 60
thrombosis *in situ*, 37
thromboxane, 37, 92, 95, 262, 266
  increase in PFC models, 110
  TXA_2, 63, 64, **95**, **96**, 208, 217, 261, 262
  TXB_2, 64, 96, 264
thromboxane synthetase, 63
tidal volume, permeability edema, 256, 257
toxicity, NO administration, 40–1, **205–8**
trachea, ET-1 synthesis of arachidonic acid metabolites, 64
transmural colloid osmotic gradient, 272
transtracheal catheter (TTC), 157, 159, 161, 162, **164**, *165*, **166**, **167–8**
transvascular oncotic gradient, 275, 276
tricuspid regurgitation, home oxygen therapy study, 164, 167
tumor necrosis factor (TNF)
  pulmonary hypertension model, cyclooxygenase inhibitors, 262–3
  TNF-α, role in lung injury, 248
type II NOS *see* inducible NOS (iNOS)
type III NOS *see* constitutive NOS (cNOS)

U46619, TXA_2 analog, 63
ultrafiltration circuits, oncotic manipulations, 279, 280, 281
ultrasonic flow probes, 172
unilung venous admixture, 173–4

vascular adhesion molecule (VCAM-1), 84
vasoconstriction, 34, *36*
  ALI and other disease states, 35, 37
  enhancement and co-administration with NO, 189–98
  mediators of, 57–71
vasodilation, 34–5, *36*
  ALI and other disease states, 35, 37
  cGMP, 18, *19*, 20, 34, *35*, 37
  intrapulmonary shunt, 148, 181
  NO-induced, 210
    schema for, 21, *22*, 23–9
  selective, COPD exacerbations, 234–6
  time-limited response limits, fetal circulation, 107
vasodilators and lung function interaction, 33–48
  implications of selective vasodilators, 37–8
  vasodilators with potential therapeutic application, 38–46
vasomotor control *see* pulmonary vascular tone; vasoconstriction; vasodilation
veins
  NO production, 26
  NO-induced venodilation, 210
venous oxygen saturation (Svo_2), dose-response curves inhaled NO, 220, *221*
ventilation, mechanical
  alkalosis-induced hyperventilation, 116
  co-administration NO and almitrine, 194–5
  cyclooxygenase inhibitors, 264–5
  effects on previously injured lungs, 256–7
  high-frequency oscillatory ventilation (HFOV), 115
    persistant pulmonary hypertension of newborn, 116
  high-pressure/high-volume, pulmonary edema, 253–5, 257–8
  inadvertant airway disconnection, 182
  pulmonary vascular tone, COPD, 229–37
  side effects, 189, 253
  total or partial liquid, 116
  see also positive end-expiratory pressure (PEEP); zero end-expiratory pressure (ZEEP)
ventilation, onset at birth, 108, 110
ventilation-perfusion (*V/Q*)
  distributions, NO inhalation in COPD, 142, *143*
  inhaled-NO-induced arteriolar vasodilation, 212, 213
  matching, endogenous NO model, 191
  mismatch, 34, 35, 171, 189, 191, 242
    almitrine, **193**, **194**, 196
    in COPD, 144
    HPV reducing, 126
    pulmonary vasodilators, 37, 40
      PGI_2, 43–4
ventricular afterload, 183, 185

ventriculography, isotopic, home oxygen therapy study, 159–60, 161
  hemodynamic response, *161*
volutrauma, 7, 198, 256, 257
  alkalosis-induced mechanical hyperventilation, 116

walking test, 6 minute, home oxygen therapy study, 158–9, 162, 163, 166–7
water reabsorption, alveolar epithelium, 243
WEB 2086, PAF receptor antagonist, 64
wedge pressure increases, 147, 152

zaprinast, 112, 116
zero end-expiratory pressure (ZEEP), 211, 212, *213*
  ventilation-induced pulmonary edema, 255–6